CURRENT CLINICAL UROLOGY

ERIC A. KLEIN, MD, SERIES EDITOR
PROFESSOR OF SURGERY
CLEVELAND CLINIC LERNER COLLEGE OF MEDICINE HEAD
SECTION OF UROLOGIC ONCOLOGY
GLICKMAN UROLOGICAL AND KIDNEY INSTITUTE
CLEVELAND, OH

For further volumes:
http://www.springer.com/series/7635

Alan J. Wein • Karl-Erik Andersson
Marcus J. Drake • Roger R. Dmochowski
Editors

Bladder Dysfunction in the Adult

The Basis for Clinical Management

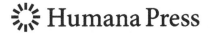 Humana Press

Editors

Alan J. Wein, M.D., Ph.D. (Hon.), F.A.C.S.
Perelman School of Medicine
University of Pennsylvania
   Health System
Philadelphia, PA, USA

Marcus J. Drake, M.A. (Cantab),
   D.M. (Oxon.), F.R.C.S. (Urol.)
University of Bristol and Bristol
   Urological Institute
Bristol, UK

Karl-Erik Andersson, M.D., Ph.D.
AIAS, Aarhus Institute of Advanced
   Studies
Aarhus University
Aarhus, Denmark

Roger R. Dmochowski, M.D., M.M.H.C.
Department of Urologic Surgery
Vanderbilt University Medical Center
Nashville, TN, USA

ISSN 2197-7194   ISSN 2197-7208 (electronic)
ISBN 978-1-4939-0852-3   ISBN 978-1-4939-0853-0 (eBook)
DOI 10.1007/978-1-4939-0853-0
Springer New York Heidelberg Dordrecht London

Library of Congress Control Number: 2014941584

Preface

The idea for this text arose from an informal discussion between the four of us at the annual ICI-RS (International Consultation on Incontinence-Research Society). The concept was to produce a series of presentations that covered virtually every topic that fell under the rubric of bladder function and dysfunction in the adult. We wanted to cover "the basics" in a manner sufficient for understanding how and why things "work", but not in an overly detailed manner that would be considered suffocating. The same concept was meant to apply to a description of the common types of dysfunctions which we encounter in clinical practice and to the methods of evaluation and therapies (non-, minimally and maximally invasive) which we commonly utilize. Hopefully, we have achieved that goal.

Philadelphia, PA   Alan J. Wein
Aarhus, Denmark   Karl-Erik Andersson
Bristol, UK   Marcus J. Drake
Nashville, TN   Roger R. Dmochowski

(Written by Alan J. Wein, M.D. for the Editors)

Acknowledgement

The editors would like to thank Mr. Michael Griffin of Springer for his advice and assistance in bringing this volume forward.

Contents

Part IV   Management

Part V   Other Considerations

Contributors

Karl-Erik Andersson, M.D., Ph.D. AIAS, Aarhus Institute of Advanced Studies Aarhus University, Aarhus, Denmark

Jonathan J. Aning, D.M., F.R.C.S. (Urol.) Southmead Hospital, Bristol Urological Institute, Bristol, UK

Andrew D. Baird, M.B., Ch.B., F.R.C.S. (Urol.) Paediatric, Adolescent and Reconstructive Urology, Alder Hey Children's Hospital, Liverpool, Merseyside, UK

Roger R. Dmochowski, M.D., M.M.H.C. Department of Urologic Surgery, Vanderbilt University Medical Center, Nashville, TN, USA

Marcus J. Drake, M.A. (Cantab), D.M. (Oxon.), F.R.C.S. (Urol.) University of Bristol and Bristol Urological Institute, Bristol, UK

Alex Gomelsky, M.D. Department of Urology, LSU Health—Shreveport, Shreveport, LA, USA

Jackie Gordon, M.A., M.B., B.Chir., M.R.C.Psych. Mental Health Liaison Service, Worthing Hospital, West Sussex, UK

Dev Mohan Gulur, M.B.B.S., M.R.C.S. Department of Urology, Aintree University Hospital NHS Foundation Trust, Liverpool, UK

Hashim Hashim, M.B.B.S., M.R.C.S. (Eng.), M.D., F.E.B.U., F.R.C.S. (Urol.) Southmead Hospital, Bristol Urological Institute, Bristol, UK

Emily J. Henderson, M.B., Ch.B., M.R.C.P. School of Social and Community Medicine, University of Bristol, Bristol, UK

Amit Mevcha, M.B.B.S., M.R.C.S., F.R.C.S. (Urol.) Department of Urology, Birmingham Heartlands Hospital, Birmingham, UK

Diane K. Newman, D.N.P., A.N.P.-B.C., F.A.A.N. Division of Urology, Department of Surgery, Perelman School of Medicine, University of Pennsylvania, Philadelphia, PA, USA

Jalesh N. Panicker, M.D., D.M., M.R.C.P. (UK) Department of Uroneurology, The National Hospital for Neurology and Neurosurgery, London, UK

Brian Andrew Parsons, B.Sc., M.B.Ch.B., M.R.C.S. Department of Urology, Cheltenham General Hospital, Cheltenham, Gloucestershire, UK

Thomas Renninson, M.B.Ch.B. Department of Medicine, Frenchay Hospital, Bristol, Avon, UK

Alan J. Wein, M.D., Ph.D. (Hon.), F.A.C.S. Perelman School of Medicine, University of Pennsylvania Health System, Philadelphia, PA, USA

Jonathan Williams, M.B.B.S., B.Sc. Department of Urology, Southmead Hospital, Bristol, UK

Part I

Basic Considerations: Normal Function

Relevant Anatomy, Physiology, and Pharmacology

Karl-Erik Andersson

Relevant Gross Anatomy

The main components of the lower urinary tract (LUT) consist of the urinary bladder and the urethra (Fig. 1.1). The main components of the bladder are the bladder body, which is located above the ureteral orifices, and the base, including the trigone, urethro-vesical junction, deep detrusor, and the anterior bladder wall. The inside of the bladder is lined by a mucous membrane consisting of the urothelium, a basal lamina, and the lamina propria (Fig. 1.2). Below the lamina propria is a layer of smooth muscle cells, which comprise the detrusor muscle, which is structurally and functionally different from, e.g., trigonal and urethral smooth muscle. The outer part of the bladder is covered partly by peritoneal serosa and partly by fascia. The urethra contains both smooth and striated muscles. The smooth muscle part consists of an inner longitudinal and an outer longitudinal part, and the striated muscle partly surrounds the urethra and forms the external sphincter. Further details on urethral structure can be found elsewhere [1, 2].

K.-E. Andersson, M.D., Ph.D. (✉)
AIAS, Aarhus Institute of Advanced Studies,
Aarhus University, Aarhus, Denmark

Institute for Regenerative Medicine, Wake Forest
University School of Medicine, Medical Center Blvd,
Winston Salem, NC 27157, USA
e-mail: keanders@wakehealth.edu

In many textbooks, three layers of smooth muscle in the bladder wall have been described: the cells of the outer and inner layers tend to be oriented longitudinally, and those of the middle layer circularly. However, these layers are often difficult to clearly separate. In the human detrusor, bundles of muscle cells of varying size are surrounded by connective tissue rich in collagen. They may be large, often a few mm in diameter, and composed of several smaller sub-bundles and are not clearly arranged in distinct layers. Within the main bundles, the smooth muscle cells may exist in groups of small functional units, or fascicles [3]. The orientation and interaction between the smooth muscle cells in the bladder are important, since this will determine how the bladder wall behaves and what effect activity in the cells will have on its shape and intraluminal pressure. In smaller animals, e.g., rabbit, the muscle bundles are less complex and the patterns of arrangement simpler than in the human detrusor.

The individual smooth muscle cells in the detrusor are similar to those in other muscular organs. They are long, spindle shaped with a central nucleus. When fully relaxed the cells are several hundred microns long, and the widest diameter is 5–6 μm. The cytoplasm contains the normal myofilaments, and the membranes exhibit regularly spaced dense bands, with membrane vesicles (caveoli) between them. There are also scattered dense bodies in the cytoplasm. Mitochondria and fairly sparse elements of sarcoplasmic reticulum (mostly near the nucleus) are also present [4].

A.J. Wein et al. (eds.), *Bladder Dysfunction in the Adult: The Basis for Clinical Management*, Current
Clinical Urology, DOI 10.1007/978-1-4939-0853-0_1, © Springer Science+Business Media New York 2014

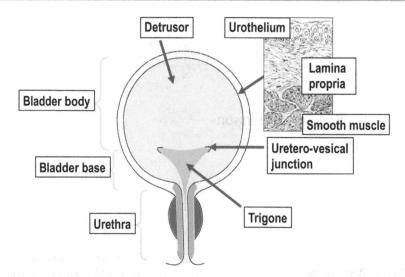

Fig. 1.1 Components of the urinary bladder

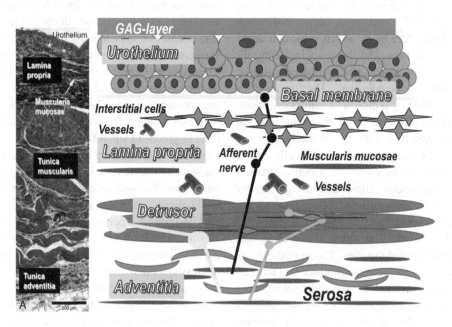

Fig. 1.2 Components of the bladder wall. Left panel: histological section

Cells with long dendritic processes can be found in the lamina propria and also within the detrusor in parallel to the smooth muscle fibers. These interstitial cells (ICs) (see below), named in various ways, contain vimentin, an intermediate filament protein expressed by cells of mesenchymal origin and non-muscle myosin, but also several other markers [5, 6].

The vascular supply to the human bladder is derived mainly from the superior and inferior vesical arteries, the latter directly connected to the internal iliac artery. To maintain the barrier function of the urothelium and contractile functions of the detrusor, an adequate supply of oxygen and nutrients from the blood is necessary. Therefore, the blood vessels in the bladder wall must be capable of adaptation to the spatial changes resulting from the filling/voiding cycle without compromising the blood flow. In a corrosion casting study of the human bladder wall, two major vascular plexuses (adventitial/serosal and mucosal) were identified and two distinct capillary networks (muscular and subepithelial) could be distinguished [7]. Almost all bladder vessels except the capillaries have a conspicuous tortuosity ranging from waviness to tight coiling. The mucosal plexus consists of some capillaries, thin arteries (50–100 μm), and more numerous, thicker veins (80–250 μm), showing a tortuous appearance and frequent interlacements; it forms a distinct vascular layer parallel to the inner surface of the bladder. This rich plexus follows the mucosal folds parallel to their surface and gives off short, straight, mostly perpendicular twigs communicating with the subepithelial capillary network. The subepithelial capillary network shows extreme density and uneven contours of the capillaries; only in less folded areas of the trigone and urethral orifice is the network looser and capillaries thinner. In contrast, the capillary system of the muscularis is poorly developed.

Mucosa

The bladder mucosa consists of the urothelium, basement membrane, and lamina propria (Fig. 1.2). The lamina propria also contains some smooth muscle cells, muscularis mucosae. Since this structure is not very well defined in the human bladder (and sometimes seems to be absent), it may be questioned whether the human bladder, unlike the gut, has a true "submucosal" layer. However, the term is sometimes used to denote the part of the lamina propria closest to the muscularis propria.

Urothelium. The uroepithelium, or urothelium, is a transitional epithelial tissue, composed of at least three layers (Fig. 1.3): a basal cell layer attached to a basement membrane, an intermediate layer, and a superficial or apical layer composed of large hexagonal cells (diameters of 25–250 μm) known as "umbrella cells" [8, 9]. The apical surface of umbrella cells possesses a unique asymmetric unit membrane (AUM). The umbrella cells, which are interconnected by tight junctions, are covered on their apical surface (nearly 70–80 %) by uroplakins, which are crystalline proteins that assemble into hexagonal plaques. Uroplakins and other urothelial cellular differentiation markers, such as cytokeratin, are not expressed in the stratified epithelium of the urethra. A urothelial glycosaminoglycan (GAG) layer covers the umbrella cells and has been suggested to contribute to urothelial barrier function.

Lamina Propria. The lamina propria lies between the basement membrane of the mucosa and the

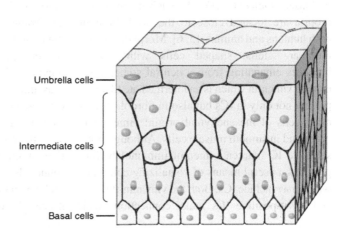

Fig. 1.3 The urothelium contains three different cell layers

Umbrella cells —

Intermediate cells ⟨

Basal cells —

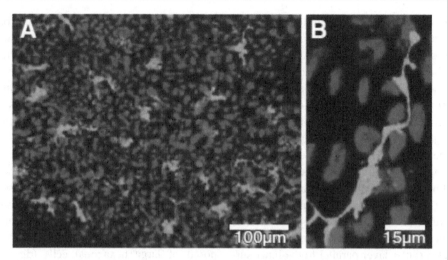

Fig. 1.4 Innervation of the human LUT. Coordination between bladder and outlet (bladder neck, urethra, and urethral sphincters) is mediated by sympathetic (hypogastric), parasympathetic (pelvic), and somatic (pudendal) nerves

detrusor muscle, and is composed of an extracellular matrix containing several types of cells, including fibroblasts, adipocytes, ICs, and sensory nerve endings. As mentioned, the lamina propria contains a rich vascular network, but also lymphatic channels, elastic fibers, and smooth muscle fascicles (muscularis mucosae). Notably, the thickness of the lamina propria varies within the bladder. The lamina propria is a functionally active structure essential for, e.g., afferent signaling [10].

Interstitial Cells. The spindle-/stellate-shaped cells in the bladder wall have been categorized heterogeneously as ICs, interstitial cells of Cajal (ICC), interstitial Cajal-like cells (ICLC), myofibroblasts, or telocytes (Fig. 1.4). ICs in the lamina propria are located close to the urothelium in both humans and animals [5, 6]. Morphologically they are stellate-shaped cells with several branches emanating from a central soma. They contain vimentin which is an intermediate filament present not only in ICs but also in fibroblasts and other cells of mesenchymal origin; vimentin is not found in smooth muscle cells. Although not a selective IC marker, vimentin immunolabelling provides a useful means of visualizing cell types which may include ICs. Both the vimentin-positive and c-Kit-positive ICs make connections with

neighboring cells to form an interconnected cellular network. This network appears to be connected by connexin 43 gap junctions, as shown by immunohistochemistry and transmission electron microscopy [11, 12]. Double labeling with nerve antibodies demonstrates that the ICs in the lamina propria are located close to nerves. Close contacts between lamina propria ICs and nerve endings have also been observed by electron microscopy [12].

The ICs in the detrusor are distinctly different from those in the lamina propria, both in distribution and morphology. c-Kit-positive cells in the detrusor comprise two subtypes: elongated cells with several lateral branches and stellate cells similar to lamina propria ICs. The elongated detrusor ICs are not networked to each other but are arranged in parallel lines in circular, longitudinal, and oblique orientation, reminiscent of the basket-weave array of detrusor smooth muscle bundles [5]. These cells have been denoted intramuscular ICs, and double-labeling studies with c-Kit and smooth muscle myosin antibodies have shown that they are located on the boundary of smooth muscle bundles and follow the orientation of the bundles [13]. This type of cells is found also within the smooth muscle bundles. Stellate-shaped ICs are found within the interstitial spaces between the detrusor smooth muscle bundles, forming regions of interconnected cells. This subtype has been denoted interbundle ICs [13]. Both subtypes of detrusor ICs make close structural connections with nerves [14].

Koh et al. [15] demonstrated in mouse bladder a subpopulation of ICs identified using antibodies against platelet-derived growth factor receptor-α (PDGFRα) and distinct from "conventional" ICs. PDGFRα(+) cells had a spindle-shaped or stellate morphology and often possessed multiple processes that contacted one another forming a loose network. PDGFRα+ cells were distributed as a densely packed network in the LP, and these cells were also distributed throughout the detrusor muscle, being located within and around the periphery of smooth muscle bundles. Many of the PDGFRα+ cells in the LP as well as the detrusor muscle co-labeled with vimentin antibodies. PDGFRα+ cells were found to be present also in human and guinea pig bladder [16]. The function of PDGFRα+ cells in the urinary bladder is unknown, but a possible neuromodulatory role in bladder function cannot be excluded.

Johnston et al. [17] found that the abundant microvessels in the lamina propria were associated with branched, elongated c-Kit positive ICs along the vessel axis, and they suggested the existence of an interstitial cell-vascular coupling.

The role of bladder ICs, including those in the lamina propria, has not been established. The ICs in the lamina propria and within the detrusor may serve different functions. Available evidence suggests that the lamina propria ICs may constitute a structural and functional link between urothelial cells and sensory nerves and/or between urothelial cells and detrusor smooth muscle cells [5, 6].

Detrusor Smooth Muscle

The bladder wall undergoes large changes in extension during normal filling and emptying, posing different demands on the detrusor during the two phases. During filling, the smooth muscle cells have to relax in order elongate and rearrange in the wall over a large length interval.

During micturition, force generation and shortening must be initiated comparatively fast, be synchronized, and occur over a large length range. These activities thus require both regulation of contraction and regulation of relaxation. To be able to respond to the nervous and hormonal control systems, each part of the urinary tract muscles has to have specific receptors for the transmitters/modulators, released from nerves or generated locally, and the associated cellular pathways for initiating contraction and relaxation.

On the basis of contractile behavior, smooth muscle can be divided in two classes, "single unit" and "multiunit." Single-unit smooth muscles are arranged in sheets or bundles, and the cell membranes have many points of close contact, gap junctions, and the low resistance pathways formed by connexin subunits, through which ions can flow from one cell to the other. Thereby, an electrical signal can be spread rapidly throughout the tissue. Action potentials can thus be conducted from one area to another by direct electrical conduction. A minority of the fibers in a single-unit muscle spontaneously generates action potentials—pacemaker cells. In single-unit smooth muscles, a contractile response can often be induced by stretching the muscle. In contrast, multiunit smooth muscle is thought to be composed of discrete muscle fibers or bundles of fibers that operate independently of each other. They are richly innervated by the autonomic nervous system, are controlled mainly by nerve signals, and rarely show spontaneous contractions. Although the detrusor muscle exhibits several of the characteristics ascribed to a single-unit smooth muscle, it also shows several features ascribed to multiunit smooth muscles, being densely innervated, and functionally requiring nervous coordination to achieve voiding. Smooth muscles can also be divided into "phasic" and "tonic" types based on membrane properties and contractile behavior [18]. The urinary bladder smooth muscle is a comparatively fast smooth muscle with characteristics of a "phasic" smooth muscle. Details on the contractile mechanisms can be found elsewhere [19].

Receptors in the LUT

Muscarinic Receptors. The neurotransmitter, acetylcholine (ACh), acts on two classes of receptors, the nicotinic and the muscarinic. While the former play a role in the signal transduction between neurons or between neurons and skeletal muscle (e.g., in the distal urethra), the signal transduction between parasympathetic nerves and smooth muscle of the detrusor involves muscarinic receptors [20–22]. Importantly, ACh is not necessarily derived only from parasympathetic nerves in the urinary bladder but can also be formed and released nonneuronally by the urothelium [22–25]. Five subtypes of muscarinic receptors have been cloned in humans and other mammalian species, which are designated M_{1-5} [26]. Based upon structural criteria and shared preferred signal transduction pathways, the subtypes can be grouped into M_1, M_3, and M_5 on the one hand and the subtypes M_2 and M_4 on the other. The former prototypically couple via pertussis toxin-insensitive G_q proteins to stimulate phospholipase C followed by elevation of intracellular calcium and activation of protein kinase C, whereas the latter couple via pertussis toxin-sensitive G_i proteins to inhibit adenylyl cyclase leading to modulation of several ion channels [26]. While sensitive molecular techniques such as reverse transcriptase polymerase chain reaction can detect mRNA for all five subtypes in the mammalian bladder [27, 28], studies at the protein level, e.g., based upon radioligand binding, have typically detected only M_2 and M_3 receptors, with the former dominating quantitatively (ratio 3:1) [22, 26, 27]. Inhibitory prejunctional muscarinic receptors have been classified as M_2 in the rabbit and rat and M_4 in the guinea pig, rat, and human bladder [22]. These receptors appear to be of the M_1 subtype in the rat and rabbit urinary bladder but have also been detected in human bladders. The muscarinic facilitatory mechanism seems to be upregulated (M_3 receptors) in overactive bladders from chronic spinal cord transected rats.

Apparently, most muscarinic receptors in the bladder are found on the smooth muscle cells of the detrusor. While the detrusor expresses far more M_2 than M_3 receptors, it appears that detrusor contraction under physiological conditions is largely if not exclusively mediated by the M_3 receptor [28–33]. Studies in knock-out mice confirm this conclusion [34–37]. Under physiological conditions, M_2 receptor-selective stimulation causes little contraction but rather appears to act mainly by inhibiting β-adrenoceptor-mediated detrusor relaxation [28, 34, 35, 37]. It has been proposed that M_2 receptors can also directly elicit bladder contraction under pathological conditions [38–43], but such observations have not been confirmed by other investigators using distinct methodological approaches [32, 33].

Based upon the prototypical signaling pathway of M_3 receptors [26] and the presence of phospholipase C stimulation by muscarinic agonists in the bladder [31–33], it was originally been believed that muscarinic receptor-mediated contraction is largely mediated by an activation of phospholipase C [44]. While some earlier data had supported this concept, it now appears clear that at least in rat, mice, and humans, muscarinic receptor-mediated bladder contraction occurs largely independent of phospholipase C [32, 33, 45, 46]. Rather, alternative signaling pathways such as opening of L-type calcium channels and activation of a Rho kinase appear to contribute to muscarinic receptor-mediated bladder contraction in a major way [47] (Fig. 1.5).

Muscarinic receptors have also been identified in the urothelium [48, 49]. Similar to the findings in bladder smooth muscle, the muscarinic receptors in the urothelium mainly belong to the M_2 and M_3 subtype, with the former dominating quantitatively [23, 24]. At present the functional role of muscarinic receptors in the urothelium has largely been studied indirectly, i.e., by investigating the effects of urothelium removal or of administration of pharmacological inhibitors. These data indicate that muscarinic stimulation of the urothelium causes release of an as yet unidentified factor which inhibits detrusor contraction [50–52]. Some data indicate that muscarinic receptors in the urothelium may partly act by releasing nitric oxide (NO) [53]. Muscarinic receptor blockade in urothelial cells may also

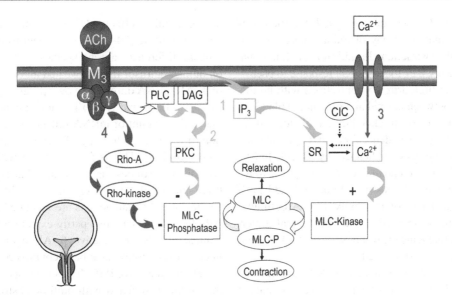

Fig. 1.5 Interstitial cells of the bladder

reduce ATP release induced by stretch [54]. Thus, it appears that muscarinic receptors in the urothelium also contribute to the regulation of overall bladder function, but their specific roles in health and disease have not been fully established.

Assuming an involvement of muscarinic receptors in physiological voiding contractions of the bladder, numerous studies have explored whether an overactivity of the muscarinic system may play a causative role in bladder dysfunction. This could involve, e.g., an enhanced expression of such receptors and/or an increased functional responsiveness. In vitro, an increased sensitivity to muscarinic receptor stimulation was found in both idiopathic and neurogenic overactive human detrusors [55]. However, according to Michel and Barendrecht [56], the overall balance of available studies suggests that the muscarinic receptor system is not hyperactive under conditions of detrusor overactivity (DO) and, if anything, can be even hypoactive [56]. This does not exclude a contribution to DO of ACh and muscarinic receptor stimulation during bladder filling. It appears that the contribution of muscarinic mechanisms to the overall regulation of bladder contractility decreases in favor of non-cholinergic

mechanisms under pathological conditions [57, 58]. These observations may help to explain the moderate efficacy of muscarinic receptor antagonists relative to placebo in controlled clinical studies [59–62].

α-Adrenoceptors. In the bladder, α-ARs can be found in the detrusor smooth muscle, the vasculature, the afferent and efferent nerve terminals, and the intramural ganglia, but their functional importance at the different sites has not been established. In the detrusor, β-ARs dominate over α-ARs, and the normal response to noradrenaline is relaxation [63]. Most investigators agree on that there is a low expression of these receptors in the detrusor muscle [64–66]. Among the high affinity receptors for prazosin, only α_{1A} and α_{1D}-mRNAs were expressed in the human bladder. The relation between the different subtypes was α_{1D}, 66 %, and α_{1A}, 34 %, with no expression of α_{1B} [64]. Even if the α-ARs have no significant role in normal bladder contraction, there is evidence that there may be changes (upregulation) after, e.g., bladder outlet obstruction [63, 67]. Nomiya and Yamaguchi [81] confirmed the low expression of α_1-AR mRNA in normal human bladder and further demonstrated that there was no upregulation of any of the adrenergic receptors with obstruction. In addition, in functional experiments, they found a small response to phenylephrine at high drug concentrations with no difference between normal and obstructed bladders. Thus, in the obstructed human bladder, there seemed to be no evidence for α_1-AR upregulation. This finding was challenged by Bouchelouche et al. [69] who found an increased response to α_1-AR stimulation in obstructed human bladders. If there is a change of sensitivity to α_1-AR stimulation in the obstructed bladder of clinical importance (influencing the response to α_1-AR blockers) remains to be established.

It has been shown that α_1-ARs are located prejunctionally on cholinergic nerve terminals in the rat urinary bladder [66]. Activation of these receptors facilitates ACh release and enhances neurogenic contractions. Trevisani et al. [70] examined the influence of α_1-ARs on neuropeptide release from primary sensory neurons of the LUT in rats and concluded that α_1-ARs are functionally expressed by capsaicin-sensitive nociceptive neurons and that activation of these neurons may contribute to signal irritative and nociceptive responses arising from this region. They suggested that parts of the beneficial effects of α_1-AR antagonists in the amelioration of storage symptoms in the LUT could be derived from their inhibitory effect on neurogenic inflammatory responses.

All α_1-adrenoceptor subtypes can be demonstrated in the urothelium, and it has been suggested, based on rat studies, that α_{1A}-adrenoceptors can modulate bladder afferent activity under both normal and pathophysiological conditions [71, 72]. A study in humans suggested a relationship between the expression of α_{1D}-AR mRNA in the bladder mucosa and storage-phase urodynamics in LUTS/BPO patients, suggesting a role of α_{1D}-ARs in bladder sensation [73].

β-Adrenoceptors. In the human detrusor, it is now generally accepted that the most important β-AR for bladder relaxation is the β_3-AR. Normal as well as neurogenic human detrusors are able to express β_1, β_2, and β_3-AR mRNA, and selective β3-AR agonists effectively relax both types of detrusor muscle [74–78]. There seem to be significant differences among species [79]. Studies on human detrusor tissue revealed an expression of β_3-AR mRNA dominating over β_1- and β_2-ARS (97 % vs. 1.5 % and 1.4 %) The author concluded that if the amount of mRNA reflects the population of receptor protein, β_3 ARs mediate bladder relaxation [68]. This is in accordance with several in vitro studies, and it seems that atypical β-AR-mediated responses reported in early studies of β-AR antagonists are mediated by β_3-ARs [74–77]. It can also partly explain why the clinical effects of selective β_2-AR agonists in bladder overactivity have been controversial and largely inconclusive [80]. It has been speculated that in DO associated with outflow obstruction, there is a lack of an inhibitory β-AR-mediated noradrenaline response, but this has never been verified in humans [81–83].

The generally accepted mechanism by which β-ARs induce detrusor relaxation in most species is activation of adenylyl cyclase with subsequent formation of cAMP. However, there is evidence suggesting that in the bladder, K+ channels, particularly BK_{Ca} channels, may be more important in β_3-AR-mediated relaxation than cAMP [47, 84, 85] (Fig. 1.6).

The normal stimulus for the activation of the micturition reflex is considered to be distension of the bladder, initiating activity in "in series"-coupled, low-threshold mechanoreceptive (Aδ) afferents [86]. If this response to distension is decreased by the detrusor muscle being relaxed and more compliant, the afferent activity needed to initiate micturition will be delayed and bladder capacity increased. Such an effect may be obtained by stimulating the β_3-ARs on the detrusor muscle. There are reasons to believe that the spontaneous contractile, phasic activity of the detrusor smooth muscle during filling not only can create tone in the detrusor muscle but also generate afferent input ("afferent noise"), contributing to OAB/DO. In fact, Aizawa et al. [87] showed that the β_3-AR selective agonist, mirabegron, could inhibit filling-induced activity not only in mechano-sensitive Aδ-fibers, but also in C-fiber primary bladder afferents. β_3-AR agonists

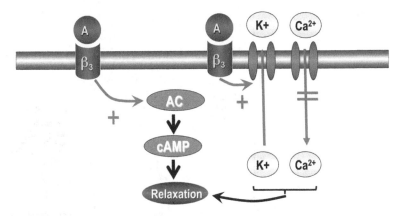

Fig. 1.6 Stimulation of the muscarinic M3 receptor: molecular mechanism of action

have a pronounced effect on autonomous contractile activity in detrusor muscle in vitro [88] and on non-voiding contractions in vivo [89], which may be an important basis for their clinical effects.

Since β_3-ARs are present in the urothelium [90], their possible role in bladder relaxation has been investigated [90, 91]. However, to what extent a urothelial signaling pathway contributes in vitro and in vivo to the relaxant effects of β-AR agonists in general, and β_3-AR agonists specifically, remains to be elucidated.

Neural Control of LUT Function

Both bladder filling and voiding are controlled by neural circuits in the brain, spinal cord, and peripheral ganglia [92–95]. These circuits coordinate the activity of the smooth muscle in the detrusor and urethra with that of the striated muscles in the urethral sphincter and pelvic floor. Suprapontine influences are believed to act as on-off switches to shift the LUT between the two modes of operation: storage and elimination. In adults, urine storage and voiding are under voluntary control and depend upon learned behavior, but in infants these switching mechanisms function in a reflex manner to produce involuntary voiding. Injuries or diseases of the central nervous system (CNS) can disrupt the voluntary control of micturition and cause the

reemergence of reflex micturition, resulting in bladder dysfunction. However, bladder dysfunction may also result from changes in the peripheral innervation or the smooth and skeletal muscle components of the LUT [19, 92, 96].

Normal micturition occurs in response to afferent signals from the LUT [93, 94, 97, 98]. However, both filling of the bladder and voiding involve a complex pattern of afferent and efferent signaling in parasympathetic (pelvic nerves), sympathetic (hypogastric nerves), and somatic (pudendal nerves) pathways, which either keep the bladder in a relaxed state, enabling urine storage at low intravesical pressure, or which initiate bladder emptying by relaxing the outflow region and contracting the detrusor (Fig. 1.7). Integration of the autonomic and somatic efferents results in the contraction of the detrusor muscle being preceded by relaxation of the outlet region, thereby facilitating bladder emptying. On the contrary, during the storage phase, the detrusor muscle is relaxed and the outlet region is contracted to maintain continence.

The sacral parasympathetic pathways mediate contraction of the detrusor smooth muscle and relaxation of the outflow region. The preganglionic parasympathetic neurons are located to the sacral parasympathetic nucleus (SPN) in the spinal cord at the level of S2–S4. The axons pass through the pelvic nerves and synapse with the postganglionic nerves in either the pelvic plexus, in ganglia on the surface of the bladder

Fig. 1.7 Stimulation of the
β_3-adrenoceptor: molecular
mechanism of action

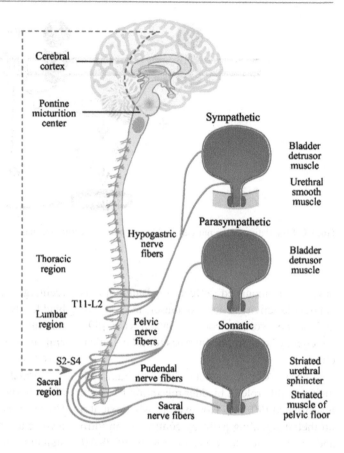

(vesical ganglia), or within the walls of the bladder and urethra (intramural ganglia). The ganglionic neurotransmission is predominantly mediated by ACh acting on nicotinic receptors, although the transmission can be modulated by adrenergic, muscarinic, purinergic, and peptidergic presynaptic receptors. The postganglionic neurons in the pelvic nerve mediate the excitatory input to the normal human detrusor smooth muscle by releasing ACh acting on muscarinic receptors. However, an atropine-resistant (non-adrenergic, non-cholinergic: NANC) contractile component is regularly found in the bladders of most animal species. Such a component can also be demonstrated in functionally and morphologically altered human bladder tissue but contributes only to a few percent to normal detrusor contraction [92]. Adenosine triphosphate (ATP) is the most important mediator of the NANC contraction, although the involvement of other transmitters

cannot be ruled out [92]. The pelvic nerve also conveys parasympathetic nerves to the outflow region and the urethra. These nerves exert an inhibitory effect on the smooth muscle, by releasing nitric oxide and other transmitters [92].

The sympathetic innervation of the bladder and urethra originates from the intermediolateral nuclei in the thoracolumbar region (T10–L2) of the spinal cord. The axons leave the spinal cord via the splanchnic nerves and either travel through the inferior mesenteric ganglia (IMF) and the hypogastric nerve or pass through the paravertebral chain to the lumbosacral sympathetic chain ganglia and enter the pelvic nerve. Thus, sympathetic signals are conveyed in both the hypogastric nerve and the pelvic nerve. Like the parasympathetic preganglionic transmission, the ganglionic sympathetic transmission is predominantly mediated by ACh acting on nicotinic receptors. Some preganglionic terminals synapse with the postganglionic cells in the paravertebral ganglia or in the IMF, while others synapse closer to the pelvic organs, and short postganglionic neurons innervate the target organs. Thus, the hypogastric and pelvic nerves contain both pre- and postganglionic fiber. The predominant effect of the sympathetic innervation is to contract the bladder base and the urethra. In addition, the sympathetic innervation inhibits the parasympathetic pathways at spinal and ganglionic levels. In the human bladder, noradrenaline is released in response to electrical stimulation in vitro, and the normal detrusor response to released noradrenaline is relaxation [63]. However, the importance of the sympathetic innervation for relaxation of the human detrusor has never been established. In contrast, in several animal species, the adrenergic innervation has been demonstrated to mediate relaxation of the detrusor during filling [19].

The somatic innervation of the urethral rhabdosphincter and of some perineal muscles (e.g., compressor urethrae and urethrovaginal sphincter) is provided by the pudendal nerve. These fibers originate from sphincter motor neurons located in the ventral horn of the sacral spinal cord (levels S2–S4) in a region called Onuf's (Onufrowicz's) nucleus [99, 100].

The afferent nerves to the bladder and urethra originate in the dorsal root ganglia at the lumbosacral level of the spinal cord and travel via the pelvic nerve to the periphery [101–103]. Afferent axons are identified primarily by their content of neuropeptide/calcitonin-gene-related peptide (CGRP), pituitary adenylate cyclase-activating peptide (PACAP), vasoactive intestinal peptide (VIP), or substance P [104]. Some afferents originate in the dorsal root ganglia at the thoracolumbar level and travel peripherally in the hypogastric nerve. The afferent nerves to the striated muscle of the external urethral sphincter travel in the pudendal nerve to the sacral region of the spinal cord.

The most important afferents for the micturition process are myelinated Aδ-fibers and unmyelinated C-fibers traveling in the pelvic nerve to the sacral spinal cord, conveying information from receptors in the bladder wall. The Aδ-fibers respond to passive distension and active contraction, thus conveying information about bladder filling. The activation threshold for Aδ-fibers is 5–15 mm H_2O. This is the intravesical pressure at which humans report the first sensation of bladder filling. C-fibers have a high mechanical threshold and respond primarily to chemical irritation of the bladder urothelium/suburothelium or to cold. Following chemical irritation, the C-fiber afferents exhibit spontaneous firing when the bladder is empty and increased firing during bladder distension. These fibers are normally inactive and are therefore termed "silent fibers." Afferent information about the amount of urine in the bladder is continuously conveyed to the mesencephalic periaqueductal gray (PAG), and from there to the pontine micturition center (PMC), also called Barrington's nucleus [105].

Bladder Filling

Storage Reflexes. As mentioned, during the storage phase, the bladder has to relax in order to maintain a low intravesical pressure. Urine storage is regulated by two separate storage reflexes, of which one is sympathetic (autonomic) and the other is somatic [100]. The sympathetic storage reflex (*pelvic-to-hypogastric reflex*) is initiated as the bladder distends (myelinated Aδ-fibers) and the generated afferent activity travels in the pelvic nerves to the spinal cord. Within the spinal cord, sympathetic firing from the lumbar region (L1–L3) is initiated, which, by effects at the ganglionic level, decreases excitatory parasympathetic inputs to the bladder. Postganglionic neurons release noradrenaline, which facilitates urine storage by stimulating β_3-adrenoceptors (ARs) in the detrusor smooth muscle. There is little evidence for a functionally important sympathetic innervation of the human detrusor, which is in contrast to what has been found in several animal species. The sympathetic innervation of the human bladder is found mainly in the outlet region, where it mediates contraction. During micturition, this sympathetic reflex pathway is markedly inhibited via supraspinal mechanisms to allow the bladder to contract and the urethra to relax. Thus, the Aδ afferents and the sympathetic efferent fibers constitute a *vesico-spinal-vesical storage reflex*, which maintains the bladder in a relaxed mode while the proximal urethra and bladder neck are contracted.

In response to a sudden increase in intra-abdominal pressure, such as during a cough, laugh, or sneeze, a more rapid somatic storage reflex (*pelvic-to-pudendal reflex*), also called the guarding or continence reflex, is initiated. The evoked afferent activity travels along myelinated Aδ afferent nerve fibers in the pelvic nerve to the sacral spinal cord, where efferent somatic ure-thral motor neurons, located in the nucleus of Onuf, are activated. Afferent information is also conveyed to the PAG and from there to the L-region of the PMC. From this center impulses are conveyed to the motor neurons in the nucleus of Onuf. Axons from these neurons travel in the pudendal nerve and release ACh which activates nicotinic cholinergic receptors on the rhabdo-sphincter, which contracts. This pathway is toni-cally active during urine storage. During sudden abdominal pressure increases, however, it becomes dynamically active to contract the rhab-dosphincter. During micturition, this reflex is strongly inhibited via spinal and supraspinal mechanisms to allow the rhabdosphincter to relax and permit urine passage through the urethra. In addition to this spinal somatic storage reflex, there is also supraspinal input from the pons, which projects directly to the nucleus of Onuf and is of importance for voluntary control of the rhabdosphincter [106, 107].

Bladder Emptying

The Vesico-bulbo-vesical Micturition Reflex. Electrophysiological experiments in animals pro-vide evidence for a voiding reflex mediated through a vesico-bulbo-vesical pathway involv-ing neural circuits in the pons, which constitute the PMC. Other regions in the brain, important for micturition, include the hypothalamus and cerebral cortex [94, 108, 109]. Bladder filling leads to increased activation of tension receptors within the bladder wall and thus to increased

afferent activity in Aδ-fibers [86]. These fibers project on spinal tract neurons mediating increased sympathetic firing to maintain conti-nence as discussed above (storage reflex). In addition, the spinal tract neurons convey the afferent activity to more rostral areas of the spinal cord and the brain. As mentioned previously, one important receiver of the afferent information from the bladder is the PAG in the rostral brain stem [94, 105]. The PAG receives information from both afferent neurons in the bladder and from more rostral areas in the brain, that is, cere-bral cortex and hypothalamus. This information is integrated in the PAG and the medial part of the PMC (the M region), which also control the descending pathways in the micturition reflex. Thus, PMC can be seen as a switch in the mictu-rition reflex, inhibiting parasympathetic activity in the descending pathways when there is low activity in the afferent fibers, and activating the parasympathetic pathways when the afferent activity reaches a certain threshold. The threshold is believed to be set by the inputs from more ros-tral regions in the brain. In cats, lesioning of regions above the inferior colliculus usually facilitates micturition by elimination of inhibi-tory inputs from more rostral areas of the brain. On the other hand, transections at a lower level inhibit micturition. Thus, the PMC seems to be under a tonic inhibitory control. A variation of the inhibitory input to PMC results in a variation of bladder capacity. Experiments on rats have shown that the micturition threshold is regulated by, for example, gamma-aminobutyric acid (GABA)-ergic inhibitory mechanisms in the PMC neurons.

The Vesico-spinal-vesical Micturition Reflex. Spinal lesions rostral to the lumbosacral level interrupt the vesico-bulbo-vesical pathway and abolish the supraspinal and voluntary control of micturition [92, 101, 102]. This results initially in an areflexic bladder accompanied by urinary retention. An automatic vesico-spinal-vesical micturition reflex develops slowly, although voiding is generally insufficient due to bladder-sphincter dyssynergia, that is, simultaneous con-traction of bladder and urethra. The recovery of bladder function after spinal cord injury is dependent in part on the plasticity of bladder afferent pathways and the unmasking of reflexes triggered by unmyelinated, capsaicin-sensitive, C-fiber bladder afferent neurons. Plasticity is associated with morphologic, chemical, and electrical changes in bladder afferent neurons and appears to be mediated in part by neurotrophic factors released in the spinal cord and the peripheral target organs [101, 102].

References

1. Williams JH, Brading AF. Urethral sphincter: normal function and changes in disease. In: Daniel EE, Tomita Y, Tsuchida S, Watanabe M, editors. Sphincters: normal function—changes in diseases. Boca Raton: CRC Press; 1992. p. 315–38.
2. Brading AF, Teramoto N, Dass N, McCoy R. Morphological and physiological characteristics of urethral circular and longitudinal smooth muscle. Scand J Urol Nephrol Suppl. 2001;207:12–8.
3. Drake MJ, Mills IW, Gillespie JI. Model of peripheral autonomous modules and a myovesical plexus in normal and overactive bladder function. Lancet. 2001;358:401–3.
4. Dixon J, Gosling JA. Ultrastructure of smooth muscle cells in the urinary system. In: Motta PM, editor. Ultrastructure of smooth muscle. Boston: Kluwer; 1990. p. 153–69.
5. McCloskey KD. Interstitial cells of Cajal in the urinary tract. Handb Exp Pharmacol. 2011;202:233–54.
6. McCloskey KD. Bladder interstitial cells: an updated review of current knowledge. Acta Physiol (Oxf). 2013;207(1):7–15.
7. Miodoński AJ, Litwin JA. Microvascular architecture of the human urinary bladder wall: a corrosion casting study. Anat Rec. 1999;254(3):375–81.
8. Apodaca G. The uroepithelium: not just a passive barrier. Traffic. 2004;5(3):117–28.
9. Khandelwal P, Abraham SN, Apodaca G. Cell biology and physiology of the uroepithelium. Am J Physiol Renal Physiol. 2009;297(6):F1477–501.
10. Andersson K-E, McCloskey K. Lamina propria: the functional center of the bladder? Neurourol Urodyn. 2014;33(1):9–16.
11. Sui GP, Rothery S, Dupont E, Fry CH, Severs NJ. Gap junctions and connexin expression in human suburothelial interstitial cells. BJU Int. 2002;90:118–29.
12. Wiseman OJ, Fowler CJ, Landon DN. The role of the human bladder lamina propria myofibroblast. BJU Int. 2003;91:89–93.
13. Brading AF, McCloskey KD. Mechanisms of disease: specialized interstitial cells of the urinary

tract—an assessment of current knowledge. Nat Clin Pract Urol. 2005;2(11):546–54.
14. Davidson RA, McCloskey KD. Morphology and localization of interstitial cells in the guinea pig bladder: structural relationships with smooth muscle and neurons. J Urol. 2005;173(4):1385–90.
15. Koh BH, Roy R, Hollywood MA, Thornbury KD, McHale NG, Sergeant GP, Hatton WJ, Ward SM, Sanders KM, Koh SD. Platelet-derived growth factor receptor-α cells in mouse urinary bladder: a new class of interstitial cells. J Cell Mol Med. 2012;16:691–700.
16. Monaghan KP, Johnston L, McCloskey KD. Identification of PDGFRα positive populations of interstitial cells in human and guinea pig bladders. J Urol. 2012;188(2):639–47.
17. Johnston L, Woolsey S, Cunningham RM, O'Kane H, Duggan B, Keane P, McCloskey KD. Morphological expression of KIT positive interstitial cells of Cajal in human bladder. J Urol. 2010;184(1):370–7.
18. Somlyo AP, Somlyo AV. Vascular smooth muscle. I. Normal structure, pathology, biochemistry, and biophysics. Pharmacol Rev. 1968;20:197–272.
19. Andersson KE, Arner A. Urinary bladder contraction and relaxation: physiology and pathophysiology. Physiol Rev. 2004;84(3):935–86.
20. Abrams P, Andersson KE. Muscarinic receptor antagonists for overactive bladder. BJU Int. 2007;100(5):987–1006.
21. Giglio D, Tobin G. Muscarinic receptor subtypes in the lower urinary tract. Pharmacology. 2009;83(5):259–69.
22. Andersson KE. Muscarinic acetylcholine receptors in the urinary tract. Handb Exp Pharmacol. 2011;202:319–44.
23. Bschleipfer T, Schukowski K, Weidner W, Grando SA, Schwantes U, Kummer W, Lips KS. Expression and distribution of cholinergic receptors in the human urothelium. Life Sci. 2007;80(24–25):2303–7.
24. Mansfield KJ, Liu L, Mitchelson FJ, Moore KH, Millard RJ, Burcher E. Muscarinic receptor subtypes in human bladder detrusor and mucosa, studied by radioligand binding and quantitative competitive RT-PCR: changes in ageing. Br J Pharmacol. 2005;144(8):1089–99.
25. Zarghooni S, Wunsch J, Bodenbenner M, Brüggmann D, Grando SA, Schwantes U, Wess J, Kummer W, Lips KS. Expression of muscarinic and nicotinic acetylcholine receptors in the mouse urothelium. Life Sci. 2007;80(24–25):2308–13.
26. Caulfield MP, Birdsall NJM. International Union of Pharmacology. XVII. Classification of muscarinic acetylcholine receptors. Pharmacol Rev. 1998;50:279.
27. Abrams P, Andersson KE, Buccafusco JJ, Chapple C, de Groat WC, Fryer AD, Kay G, Laties A, Nathanson NM, Pasricha PJ, Wein AJ. Muscarinic receptors: their distribution and function in body systems, and the implications for treating overactive bladder. Br J Pharmacol. 2006;148(5):565–78.

28. Hegde SS. Muscarinic receptors in the bladder: from basic research to therapeutics. Br J Pharmacol. 2006;147:S80.

29. Chess-Williams R, Chapple CR, Yamanishi T, Yasuda K, Sellers DJ. The minor population of M3-receptors mediate contraction of human detrusor muscle in vitro. J Auton Pharmacol. 2001;21(5–6):243–8.

30. Fetscher C, Fleichman M, Schmidt M, Krege S, Michel MC. M(3) muscarinic receptors mediate contraction of human urinary bladder. Br J Pharmacol. 2002;136(5):641–3.

31. Kories C, Czyborra C, Fetscher C, Schneider T, Krege S, Michel MC. Gender comparison of muscarinic receptor expression and function in rat and human urinary bladder: differential regulation of M2 and M3 receptors? Naunyn Schmiedebergs Arch Pharmacol. 2003;367(5):524–31.

32. Schneider T, Hein P, Michel MC. Signal transduction underlying carbachol-induced contraction of rat urinary bladder. I. Phospholipases and Ca^{2+} sources. Pharmacol Exp Ther. 2004;308(1):47–53.

33. Schneider T, Fetscher C, Krege S, Michel MC. Signal transduction underlying carbachol-induced contraction of human urinary bladder. J Pharmacol Exp Ther. 2004;309(3):1148–53.

34. Matsui M, Motomura D, Karasawa H, Fujikawa T, Jiang J, Komiya Y, Takahashi S, Taketo MM. Multiple functional defects in peripheral autonomic organs in mice lacking muscarinic acetylcholine receptor gene for the M3 subtype. Proc Natl Acad Sci U S A. 2000;97(17):9579–84.

35. Matsui M, Motomura D, Fujikawa T, Jiang J, Takahashi S, Manabe T, Taketo MM. Mice lacking M2 and M3 muscarinic acetylcholine receptors are devoid of cholinergic smooth muscle contractions but still viable. J Neurosci. 2002;22(24):10627–32.

36. Stengel PW, Yamada M, Wess J, Cohen ML. M(3)-receptor knockout mice: muscarinic receptor function in atria, stomach fundus, urinary bladder, and trachea. Am J Physiol Regul Integr Comp Physiol. 2002;282(5):R1443–9.

37. Ehlert FJ, Ahn S, Pak KJ, Park GJ, Sangnil MS, Tran JA, Matsui M. Neuronally released acetylcholine acts on the M2 muscarinic receptor to oppose the relaxant effect of isoproterenol on cholinergic contractions in mouse urinary bladder. J Pharmacol Exp Ther. 2007;322(2):631–7.

38. Braverman AS, Luthin GR, Ruggieri MR. M2 muscarinic receptor contributes to contraction of the denervated rat urinary bladder. Am J Physiol. 1998;275:R1654.

39. Braverman AS, Kohn IJ, Luthin GR, et al. Prejunctional M1 facilitatory and M2 inhibitory muscarinic receptors mediate rat bladder contractility. Am J Physiol. 1998;274:R517.

40. Braverman AS, Karlovsky M, Pontari MA, et al. Aging and hypertrophy change the muscarinic receptor subtype mediating bladder contraction from M3 towards M2. J Urol. 2002;167 Suppl.:43. Abstract #170.

41. Braverman AS, Ruggieri Sr MR. Hypertrophy changes the muscarinic receptor subtype mediating bladder contraction from M3 toward M2. Am J Physiol. 2003;285:R701.

42. Braverman AS, Doumanian LR, Ruggieri Sr MR. M2 and M3 muscarinic receptor activation of urinary bladder contractile signal transduction. II. Denervated rat bladder. J Pharmacol Exp Ther. 2006;316:875.

43. Pontari MA, Braverman AS, Ruggieri Sr MR. The M2 muscarinic receptor mediates in vitro bladder contractions from patients with neurogenic bladder dysfunction. Am J Physiol Regul Integr Comp Physiol. 2004;286(5):R874–80.

44. Ouslander JG. Management of overactive bladder. N Engl J Med. 2004;350:786.

45. Wegener JW, Schulla V, Lee TS, Koller A, Feil S, Feil R, Kleppisch T, Klugbauer N, Moosmang S, Welling A, Hofmann F. An essential role of CaV1.2 L-type calcium channel for urinary bladder function. FASEB J. 2004;18:1159–61.

46. Frazier EP, Braverman AS, Peters SL, Michel MC, Ruggieri Sr MR. Does phospholipase C mediate muscarinic receptor-induced rat urinary bladder contraction? J Pharmacol Exp Ther. 2007;322:998.

47. Frazier EP, Peters SL, Braverman AS, Ruggieri Sr MR, Michel MC. Signal transduction underlying the control of urinary bladder smooth muscle tone by muscarinic receptors and beta-adrenoceptors. Naunyn Schmiedebergs Arch Pharmacol. 2008;377(4–6):449–62.

48. Chess-Williams R. Muscarinic receptors of the urinary bladder: detrusor, urothelial and prejunctional. Auton Autacoid Pharmacol. 2002;22(3):133–45.

49. Kumar V, Cross RL, Chess-Williams R, Chapple CR. Recent advances in basic science for overactive bladder. Curr Opin Urol. 2005;15:222.

50. Hawthorn MH, Chapple CR, Cock M, Chess-Williams R. Urothelium-derived inhibitory factor(s) influences on detrusor muscle contractility in vitro. Br J Pharmacol. 2000;129:416.

51. Wuest M, Kaden S, Hakenberg OW, Wirth MP, Ravens U. Effect of rilmakalim on detrusor contraction in the presence and absence of urothelium. Naunyn Schmiedebergs Arch Pharmacol. 2005;372:203.

52. Sadananda P, Chess-Williams R, Burcher E. Contractile properties of the pig bladder mucosa in response to neurokinin A: a role for myofibroblasts? Br J Pharmacol. 2008;153:1465.

53. Andersson MC, Tobin G, Giglio D. Cholinergic nitric oxide release from the urinary bladder mucosa in cyclophosphamide-induced cystitis of the anaesthetized rat. Br J Pharmacol. 2008;153:1438.

54. Young JS, Matharu R, Carew MA, Fry CH. Inhibition of stretching-evoked ATP release from bladder mucosa by anticholinergic agents. BJU Int. 2012;110(8 Pt B):E397–401.

55. Stevens LA, Chapple CR, Chess-Williams R. Human idiopathic and neurogenic overactive bladders and the role of M2 muscarinic receptors in contraction. Eur Urol. 2007;52(2):531–8.
56. Michel MC, Barendrecht MM. Physiological and pathological regulation of the autonomic control of urinary bladder contractility. Pharmacol Ther. 2008;117:297.
57. Yoshida M, Homma Y, Inadome A, Yono M, Seshita H, Miyamoto Y, Murakami S, Kawabe K, Ueda S. Age-related changes in cholinergic and purinergic neurotransmission in human isolated bladder smooth muscles. Exp Gerontol. 2001;36(1):99.
58. Yoshida M, Masunaga K, Satoji Y, Maeda Y, Nagata T, Inadome A. Basic and clinical aspects of non-neuronal acetylcholine: expression of non-neuronal acetylcholine in urothelium and its clinical significance. J Pharmacol Sci. 2008;106(2):193–8.
59. Herbison P, Hay-Smith J, Ellis G, Moore K. Effectiveness of anticholinergic drugs compared with placebo in the treatment of overactive bladder: systematic review. Br Med J. 2003;326:841.
60. Chapple CR, Khullar V, Gabriel Z, Muston D, Bitoun CE, Weinstein D. The effects of antimuscarinic treatments in overactive bladder: an update of a systematic review and meta-analysis. Eur Urol. 2008;54(3):543.
61. Novara G, Galfano A, Secco S, D'Elia C, Cavalleri S, Ficarra V, Artibani W. Systematic review and meta-analysis of randomized controlled trials with antimuscarinic drugs for overactive bladder. Eur Urol. 2008;54(4):740–63.
62. Shamliyan TA, Kane RL, Wyman J, Wilt TJ. Systematic review: randomized, controlled trials of nonsurgical treatments for urinary incontinence in women. Ann Intern Med. 2008;148:459.
63. Andersson KE. Pharmacology of lower urinary tract smooth muscles and penile erectile tissues. Pharmacol Rev. 1993;45(3):253–308.
64. Malloy BJ, Price DT, Price RR, Bienstock AM, Dole MK, Funk BL, Rudner XL, Richardson CD, Donatucci CF, Schwinn DA. Alpha1-adrenergic receptor subtypes in human detrusor. J Urol. 1998;160:937–43.
65. Michel MC, Vrydag W. Alpha1-, alpha2- and beta-adrenoceptors in the urinary bladder, urethra and prostate. Br J Pharmacol. 2006;147 Suppl 2:S88–119.
66. Andersson KE, Gratzke C. Pharmacology of alpha1-adrenoceptor antagonists in the lower urinary tract and central nervous system. Nat Clin Pract Urol. 2007;4(7):368–78.
67. Hampel C, Dolber PC, Smith MP, Savic SL, Throff JW, Thor KB, Schwinn DA. Modulation of bladder alpha1-adrenergic receptor subtype expression by bladder outlet obstruction. J Urol. 2002;167(3):1513–21.
68. Yamaguchi O. Beta3-adrenoceptors in human detrusor muscle. Urology. 2002;59:25–9.
69. Bouchelouche K, Andersen L, Alvarez S, Nordling J, Bouchelouche P. Increased contractile response to phenylephrine in detrusor of patients with bladder outlet obstruction: effect of the alpha1A and alpha1D-adrenergic receptor antagonist tamsulosin. J Urol. 2005;173(2):657–61.
70. Trevisani M, Campi B, Gatti R, André E, Materazzi S, Nicoletti P, Gazzieri D, Geppetti P. The influence of alpha1-adrenoreceptors on neuropeptide release from primary sensory neurons of the lower urinary tract. Eur Urol. 2007;52(3):901–8.
71. Yokoyama O, Ito H, Aoki Y, Oyama N, Miwa Y, Akino H. Selective α1A-blocker improves bladder storage function in rats via suppression of C-fiber afferent activity. World J Urol. 2010;28(5):609–14.
72. Yazaki J, Aikawa K, Shishido K, Yanagida T, Nomiya M, Ishibashi K, Haga N, Yamaguchi O. Alpha1-adrenoceptor antagonists improve bladder storage function through reduction of afferent activity in rats with bladder outlet obstruction. Neurourol Urodyn. 2011;30(3):461–7.
73. Kurizaki Y, Ishizuka O, Imamura T, Ichino M, Ogawa T, Igawa Y, Nishizawa O, Andersson KE. Relation between expression of α(1)-adrenoceptor mRNAs in bladder mucosa and urodynamic findings in men with lower urinary tract symptoms. Scand J Urol Nephrol. 2011;45(1):15–9.
74. Igawa Y, Yamazaki Y, Takeda H, Hayakawa K, Akahane M, Ajisawa Y, Yoneyama T, Nishizawa O, Andersson KE. Functional and molecular biological evidence for a possible beta3-adrenoceptor in the human detrusor muscle. Br J Pharmacol. 1999;126:819–25.
75. Takeda M, Obara K, Mizusawa T, Tomita Y, Arai K, Tsutsui T, Hatano A, Takahashi K, Nomura S. Evidence for beta3-adrenoceptor subtypes in relaxation of the human urinary bladder detrusor: analysis by molecular biological and pharmacological methods. J Pharmacol Exp Ther. 1999;288:1367–73.
76. Igawa Y, Aizawa N, Homma Y. Beta3-adrenoceptor agonists: possible role in the treatment of overactive bladder. Korean J Urol. 2010;51(12):811–8.
77. Michel MC. β-Adrenergic receptor subtypes in the urinary tract. Handb Exp Pharmacol. 2011;(202):307–18.
78. Igawa Y, Michel MC. Pharmacological profile of β(3)-adrenoceptor agonists in clinical development for the treatment of overactive bladder syndrome. Naunyn Schmiedebergs Arch Pharmacol. 2013;386(3):177.
79. Yamazaki Y, Takeda H, Akahane M, Igawa Y, Nishizawa O, Ajisawa Y. Species differences in the distribution of beta-adrenoceptor subtypes in bladder smooth muscle. Br J Pharmacol. 1998;124:593–9.
80. Andersson KE, Chapple C, Wein A. The basis for drug treatment of the overactive bladder. World J Urol. 2001;19:294–8.
81. Nomiya M, Yamaguchi O. A quantitative analysis of mRNA expression of alpha 1 and beta-adrenoceptor subtypes and their functional roles in human normal

and obstructed bladders. J Urol. 2003;170 (2 Pt 1):649–53.

82. Rohner TJ, Hannigan JD, Sanford EJ. Altered in vitro adrenergic responses of dog detrusor muscle after chronic bladder outlet obstruction. Urology. 1978;11:357–61.

83. Tsujii T, Azuma H, Yamaguchi T, Oshima H. A possible role of decreased relaxation mediated by beta-adrenoceptors in bladder outlet obstruction by benign prostatic hyperplasia. Br J Pharmacol. 1992;107:803–7.

84. Frazier EP, Mathy MJ, Peters SL, Michel MC. Does cyclic AMP mediate rat urinary bladder relaxation by isoproterenol? J Pharmacol Exp Ther. 2005; 313(1):260–7.

85. Uchida H, Shishido K, Nomiya M, Yamaguchi O. Involvement of cyclic AMP-dependent and -independent mechanisms in the relaxation of rat detrusor muscle via beta-adrenoceptors. Eur J Pharmacol. 2005;518(2–3):195–202.

86. Iggo A. Tension receptors in the stomach and the urinary bladder. J Physiol. 1955;128(3):593–607.

87. Aizawa N, Homma Y, Igawa Y. Effects of mirabegron, a novel β3-adrenoceptor agonist, on primary bladder afferent activity and bladder microcontractions in rats compared with the effects of oxybutynin. Eur Urol. 2012;62(6):1165–73.

88. Biers SM, Reynard JM, Brading AF. The effects of a new selective beta3-adrenoceptor agonist (GW427353) on spontaneous activity and detrusor relaxation in human bladder. BJU Int. 2006;98(6):1310–4.

89. Gillespie JI, Palea S, Guilloteau V, Guerard M, Lluel P, Korstanje C. Modulation of non-voiding activity by the muscarinergic antagonist tolterodine and the β(3)-adrenoceptor agonist mirabegron in conscious rats with partial outflow obstruction. BJU Int. 2012;110(2 Pt 2):E132–42.

90. Otsuka A, Shinbo H, Matsumoto R, Kurita Y, Ozono S. Expression and functional role of beta-adrenoceptors in the human urinary bladder urothelium. Naunyn Schmiedebergs Arch Pharmacol. 2008;377(4–6):473–81.

91. Murakami S, Chapple CR, Akino H, Sellers DJ, Chess-Williams R. The role of the urothelium in mediating bladder responses to isoprenaline. BJU Int. 2007;99(3):669–73.

92. Andersson KE, Wein AJ. Pharmacology of the lower urinary tract: basis for current and future treatments of urinary incontinence. Pharmacol Rev. 2004;56(4):581–631 [PMID: 15602011].

93. de Groat WC. Integrative control of the lower urinary tract: preclinical perspective. Br J Pharmacol. 2006;147 Suppl 2:S25–40.

94. Fowler CJ, Griffiths D, de Groat WC. The neural control of micturition. Nat Rev Neurosci. 2008;9(6):453–66.

95. Beckel JM, Holstege G. Neurophysiology of the lower urinary tract. Handb Exp Pharmacol. 2011; 202:149–69.

96. Banakhar MA, Al-Shaiji TF, Hassouna MM. Pathophysiology of overactive bladder. Int Urogynecol J. 2012;23(8):975–82.

97. Birder L, de Groat W, Mills I, Morrison J, Thor K, Drake M. Neural control of the lower urinary tract: peripheral and spinal mechanisms. Neurourol Urodyn. 2010;29(1):128–39.

98. Daly DM, Collins VM, Chapple CR, Grundy D. The afferent system and its role in lower urinary tract dysfunction. Curr Opin Urol. 2011;21(4): 268–74.

99. Thor KB, de Groat WC. Neural control of the female urethral and anal rhabdosphincter and pelvic floor muscles. Am J Physiol Regul Integr Comp Physiol. 2010;299(2):R416–38.

100. Thor KB, Donatucci C. Central nervous system control of the lower urinary tract: new pharmacological approaches to stress urinary incontinence in women. J Urol. 2004;172(1):27–33.

101. de Groat WC, Yoshimura N. Changes in afferent activity after spinal cord injury. Neurourol Urodyn. 2010;29(1):63–76.

102. de Groat WC, Yoshimura N. Plasticity in reflex pathways to the lower urinary tract following spinal cord injury. Exp Neurol. 2012;235(1):123–32.

103. Kanai A, Andersson KE. Bladder afferent signaling: recent findings. J Urol. 2010;183(4):1288–95.

104. Smet PJ, Moore KH, Jonavicius J. Distribution and colocalization of calcitonin gene-related peptide, tachykinins, and vasoactive intestinal peptide in normal and idiopathic unstable human urinary bladder. Lab Invest. 1997;77:37–49.

105. Kuipers R, Mouton LJ, Holstege G. Afferent projections to the pontine micturition center in the cat. J Comp Neurol. 2006;494(1):36–53.

106. Sugaya K, Nishijima S, Miyazato M, Ogawa Y. Central nervous control of micturition and urine storage. J Smooth Muscle Res. 2005;41(3): 117–32.

107. Blok BF, de Weerd H, Holstege G. The pontine micturition center projects to sacral cord GABA immunoreactive neurons in the cat. Neurosci Lett. 1997;233(2–3):109–12.

108. Griffiths DJ. Cerebral control of bladder function. Curr Urol Rep. 2004;5(5):348–52.

109. Griffiths D, Derbyshire S, Stenger A, Resnick N. Brain control of normal and overactive bladder. J Urol. 2005;174(5):1862–7.

Normal and Abnormal Function: An Overview

2

Alan J. Wein

The bladder (reservoir) and its outlet function as a pair of interrelated structures whose coordinated actions in the adult normally bring about (1) low-pressure reservoir filling and urine storage without involuntary leakage and (2) periodic voluntary emptying of the system, again at low pressure [1, 2]. The neuroanatomic, physiologic, and pharmacologic milieu which normally serves as a background and operating system for this simple sounding cycle is well described in the previous chapter. For conceptualization and a framework for evaluation, categorization, and management of abnormal function, it is logical to consider these two phases as relatively discrete: bladder filling and urine storage, and bladder emptying/voiding [3]. This micturition cycle normally displays these two modes of operation in a simple on-off fashion [4–6] which involves (1) activation of storage reflexes affecting the outlet and inhibiting the detrusor contraction reflex and (2) switching to inhibition of the storage reflexes and concomitant activation of the voiding reflex—and back again. As an easy to understand framework for subsequent discussion of evaluation, categorization, and management, the basics of these two phases are summarized followed by a brief description of what can and does malfunction.

A.J. Wein, M.D., Ph.D. (Hon.), F.A.C.S. (✉)
Perelman School of Medicine,
University of Pennsylvania Health System,
Philadelphia, PA 19104, USA
e-mail: alan.wein@uphs.upenn.edu

Normal Function [4, 6–9]

The normal adult bladder response to filling at a physiologic rate is an almost imperceptible change in content pressure. During at least the initial stages of bladder filling, this very high compliance (Δ volume/Δ pressure) is due primarily to the elastic and viscoelastic properties of the bladder wall which allow it to stretch to a certain degree without any increase in tension exerted on its contents. The viscoelastic properties of the stroma (bladder wall less smooth muscle and epithelium) are due to its primary components, collagen and elastin. There may also be an active but non-neurogenic component to the filling/storage properties of the bladder. Some have suggested that an as yet unidentified relaxing factor is released from the urothelium, and others have suggested urothelium released nitric oxide may exert an inhibitory effect on the afferent mechanisms during filling. At physiologic filling rates, intravesical pressure remains essentially unchanged. In the clinical setting, filling cystometry normally shows a slight increase in detrusor pressure, but this pressure rise is a function of the fact that clinic cystometry filling is always carried out at a greater than normal physiologic rate.

At a certain level of bladder filling, spinal sympathetic reflexes are evoked in many animals, and there is evidence to support such a role for at least some components of these in humans. There are three limbs to this sympathetic reflex (see Fig. 2.1).

A.J. Wein et al. (eds.), *Bladder Dysfunction in the Adult: The Basis for Clinical Management*, Current Clinical Urology, DOI 10.1007/978-1-4939-0853-0_2, © Springer Science+Business Media New York 2014

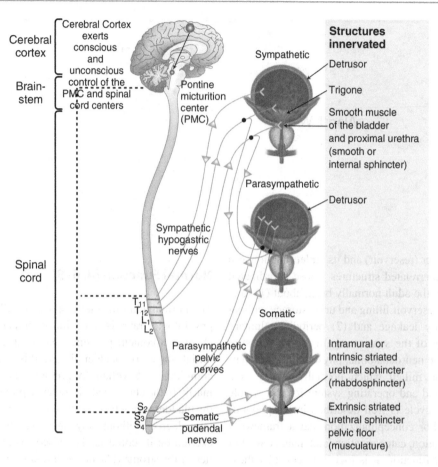

Fig. 2.1 Current conceptualization of lower urinary tract innervation by somatic (pudendal nerve) and autonomic (sympathetic and parasympathetic) nervous systems (modified after Newman and Wein [10]; courtesy of Robin Noel)

One is neurally mediated stimulation of the predominantly α-1a adrenergic receptors in the area of the bladder neck and proximal urethra, the net result of which would be to cause an increase of resistance in that area. One is neurally mediated stimulation of the predominantly β-3 adrenergic receptors in the bladder body smooth musculature, causing a decrease in tension. The third is an inhibitory effect on bladder contractility thought to be mediated primarily by sympathetic modulation of parasympathetic ganglionic transmission. Good evidence seems to also support a strong tonic inhibitory effect of endogenous opioids and other transmitters on bladder activity at the level of the spinal cord, the parasympathetic ganglia, and the brain stem as well. Finally, bladder filling and wall distention may release autocrine-like factors which themselves influence contractility, either by stimulation or inhibition.

There is a gradual increase in urethral pressure during bladder filling primarily contributed by a striated sphincter reflex. The rise in urethral pressure seen during the filling and storage phase of micturition can be correlated with an increase in efferent pudendal nerve impulse frequency. This constitutes the efferent limb of a spinal somatic reflex that is initiated when a certain critical intravesical pressure is reached, the so-called guarding reflex, which results in an increase in striated sphincter activity.

The passive properties of the urethral wall also undoubtedly play a large role in the maintenance of continence. Urethral wall tension develops within the outer layers of the urethra; however, it is a product not only of the active characteristics of smooth and striated muscle but also of the passive characteristics of the elastic and collagenous tissues that make up the urethral wall. In addition, this tension must be exerted on a soft, plastic inner layer capable of being compressed to a closed configuration—the "filler material" representing the submucosal portion of the urethra. The softer and more plastic this area is, the less pressure required by the tension-producing layers to produce continence. Finally, whatever the compressive forces, the lumen of the urethra must be capable of being obliterated by a watertight seal. This mucosal seal mechanism explains why a very thin-walled rubber tube requires less pressure to close an open end when the inner layer is coated with a fine layer of grease than when it is not—the latter case being analogous to scarred or atrophic urethral mucosa [11].

Continence during increases in intra-abdominal pressure is maintained by (1) the effects of the spinal somatic and sympathetic reflexes on the striated and smooth sphincter areas, the intrinsic competence of the bladder outlet, and, in the female, urethral compression against a suburethral supporting layer. A further increase in striated sphincter activity on a reflex basis (the cough reflex) is also contributory.

Normally, it is increased detrusor pressure producing the sensation of fullness that is primarily responsible for the initiation of voluntary induced bladder emptying. Although the origin of the parasympathetic neural outflow to the bladder, the pelvic nerve, is in the sacral spinal cord, the actual organizational center for the micturition reflex in an intact neural axis is in the brain stem (pontine-mesencephalic formation), and the complete neural circuit for normal micturition includes the ascending and descending spinal cord pathways to and from this area and the facilitatory and inhibitory influences from other parts of the brain.

The final step in voluntarily induced micturition initially involves inhibition of the reflex responsible for increased somatic neural efferent activity to the striated sphincter and an inhibition of all aspects of any spinal sympathetic reflexes evoked during filling. Efferent parasympathetic pelvic nerve activity is ultimately what is responsible for a highly coordinated and sustained contraction of the bulk of the bladder smooth musculature. A decrease in outlet resistance occurs with adaptive shaping or funneling of the relaxed bladder outlet. In addition to the inhibition of any continence-promoting reflexes that have occurred during bladder filling, the change in outlet resistance may also involve an active relaxation of the smooth muscle sphincter area through a mechanism mediated by nitric oxide. The adaptive changes that occur in the outlet area are also in part due to the anatomic interrelationships of the smooth muscle of the bladder base and proximal urethra (continuity). Other reflexes elicited by bladder contraction and by the passage of urine through the urethra may reinforce and facilitate complete bladder emptying. Superimposed on these autonomic and somatic reflexes are complex modifying supraspinal inputs from other central neuronal networks. These facilitatory and inhibitory impulses originate from several areas of the nervous system and allow for the full conscious control of micturition in the adult.

Abnormal Function [1–3, 12]

Whatever disagreements exist regarding the details of the anatomy, morphology, physiology, pharmacology, and mechanics involved in both the storage and expulsion of urine by the bladder, agreement is found regarding certain points. First, the micturition cycle involves two relatively discrete processes: bladder filling/storage and bladder emptying/voiding. Second, whatever the details involved, these processes can be summarized succinctly from a conceptual point of view (Tables 2.1 and 2.2).

Any type of voiding dysfunction must result from an abnormality of one or more of the factors previously listed regardless of the exact pathophysiology involved. This division, with its implied subdivision under each category into causes related to the bladder and the outlet, provides a logical rationale for discussion and classification of all types of voiding dysfunction and disorders as related primarily to bladder

Table. 2.1 Bladder filling/storage: the essentials

1. Accommodation of increasing volumes of urine at a low intravesical pressure (normal compliance) with appropriate sensation
2. Bladder outlet closed at rest; remains so during increases in intra-abdominal pressure
3. Absence of involuntary bladder contractions (detrusor overactivity, DO)

Table. 2.2 Bladder emptying/voiding: the essentials

1. Sustained coordinated bladder contraction of adequate magnitude and duration
2. Concomitant adequate lowering of resistance at the level of the smooth and striated sphincter (no functional obstruction)
3. Absence of anatomic outlet obstruction

Table. 2.3 Abnormal lower urinary tract function: simple functional classification

Failure to store

Because of the bladder

Because of the outlet

Failure to empty

Because of the bladder

Because of the outlet

Table. 2.4 Abnormal lower urinary tract function: expanded functional classification of dysfunction

I. Failure to store
A. Because of the bladder
    1. Overactivity
        a. Involuntary contractions (detrusor overactivity, DO)
           Neurologic disease or injury
           Bladder outlet obstruction (myogenic)
           Decreased pelvic floor activity
           Inflammation
           Idiopathic
        b. Decreased compliance
           Neurologic disease or injury
           Fibrosis
           Idiopathic
        c. Combination
    2. Hypersensitivity
        a. Inflammatory/infectious
        b. Neurologic
        c. Psychologic
        d. Idiopathic

    3. Underactivity (with retention and overflow incontinence)
B. Because of the outlet
    1. Stress urinary incontinence (SUI)
        a. Lack of suburethral support
        b. Pelvic floor laxity, hypermobility
    2. Intrinsic sphincter deficiency (ISD)
        a. Neurologic disease or injury
        b. Fibrosis
    3. Combination (SUI and ISD)
C. Combination (bladder and outlet factors)
D. Fistula
II. Failure to empty
A. Because of the bladder (underactivity)
    1. Neurogenic
    2. Myogenic
    3. Psychogenic
    4. Idiopathic
B. Because of the outlet
    1. Anatomic
        a. Prostatic obstruction
        b. Bladder neck contracture
        c. Urethral stricture, fibrosis
        d. Urethral compression
    2. Functional
        a. Smooth sphincter dyssynergia (bladder neck dysfunction)
        b. Striated sphincter dyssynergia
        c. Combination (bladder and outlet factors)
III. Combination

filling/urine storage or to bladder emptying/voiding (Tables 2.3 and 2.4). There are some types of voiding dysfunction that represent combinations of filling and storage and emptying and voiding abnormalities. Within this scheme, however, these become readily understandable, and their detection and treatment can be logically described. For example, the type of abnormal function seen in a patient with suprasacral spinal cord injury after spinal shock has passed represents a combined filling/storage problem (detrusor overactivity) and an emptying one (striated sphincter dyssynergia). Further, using this simple-minded scheme, all aspects of urodynamic, radiologic, and video urodynamic evaluation can be conceptualized as to exactly what they evaluate in terms of either bladder or outlet activity during filling and storage or emptying and voiding (see Table 2.5). Treatments for voiding dysfunction can be classified as under broad categories according to whether they facilitate filling and storage or emptying and voiding and whether they do so by acting primarily on the bladder or on one or more of the components of the bladder outlet (see Tables 2.6 and 2.7).

Table. 2.5 Using the functional schema to simply categorize urodynamic studies (after Wein [2])

	Bladder	Outlet
Filling/storage	P^a_{ves} P^b_{det} (FCMG[c])	ALPP[d]
	DLPP[e]	UPP[f]
		FLUORO[g]
Emptying/voiding	P^a_{ves} P^b_{det} (VCMG[h])	FLUORO[g]
		MUPP[i]
		EMG[j]
	Uroflowmetry	
	Residual urine	

In this representation uroflowmetry and residual urine volume integrate the activity of the bladder and outlet during the emptying/voiding phases of micturition
[a]Total intravesical pressure
[b]Detrusor pressure
[c]Filling cystometrogram
[d]Abdominal leak point pressures
[e]Detrusor leak point pressure
[f]Urethral pressure profile
[g]Fluoroscopy of outlet
[h]Voiding cystometrogram
[i]Micturitional urethral pressure profile
[j]Electromyography of striated sphincter

Table. 2.6 Functional categorization of therapy to facilitate urine storage/bladder filling

I. Bladder
  A. Behavioral therapy including any or all of
    1. Education
    2. Bladder training
    3. Timed bladder emptying or prompted voiding
    4. Fluid restriction
    5. Pelvic floor physiotherapy ± biofeedback
  B. Pharmacologic therapy (oral, intravesical, intradetrusor)
    1. Antimuscarinic agents
    2. Drugs with mixed actions
    3. β-Adrenergic agonists
    4. Botulinum toxin
    5. Calcium antagonists
    6. Potassium channel openers
    7. Prostaglandin inhibitors
    8. α-Adrenergic antagonists
    9. Tricyclic antidepressants, serotonin and norepinephrine reuptake inhibitors
    10. Dimethyl sulfoxide (DMSO)
    11. Polysynaptic inhibitors
    12. Capsaicin, resiniferatoxin, and like agents
  C. Bladder overdistention
  D. Electrical stimulation (sacral neuromodulation, posterior tibial and other peripheral nerve stimulation)
  E. Acupuncture and electroacupuncture
  F. Interruption of innervation
    1. Very central (subarachnoid block)
    2. Less central (sacral rhizotomy, selective sacral rhizotomy)
    3. Peripheral motor or/and sensory
  G. Augmentation cystoplasty (auto, bowel, tissue engineering)
II. Outlet related (increasing outlet resistance)
  A. Behavioral therapy (see I, A)
  B. Electrical stimulation
  C. Pharmacologic therapy
    1. α-Adrenergic agonists
    2. Tricyclic antidepressants, serotonin and norepinephrine reuptake inhibitors
    3. β-Adrenergic antagonists, agonists
  D. Vaginal and perineal occlusive and/or supportive devices, urethral plugs
  E. Nonsurgical periurethral bulking
    1. Synthetics
    2. Tissue engineering
  F. Retropubic vesicourethral suspension ± prolapse repair (female)
  G. Sling procedures ± prolapse repair (female)
  H. Mid-urethral tapes ± prolapse repair (female)
  I. Perineal sling procedure (male)
  J. Artificial urinary sphincter
  K. Myoplasty (muscle transposition)
  L. Bladder outlet closure
III. Circumventing the problem
  A. Absorbent products
  B. External collecting devices
  C. Antidiuretic hormone-like agents
  D. Short-acting diuretics
  E. Intermittent catheterization
  F. Continuous catheterization
  G. Urinary diversion

Table. 2.7 Functional categorization of therapy to facilitate bladder emptying/voiding (after Wein [2])

I. Bladder related (increasing intravesical pressure or facilitating or augmenting bladder contractility)
  A. External compression, Valsalva
  B. Promotion or initiation of reflex contraction
    1. Trigger zones or maneuvers
    2. Bladder "training," tidal drainage
  C. Pharmacologic therapy (oral, intravesical)
    1. Parasympathomimetic agents
    2. Prostaglandins
    3. Blockers of inhibition
      a. α-Adrenergic antagonists
      b. Opioid antagonists
      c. Electrical stimulation
    1. Directly to the bladder or spinal cord
    2. Directly to the nerve roots
    3. Intravesical (transurethral)
    4. Sacral Neuromodulation
  E. Reduction cystoplasty
  F. Bladder myoplasty (muscle wrap)
II. Out related (decreasing outlet resistance)
  A. At a site of anatomic obstruction
    1. Pharmacologic therapy—decrease prostate size or tone
      a. α-Adrenergic antagonists
      b. 5 α-reductase inhibitors
      c. Luteinizing hormone releasing hormone-agonists/antagonists
      d. Antiandrogens
    2. Prostatectomy, prostatotomy (diathermy, heat, laser), dilation, and fixation
    3. Bladder neck incision, resection, dilation, reconstruction
    4. Urethral stricture repair, dilation
    5. Intraurethral stent
  B. At level of smooth sphincter (functional obstruction)
    1. Pharmacologic therapy
      a. α-Adrenergic antagonists
      b. β-Adrenergic agonists
    2 Resection, incision, reconstruction
  C. At level of striated sphincter (functional obstruction)
    1. Behavioral therapy ± biofeedback
    2. Pharmacologic therapy
      a. α-Adrenergic antagonists
      b. Botulinum toxin (injection)
      c. Benzodiazepines
      d. Baclofen
      e. Dantrolene
    3. Urethral overdilation
    4. Surgical sphincterotomy

    5. Urethral stent
    6. Pudendal nerve interruption
III. Circumventing the problem
  A. Intermittent catheterization
  B. Continuous catheterization
  C. Urinary diversion

References

1. Wein AJ, Barrett DM. Voiding D+function and dysfunction: a logical and practical approach. Chicago, IL: Year Book Medical; 1988.
2. Wein AJ. Pathophysiology and classification of lower urinary tract dysfunction. In: Wein AJ, Kavoussi LR, Novick AC, Parlin AW, Peters CA, editors. Campbell-Walsh urology. Philadelphia, PA: Elsevier/Saunders; 2012. p. 1834–46.
3. Wein AJ. Classification of neurogenic voiding dysfunction. J Urol. 1981;125:605–9.
4. de Groat WC, Booth AM, Yoshimura N. Neurophysiology of micturition and its modifications in animal modules of human disease. In: Maggi CA, editor. Autonomic nervous system. London: Harwood Academic; 1993. p. 227–90.
5. de Groat WC, Downie JW, Levin RM, et al. Basic neurophysiology and neuropharmacology. In: Abrams P, Khoury S, Wein AJ, editors. International consultation on incontinence. Plymouth, UK: Health Publications; 1999. p. 105–54.
6. Fowler CJ, Griffiths D, de Groat WC. The neural control of micturition. Nat Rev Neurosci. 2008;9:453–66.
7. Andersson K-E, Arner A. Urinary bladder contraction and relaxation: physiology and pathophysiology. Physiol Rev. 2004;84:935–88.
8. Yoshimura N, Chancellor MB. Physiology and pharmacology of the bladder and urethra. In: Wein AJ, Kavoussi LR, Novick AC, Partin AW, Peters CA, editors. Campbell-Walsh urology. Philadelphia, PA: Elsevier/Saunders; 2012. p. 1786–833.
9. Zderic SA, Levin RM, Wein AJ. Voiding function: relevant anatomy, physiology, pharmacology and molecular aspects. In: Gillenwater JY, Grayhack JT, Howard SS, Ducket Jr JW, editors. Adult and pediatric urology. Chicago, IL: Chicago Year Book Medical; 2002. p. 1159–219.
10. Newman DK, Wein AJ. Managing and treating urinary incontinence. Baltimore and London: Health Professions Press; 2009.
11. Zinner NR, Sterling AM, Ritter R. Structure and forces of continence. In: Raz S, editor. Female urology. Philadelphia, PA: WB Saunders; 1983. p. 33–41.
12. Wein AJ, Moy ML. Voiding function and dysfunction: urinary incontinence. In: Hanno PM, Malkowicz SB, Wein AJ, editors. Penn clinical manual of urology. Philadelphia, PA: Elsevier/Saunders; 2007. p. 341–478.

The Impact of Neurologic Insult on the Lower Urinary Tract

Roger R. Dmochowski and Alex Gomelsky

Introduction

The function of the urinary bladder is relatively straightforward: safely and efficiently store and empty urine. However, these two actions are contingent on intimate interaction between the central and peripheral nervous systems and the bladder and outlet. Any injury or insult to the connections between these entities may result in a problem with storage, emptying, or both. The duration, location, and severity of the insult can cause a significant impact on the person's overall health and quality of life. "Neurogenic bladder" may be effectively classified into a problem with the bladder or outlet and then further subclassified as a problem with overactivity or underactivity [1]. A successful therapeutic outcome depends on the rapid and correct diagnosis through history, physical examination, urinalysis assessment, urodynamic evaluation, and, when appropriate, radiographic imaging. The goals of this chapter are to describe the deviations in the micturition cycle produced by various types of neuromuscular dysfunction and to describe the treatment options for the particular micturition dysfunction. It is beyond the limits of this chapter to delve in detail into every neurologic process that has been associated with a defect in urinary storage or emptying. The reader is referred to a state-of-the-art review for further information [2]. While a brief summary of neuroanatomy is provided below, the reader is additionally referred to a review of normal bladder physiology elsewhere [3].

Review of Neuroanatomy

The frontal lobe houses the micturition control center which primarily has an inhibitory function to the bladder by preventing detrusor contraction. The pontine micturition center (PMC) is responsible for coordinating the functions of the bladder and sphincters so that they work in synergy. During micturition, the PMC coordinates sphincter relaxation and detrusor contraction. During bladder filling, detrusor stretch receptors update the PMC of the bladder's status, and the PMC, in turn, notifies the brain. Under normal situations, the brain will send inhibitory messages to the PMC, which will inhibit detrusor contraction (and sensation of urgency) until a socially acceptable time and location. Excitatory signals to the PMC result in relaxation and opening of the sphincters and detrusor contraction. The spinal cord allows the PMC and sacral micturition center (SMC) to communicate with each other. The spinal cord relays messages from the bladder to pontine

R.R. Dmochowski, M.D., M.M.H.C. (✉)
Department of Urologic Surgery, Vanderbilt University Medical Center, A1302 Medical Center North, Nashville, TN 37232-2765, USA
e-mail: roger.dmochowski@vanderbilt.edu

A. Gomelsky, M.D.
Department of Urology, LSU Health–Shreveport, Shreveport, LA, USA

A.J. Wein et al. (eds.), *Bladder Dysfunction in the Adult: The Basis for Clinical Management*, Current Clinical Urology, DOI 10.1007/978-1-4939-0853-0_3, © Springer Science+Business Media New York 2014

and cortical centers and messages from higher centers to the SMC and the bladder. An injury to or interruption of signals from the spinal cord typically results in a defect in urinary storage (detrusor overactivity; DO) and defect in emptying (detrusor external sphincter dyssynergia; DESD). The sacral or terminal portion of the spinal cord is in the lumbar area and houses the SMC, which is also the location of the primitive reflex voiding center. This reflex center is active in infants prior to maturation of higher integrative cortical and pontine centers. A sensation of bladder fullness in infants is transmitted to the SMC which leads to an involuntary detrusor contraction and coordinated bladder emptying. As the child's brain matures, they become able to inhibit involuntary voiding. Injury to the sacral cord typically results in detrusor areflexia and urinary retention.

The peripheral nervous system is divided into the autonomic nervous system (ANS) and the somatic nervous system (SNS), both of which are responsible for receiving and sending information from the bladder and sphincters to the spinal cord and higher centers. The ANS is comprised of paired sympathetic and parasympathetic nerves. During bladder filling, the detrusor and internal sphincter are under sympathetic control. The bladder is relaxed and accommodates increasing amounts of urine without unstable detrusor contractions or impairments in compliance, while the internal sphincter is tightly closed. Sympathetic innervation also serves to inhibit parasympathetic stimulation during bladder filling. Once again, the end result is detrusor relaxation and outlet excitation. During voiding, parasympathetic innervation stimulates detrusor contraction and suppresses internal sphincter contraction, thereby facilitating bladder emptying. Additionally, parasympathetic innervation inhibits the pudendal nerve, thereby facilitating relaxation of the SNS and the external sphincter. The SNS regulates voluntary or skeletal musculature. Activation of the pudendal nerves leads to contraction of the external sphincter and pelvic floor.

Pathophysiology of Neurogenic Bladder Conditions

In any discussion of neurogenic bladder, the expected status of the following urodynamic parameters should be described: sensation (normal, absent, impaired), detrusor activity (normal, overactive, areflexic, impaired contractility), compliance (normal, decreased, increased), smooth sphincter activity (synergic, dyssynergic), and striated sphincter activity (synergic, dyssynergic, bradykinetic, impaired voluntary control, fixed tone) [3]. These descriptions will allow a typical grouping of the neurologic insult and subsequent voiding dysfunction. Special case will be commented on separately. This chapter will, in general, limit itself to conditions afflicting adults.

Discrete neurologic lesions generally affect the storage and emptying phases of lower urinary tract function in a relatively consistent manner. The impact is dependent on the areas of the nervous system affected, the physiologic functions of the areas affected, and whether the process is destructive, inflammatory, or irritative. It is also important to note that the acute dysfunction produced may be different from the chronic one [2].

Lesions above the Brainstem

If a neurologic lesion above the brainstem affects the micturition cycle, the typical result is DO with urgency urinary incontinence (UUI). The smooth and striated sphincters are synergic (coordinated), while sensation may be deficient or delayed.

Cerebrovascular Accident

Cerebrovascular Accident (CVA) is a common cause of death and debilitating disability, with an annual incidence in the USA recently cited as approximately 795,000 and 15 million worldwide (www.strokecenter.org). The prevalence of CVA increases with age and is estimated to be 95 per 1,000 persons 75 years of age and older [4]. The prevalence of urinary incontinence ranges from 32 to 79 % on hospital admission for CVA, 25–28 % on discharge, and 12–19 % several months later [5]. Sakakibara et al. estimated that some element of voiding dysfunction occurs in 20–50 % of patients with brain tumor and CVA, with nocturnal frequency being the most common (36 %) [6]. UUI occurred in 29 %, "voiding difficulty" in 25 %, urgency without incontinence in 25 %, diurnal frequency in 13 %, and enuresis in 6 %. Acute urinary retention occurred in only 6 %.

Detrusor are flexia and subsequent urinary retention are often the first urologic sequelae following an acute CVA. Phasic DO is the most common long-term outcome and develops over the next few weeks or months [4, 7–10]. Sensation is most typically intact. The smooth sphincter is unaffected (synergic) and true DESD does not occur. If the patient can voluntarily contract their external sphincter in response to DO, then they may only manifest urinary urgency and frequency. Otherwise, the result is UUI. While infrequent, the incidence of chronic and persistent detrusor hypocontractility or areflexia after CVA is estimated to be up to 20 % in some studies [11].

Dementia

Alzheimer's disease is the principal cause of dementia in the elderly [10], a poorly understood disease complex involving atrophy and the loss of both gray and white matter of the brain [2]. The loss is most prominent in the frontal lobes and results in deficits with memory and cognition. Urinary dysfunction does not always accompany dementia; however, when it is present, the result is typically urinary incontinence. It is unclear whether the pathophysiology is similar to that seen in CVA or whether the patient becomes incontinent because they have lost the awareness or desire to control their urine. Such activity may be caused by DO or an otherwise normal, but inappropriately timed, micturition reflex.

Brain Trauma

As with many neurologic insults that result in voiding dysfunction, there may be an initial period of detrusor areflexia after brain trauma. With lesions above the PMC, DO and coordinated sphincters are the most common chronic lower urinary tract findings. DESD may be seen in patients with more isolated brainstem injuries below the PMC. Upon admission, Chua et al. observed that 62 % of 84 patients had incontinence on admission and approximately 10 % had urinary retention [12]. After rehabilitation, 36 % remained incontinent.

Brain Tumor

Urinary dysfunction may occur with both primary and metastatic brain tumors, and, when dysfunction results, it is related to the tumor location involved rather than the tumor type. The areas that are most frequently involved with micturition dysfunction are the superior aspects of the frontal lobe [13], and voiding dysfunction typically consists of DO and UUI. Smooth and striated sphincters are generally synergic, while pseudodyssynergia may be seen on urodynamics [2]. Urinary retention has also been described in patients with space-occupying lesions of the frontal cortex, in the absence of other associated neurologic deficits [14]. Posterior fossa tumors may be associated with voiding dysfunction in 32–70 % of patients, with urinary retention being the most common finding [8].

Parkinson's Disease

Parkinson's disease (PD) is a neurodegenerative disorder that affects primarily the dopaminergic neurons of the substantia nigra, the origin of the dopaminergic nigrostriatal tract to the caudate nucleus and putamen [15]. PD affects both sexes equally and the prevalence is as high as 3 % of people >65 years of age [10]. Dopamine deficiency in the nigrostriatal pathway accounts for most of the clinical motor features of parkinsonism, a symptom complex consisting of tremor, skeletal rigidity, and bradykinesia. Parkinsonian symptoms are not enough by themselves to diagnose a patient with PD, as patients with conditions such as multiple system atrophy (MSA) may present similarly. The combination of asymmetry of symptoms and signs, the presence of a resting tremor, and a good response to levodopa favors the diagnosis of PD [15], while urinary symptoms preceding or present with onset of parkinsonism, the presence of urinary incontinence, significantly elevated postvoid residual, initial erectile dysfunction, and abnormal striated sphincter EMG may favor MSA [10]. The "gold standard" for the diagnosis of PD is the characteristic pattern of the loss of selected populations of neurons and the presence of Lewy bodies, intracytoplasmic eosinophilic hyaline inclusions consistently observed in selectively vulnerable neuronal populations.

The range of micturition dysfunction seen with PD ranges from 35 to 70 % in the literature [10, 16–19], and urinary storage symptoms represent 50–75 % of the dysfunction when it occurs. The remainder of patients has voiding symptoms or a combination of storage and voiding symptoms. The most common urodynamic finding is DO and the smooth sphincter is synergic. Sporadic involuntary activity in the striated sphincter during DO has been reported in as many as 60 % of patients; however, this does not cause obstruction and true DESD does not occur [2]. Pseudodyssynergia may occur, as well as a delay in striated sphincter relaxation (bradykinesia) at the onset of voluntary micturition. Impaired detrusor contractility may also occur, while detrusor areflexia is relatively uncommon in PD [2]. It has been noted that PD may have been mistaken for MSA in some of the older studies, and, thus, symptoms and urodynamic findings may not be completely accurate.

Multiple System Atrophy

The symptoms of MSA include parkinsonism and cerebellar, autonomic, and pyramidal cortical dysfunction [2]. The neurologic lesions of MSA consist of cell loss and gliosis in widespread areas, occurring to a significantly greater degree than with PD and potentially accounting for the earlier and more severe urinary symptoms compared to PD [20–22]. Males and females are equally affected, with the onset in middle age. MSA is generally progressive and associated with a poor prognosis [2].

Urinary storage symptoms may precede the diagnosis of MSA by several years, and DO is typically found on urodynamics. However, decreased compliance may also occur, reflecting distal spinal involvement of the cell bodies of autonomic neurons innervating the lower urinary tract [2]. Disease progression is often accompanied by difficulty in initiating and maintaining voiding, likely from an effect on pontine and sacral cord lesions. Abnormalities in the smooth sphincter (open bladder neck on cystourethrography) and evidence of striated sphincter denervation on EMG are associated significantly with the diagnosis of MSA and may predispose women to stress incontinence (SUI) and make prostatectomy hazardous in men [2].

Conditions Affecting the Spinal Cord

A period of spinal shock and urinary retention is common. Patients with complete lesions of the spinal cord between spinal cord level T6 and S2 generally demonstrate DO, while sensation is absent. The smooth sphincter is synergic, but DESD is present. Lesions above spinal cord level T6 may also experience smooth sphincter dyssynergia and autonomic hyperreflexia. Urinary incontinence may result from DO; however, DESD may result in bladder outlet obstruction (BOO), urinary retention, and overflow incontinence. Furthermore, DESD may result in an unhealthy buildup of pressure in the bladder with potential compromise of the upper urinary tracts.

An insult below spinal cord level S2 is generally not accompanied by DO. As with other spinal cord injuries, initial spinal shock and urinary retention may be present; however, persistent detrusor areflexia is the typical outcome. Other findings may include low bladder compliance during filling and a relatively incompetent smooth sphincter and will depend on the type and extent of neurologic injury. Additionally, an injury in this area is associated with a fixed residual resting tone in the external sphincter. The sphincter does not relax voluntarily, which differentiates it from true DESD. Conditions or injuries that interrupt communication and coordination between the spine, bladder, and outlet (peripheral reflex arc) may cause storage or emptying dysfunctions that resemble those seen after distal spinal cord or nerve root injury.

Multiple Sclerosis

Multiple sclerosis (MS) has a prevalence of 1 in 1,000 Americans and is primarily found in young women [23]. This condition is characterized by neural demyelination in the brain and spinal cord, typically with axonal sparing [24]. This demyelination impairs conduction velocity in axonal pathways, resulting in various neurologic abnormalities that are subject to exacerbation and remission [2]. Voiding dysfunction and sphincter dysfunction is common due to demyelination of the lateral corticospinal (pyramidal) and reticulospinal columns of the cervical spinal cord. Fifty to 90 % of patients with MS complain of voiding symptoms at some time and the prevalence of incontinence ranges between 37 and 72 % [10]. Up to 15 % of MS patients present with urinary dysfunction as their only or primary complaint, typically presenting with acute urinary retention of "unknown" origin or acute onset of urinary storage symptoms [10].

DO is the most common finding on urodynamics, occurring in up to 99 % of patients [23, 25–27]. Coexistent DESD is found in 30–65 %, while impaired or absent detrusor contractility is found in 12–38 % [10]. Recent studies estimate that 62 % of MS patients have DO with BOO; however, the variability and potential multiplicity of MS lesions may prohibit accurate diagnosis based upon urodynamics alone [2]. The smooth sphincter is typically synergic. Sensation is frequently intact in these patients. While there is no consensus regarding optimal bladder management for MS patients, the likely presence of both storage and voiding dysfunction may necessitate multicomponent therapy.

Spinal Cord Injury

There are approximately 12,000 new cases of spinal cord injury (SCI) in the USA yearly, with males accounting for 71–81 % of the injuries [28]. The most common mechanisms are motor vehicle accidents (39.2 %), violence (14.6 %), falls (28.3 %), and sport-related injuries (8.2 %). Since 2005, the most frequent neurologic category at discharge of persons reported to the database is incomplete tetraplegia (40.8 %), followed by complete paraplegia (21.6 %), incomplete paraplegia (21.4 %), and complete tetraplegia (15.8 %). Less than 1 % of persons experienced complete neurologic recovery by hospital discharge. The majority of SCI occur at or above the T12 spinal column (vertebral) level, with injury to one of the eight cervical segments accounting for the patients with tetraplegia and patients with paraplegia having injury in the thoracic, lumbar, or sacral regions of the spinal cord.

SCI is frequently responsible for altered lower urinary tract and sexual function and may have a significant impact on quality of life. SCI patients are at risk for urinary tract infection, sepsis, upper and lower urinary tract deterioration, urinary tract calculi, autonomic hyperreflexia, skin complications, and depression [2]. The degree of neurologic deficit and subsequent impact on the urinary tract varies with the level and severity of the injury. It is important to note that spinal column (bone) segments are numbered by the vertebral level, and these have a different relationship to the spinal cord segmental level at different locations [2]. The sacral spinal cord begins approximately at spinal column level T12 to L1. The spinal cord terminates in the cauda equina at approximately the spinal column level L2.

Complete SCI above the sacral spinal cord, but below the area of the sympathetic outflow, typically results in DO, absent sensation below the level of the lesion, synergic smooth sphincter, and DESD [29–31]. The urodynamic and upper tract consequences of the DESD are usually worse in males and in patients with complete lesions rather than incomplete ones [32]. Neurologic examination shows spasticity of skeletal muscle distal to the lesion, hyperreflexic deep-tendon reflexes (DTRs), and abnormal plantar responses [2]. There is impairment of superficial and deep sensation. Lesions at or above spinal cord level of T7–T8 (spinal column level T6) may result in smooth sphincter dyssynergia, as well. As the correlation between neurologic and urodynamic findings it is not perfect, urodynamics are paramount in determining risk factors and guiding treatment. As with MS, suprasacral SCI represents both a failure of urinary storage and emptying and both components should be anticipated and addressed during therapeutic intervention.

In a patient with sacral SCI who has recovered from spinal shock, there is typically a depression of DTRs below the level of a complete lesion with varying degrees of flaccid paralysis [2]. Sensation is generally absent below the lesion level and detrusor areflexia with high or normal compliance is the common initial result; however, decreased compliance may also develop [33–35]. The classic outlet findings are described as a competent but nonrelaxing smooth sphincter and a striated sphincter that retains some fixed tone but is not under voluntary control [2]. As with suprasacral SCI, the possibility of multiple lesions present at different spinal cord levels, as well as the differences seen with complete vs. incomplete lesions, makes the correlation between neurologic examination and urodynamic findings imperfect. Urodynamic principles should guide treatment, with strategies generally directed toward producing or maintaining low-pressure storage while facilitating emptying.

The American Paraplegic Society (APS) Guidelines for urologic care of SCI recommend annual follow-up for the first 5–10 years after injury, with biennial follow-up afterwards for those patients who are doing well [36]. The APS recommended upper and lower tract evaluation and urodynamics annually for 5–10 years and biennially thereafter. Cystoscopy was recommended annually in those with an indwelling catheter.

Transverse Myelitis

Acute transverse myelitis is a rapidly developing condition with motor, sensory, and sphincter abnormalities, generally with a well-defined upper sensory limit and no signs of spinal cord compression or other neurologic disease [37]. The condition may result from a variety of mechanisms and usually stabilizes within 2–4 weeks; however, recovery may be variable and some residual neurologic deficits are possible [38]. Although recovery is more variable, the development and nature of voiding dysfunction is similar by level to that of SCI [37, 39]. The prognosis is usually favorable; however, as in SCI, urodynamics are necessary to guide irreversible therapy because the activity of the bladder and outlet during storage and emptying does not always correspond to the expected pattern based on the level of pathology [2].

Conditions Distal to the Spinal Cord

Lumbar Disk Disease

The sacral segments of the adult spinal cord, also called the conus medullaris, are at the level of the L1 and L2 vertebral bodies. Thus, all of the sacral nerves that originate at the L1 and L2 spinal column levels run posterior to the lumbar vertebral bodies until they reach their appropriate site of exit from the spinal canal. This group of nerve roots running at the distal end of the spinal cord is commonly referred to as the cauda equina [40]. Disk protrusion anywhere in the lumbar spine could cause compression of the cauda equina and interfere with the parasympathetic and somatic innervation of the lower urinary tract, striated sphincter, and other pelvic floor musculature, as well as afferent activity from the bladder and affected somatic segments to the spinal cord [2]. Most disk protrusions compress the spinal roots in the L4–L5 or L5–S1 vertebral interspaces.

The clinical presentation typically consists of low back pain radiating in a girdle-like fashion along the involved spinal root areas, and sensory loss in the perineum or perianal area (S2–S4 dermatomes) and/or sensory loss on the lateral foot

(S1–S2 dermatomes) is frequently found on physical examination. The incidence of voiding dysfunction associated with lumbar disk disease ranges from 27 to 92 % in the literature, with the majority of patients presenting with urinary retention [40]. Several studies have cited detrusor areflexia in 25–30 % of patients, with the remainder having normal detrusor function [41, 42]. Compliance is typically normal, and DO is infrequent [43]. In many patients, decompressive laminectomy may not improve bladder function and prelaminectomy urodynamics are useful to differentiate voiding dysfunction due to the disk herniation from changes secondary to the surgery [2, 44].

Radical Pelvic Surgery

The paired inferior hypogastric (pelvic) plexus innervates the pelvic viscera and is located on the side of the rectum in males and at the sides of the rectum and vagina in females [2]. The incidence of voiding dysfunction after pelvic plexus injury is reported to be 20–68 % after abdominoperineal resection (APR), 16–80 % after radical hysterectomy, 20–25 % after anterior resection, and 10–20 % after proctocolectomy [45]. The injury may occur from denervation, tethering of the nerves or encasement in scar, direct bladder or urethral injury, or bladder devascularization, and chemotherapy or radiation may compound the damage. The type of voiding dysfunction is dependent on the specific nerves involved, the degree of injury, and any reinnervation or altered innervation that occurs over time. Voiding dysfunction may become permanent in 15–20 % of those affected [46, 47].

Impaired bladder contractility, or a failure of the bladder to voluntarily contract, generally represents the postoperative voiding dysfunction [2]. Urodynamically, obstruction may be seen from residual fixed striated sphincter tone which is not able to be relaxed voluntarily. Often, the smooth sphincter is open and nonfunctional. Decreased compliance is common in these patients, and, coupled with the fixed residual striated sphincter tone, storage and emptying failure may result [2]. Thus, patients may present with either retention,

incontinence, or both. The primary therapeutic goals remain the same: achieve low-pressure storage with periodic emptying to protect the upper tracts. As much of the bladder dysfunction after radical pelvic surgery may be transient, a secondary goal is to resist the desire to perform potentially irreversible surgery in these patients to treat the voiding dysfunction.

Diabetes Mellitus

Diabetes mellitus (DM) is a systemic disease that has a US prevalence of approximately 7 % [48]. The effect of DM on bladder function has been termed diabetic cystopathy (DC) and clinically manifests as decreased bladder sensation, increased residual urine, and detrusor overactivity [49, 50]. Progressively, detrusor distention, overdistention, and decompensation ultimately occur. As with many neurologic conditions impacting bladder function, the exact incidence of voiding dysfunction caused by DM varies widely (5–59 %) [2], while some have estimated that up to 80 % of patients with DM will eventually develop some manifestation of diabetic cystopathy [48]. The classic urodynamic findings include impaired bladder sensation, increased cystometric bladder capacity, decreased bladder contractility, impaired uroflow, and increased residual urine volume [2]. Low urinary flow due to BOO in men may be ruled out by pressure/flow studies. Smooth or striated sphincter dyssynergia generally is not seen in classic diabetic cystopathy [2]. Other authors have cited urodynamic evidence of DO in over 55 % of patients with diabetic cystopathy [51, 52]. Thus, the importance of urodynamic study in diabetic patients before the institution of therapy cannot be overemphasized.

Treatment of Neurogenic Bladder

The overall goals of managing patients with neurogenic bladder dysfunction are relatively straightforward: facilitate timely bladder emptying; protect upper urinary tracts from damage due to high filling pressures; minimize adverse sequelae such as calculi, UTIs, and urinary incontinence; champion independence in bladder management; and improve quality of life. Treatment options may be neatly categorized into those that address urinary storage or emptying and may be further subcategorized into those that primarily act on the bladder or outlet. If possible, the least invasive, most conservative, and least irreversible options should be employed initially, with more complex options reserved for treatment failures.

Treatment options that address the bladder as the culprit in failing to store urine include behavioral training with timed voiding, pelvic floor physical therapy with or without biofeedback (PFMT), pharmacotherapy (most commonly antimuscarinics and β-3 adrenergic agonists), intravesical onabotulinumtoxinA injection, neuromodulation (sacral, posterior tibial, pudendal, and dorsal genital nerves), sacral deafferentation and anterior root stimulator implantation, and enterocystoplasty. Options addressing the outlet in patients failing to store urine are external collection devices or penile clamps, PFMT, bladder suspension or sling surgery, periurethral bulking, artificial urinary sphincter, and bladder neck closure. Treatments aimed at improving emptying from the bladder standpoint include crédé voiding, intermittent catheterization, indwelling urethral or suprapubic catheter drainage, and neuromodulation, while sphincterotomy, urethral stenting, and sphincteric onabotulinumtoxinA injection can facilitate emptying from the outlet standpoint. Indwelling urethral catheters and urinary diversion to divert the urinary stream may address both storage and emptying failure concurrently.

Absolute or relative indications for changing or augmenting a particular treatment regimen exist and are summarized elsewhere [2]. Non-urologic factors such as impaired mobility, poor dexterity, adverse effects of polypharmacy, cognitive impairment, and inadequate social support may significantly complicate treatment. As with all patients with neurologic impairment, a careful initial evaluation and periodic, routine follow-up evaluation must be performed to identify and correct potential complications [2]. Since no treatment option is perfect, interventions should be individualized and informed consent

regarding the pros and cons of each therapeutic intervention is paramount to achieving the goals of bladder management stated above.

References

1. Wein AJ. Pathophysiology and classification of lower urinary tract dysfunction: overview. In: Wein AJ, Kavoussi LR, Novick AC, Partin AW, Peters CA, editors. Campbell-Walsh urology. 10th ed. Philadelphia, PA: Elsevier Saunders; 2012.
2. Wein AJ, Dmochowski RR. Neuromuscular dysfunction of the lower urinary tract. In: Wein AJ, Kavoussi LR, Novick AC, Partin AW, Peters CA, editors. Campbell-Walsh urology. 10th ed. Philadelphia, PA: Elsevier Saunders; 2012.
3. Yoshimura N, Chancellor MB. Physiology and pharmacology of the bladder and urethra. In: Wein AJ, Kavoussi LR, Novick AC, Partin AW, Peters CA, editors. Campbell-Walsh urology. 10th ed. Philadelphia, PA: Elsevier Saunders; 2012.
4. Khan Z, Starer P, Yang WC, et al. Analysis of voiding disorders in patients with cerebrovascular accidents. Urology. 1990;35:265–70.
5. Brittain KR, Peet SM, Castleden CM. Stroke and incontinence. Stroke. 1998;29:524–8.
6. Sakakibara R, Fowler CJ, Yasuda K, et al. Voiding and MRI analysis of the brain. Int Urogynecol J Pelvic Floor Dysfunct. 1999;10:192–9.
7. Wein AJ, Barrett D. Voiding function and dysfunction-a logical and practical approach. Year Book Medical: Chicago, IL; 1988.
8. Fowler CJ. Neurological disorders of micturition and their treatment. Brain. 1999;122:1213–31.
9. Kolominsky-Rabas PL, Hilz MJ, Neundoerfer B, et al. Impact of urinary incontinence after stroke: results from a prospective population-based stroke register. Neurourol Urodyn. 2003;22:322–7.
10. Wyndaele JJ, Castro D, Madersbacher H, et al. Neurogenic and faecal incontinence. In: Abrams P, editor. Incontinence. Paris: Health Publications; 2005. p. 1059–162.
11. Arunable MB, Badlani G. Urologic problems in cerebrovascular accidents. Probl Urol. 1993;7:41–53.
12. Chua K, Chuo A, Kong KH. Urinary incontinence after traumatic brain injury: incidence, outcomes and correlates. Brain Inj. 2003;17:469–78.
13. Blaivas JG. Non-traumatic neurogenic voiding dysfunction in the adult. AUA Update Series. 1985;4:1–15.
14. Lang EW, Chesnut RM, Hennerici M. Urinary retention and space-occupying lesions of the frontal cortex. Eur Neurol. 1996;36:43–7.
15. Lang AE, Lozano AM. Parkinson's disease. N Engl J Med. 1998;339:1044–53.
16. Berger Y, Salinas J, Blaivas JG. Urodynamic differentiation of Parkinson disease and the Shy-Drager syndrome. Neurourol Urodyn. 1990;9:117–21.
17. Sotolongo JR, Chancellor M. Parkinson's disease. Probl Urol. 1993;7:54–67.

18. Blaivas JG, Chaikin DC, Chancellor MB, et al. Bladder dysfunction with neurologic disease. Continuum: lifelong learning in neurology. 1998;4:79–124.
19. Wein AJ, Rovner E. Adult voiding dysfunction secondary to neurologic disease or injury. AUA Update Series. 1999;18:42–7.
20. Kirby R, Fowler C, Gosling J, Bannister R. Urethrovesical dysfunction in progressive autonomic failure with multiple system atrophy. J Neurol Neurosurg Psychiatry. 1986;49:554–60.
21. Beck R, Fowler CJ, Mathias CJ. Genitourinary dysfunction in disorders of the autonomic nervous system. In: Ruston D, editor. Handbook of neuro-urology. New York: Marcel Dekker; 1994. p. 281–301.
22. Chandiramani VA, Palace J, Fowler CJ. How to recognize patients with parkinsonism who should not have urological surgery. Br J Urol. 1997;80:100–4.
23. Litwiller SE, Frohman EM, Zimmern PE. Multiple sclerosis and the urologist. J Urol. 1999;161:743–57.
24. Noseworthy JH, Lucchinetti C, Rodriguez M, et al. Multiple sclerosis. N Engl J Med. 2000;343:938–52.
25. Blaivas JG, Kaplan SA. Urologic dysfunction in patients with multiple sclerosis. Semin Neurol. 1988;8:159–65.
26. Chancellor MB, Blaivas JG. Multiple sclerosis. Probl Urol. 1993;7:15–33.
27. Sirls LT, Zimmern PE, Leach GE. Role of limited evaluation and aggressive medical management in multiple sclerosis: a review of 113 patients. J Urol. 1994;151:946–50.
28. National Spinal Cord Injury Statistical Center, Birmingham, AL. Office of Special Education and Rehabilitative Services. Washington, DC: U.S. Department of Education; 2012.
29. Sullivan M, Yalla S. Spinal cord injury and other forms of myeloneuropathies. Probl Urol. 1992;6:643–58.
30. Thomas DG, O'Flynn KJ. Spinal cord injury. In: Mundy AR, Stephenson T, Wein AJ, editors. Urodynamics: principles, practice and application. London: Churchill Livingstone; 1994. p. 345–58.
31. Chancellor MB, Blaivas JG. Spinal cord injury. In: Chancellor MB, Blaivas JG, editors. Practical neurourology. Boston, MA: Butterworth-Heinemann; 1995. p. 22–118.
32. Linsenmeyer TA, Bagaria SP, Gendron B. The impact of urodynamic parameters on the upper tracts of spinal cord injured men who void reflexively. J Spinal Cord Med. 1998;21:15–20.
33. Fam B, Yalla SV. Vesicourethral dysfunction in spinal cord injury and its management. Semin Neurol. 1988;8:150–5.
34. de Groat WC, Kruse M, Vizzard MA, et al. Modification of urinary bladder function after spinal cord injury. Adv Neurol. 1997;72:347–64.
35. Blaivas JG, Chaikin DC, Chancellor MB, et al. Pathophysiology of the neurogenic bladder. Continuum: lifelong learning in neurology. 1998;4:21–8.
36. Linsenmeyer TA, Culkin D. APS recommendations for the urological evaluation of patients with spinal cord injury. J Spinal Cord Med. 1999;22:139–42.
37. Kalita J, Shah S, Kapoor R, et al. Bladder dysfunction in acute transverse myelitis: magnetic resonance imaging and neurophysiological and urodynamic correlations. J Neurol Neurosurg Psychiatry. 2002;73:154–9.
38. Ganesan V, Borzyskowski M. Characteristics and course of urinary tract dysfunction after acute transverse myelitis in. Dev Med Child Neurol. 2001;43:473–5.
39. Sakakibara R, Hattori T, Tojo M, et al. Micturitional disturbance in myotonic dystrophy. J Auton Nerv Syst. 1995;52:17–21.
40. Goldman H, Appell RA. Lumbar disc disease. In: Appell RA, editor. Voiding dysfunction. Totowa, NJ: Humana; 2000.
41. Bartolin Z, Gilja I, Bedalov G, et al. Bladder function in patients with lumbar intervertebral disk protrusion. J Urol. 1998;159:969–71.
42. Bartolin Z, Savic I, Persec Z. Relationship between clinical data and urodynamic findings in patients with lumbar intervertebral disc protrusion. Urol Res. 2002;30:219–22.
43. O'Flynn KJ, Murphy R, Thomas DG. Neurogenic bladder dysfunction in lumbar intervertebral disc prolapse. Br J Urol. 1992;69:38–40.
44. Bartolin Z, Vilendecic M, Derezic D. Bladder function after surgery for lumbar intervertebral disk protrusion. J Urol. 1999;161:1885–7.
45. Blaivas JG, Chancellor M. Cerebrovascular accidents and other intracranial lesions. In: Chancellor MB, Blaivas JG, editors. Practical Neurourology. Boston, MA: Butterworth-Heinemann; 1995. p. 119–26.
46. McGuire EJ. Clinical evaluation and treatment of neurogenic vesical dysfunction. In: Leslie JA, editor. International perspectives in urology. Baltimore: Williams & Wilkins; 1984. p. 43–56.
47. Mundy AR. Pelvic plexus injury. In: Stephenson T, Mundy AR, Wein AJ, editors. Urodynamics: principles, practice, and application. London: Churchill Livingstone; 1984. p. 273–7.
48. Nanigian DK, Keegan KA, Stone AR. Diabetic cystopathy. Curr Blad Dysf Rep. 2007;2:197–202.
49. Bradley WE. Diagnosis of urinary bladder dysfunction in diabetes mellitus. Ann Intern Med. 1980;92:323–6.
50. Frimodt-Moller C. Diabetic cystopathy: a review of the urodynamic and clinical features of neurogenic bladder dysfunction in diabetes mellitus. Dan Med Bull. 1978;25:49–60.
51. Starer P, Libow L. Cystometric evaluation of bladder dysfunction in elderly diabetic patients. Arch Intern Med. 1990;150:810–3.
52. Kaplan SA, Te AE, Blaivas JG. Urodynamic findings in patients with diabetic cystopathy. J Urol. 1995;153:342–4.

Dysfunction in Anatomic Outlet Obstruction in Men

4

Thomas Renninson, Marcus J. Drake, and Brian Andrew Parsons

The primary physiological functions of the lower urinary tract (LUT) are the storage of urine at relatively low pressure and its expulsion (voiding) at appropriate times. LUT dysfunction is a common problem and one which increases in prevalence with ageing. It may result from a failure to store urine, a failure to empty or a combination of both [1]. Under normal conditions, voiding should result in complete emptying of the bladder. This requires a coordinated contraction of the detrusor smooth muscle with a concomitant lowering of bladder outlet resistance.

Compression, distortion or occlusion of the bladder outlet impedes flow of urine during voiding, leading to characteristic symptoms of hesitancy, poor stream, dribbling and incomplete emptying. Anatomic bladder outlet obstruction (BOO) signifies the existence of abnormal tissue that alters the configuration of the bladder outlet, whether by compression, distortion or occlusion, thereby impeding the flow of urine at the time of voiding. This is progressively associated with lower urinary tract symptoms (LUTS), during voiding

and soon after micturition (post-micturition LUTS), as set out in Table 4.1. LUTS can be caused by a variety of different pathologies, and consequently the term LUTS has superseded the word 'prostatism', as the latter implies causality [3].

In men, the commonest processes responsible for BOO are BPE or urethral stricture disease. The symptomatic consequences of lesser degrees of obstruction may be slight, likely because compensatory responses, such as enhanced bladder contractility, may overcome the hindrance. Men with low-level obstruction usually do not attend for medical review, as they may be unaware of the issue or have only minor symptom bother without detrimental effect on quality of life. However, progression of obstruction, a potential feature with ageing in BPE, leads to evident voiding and post-micturition LUTS, and potentially the man affected might then seek medical advice. Crucially, the emergence of LUTS reflects a relative inadequacy in the expulsive capacity of the bladder. This could be a consequence of detrusor underactivity (DUA), which is to say that the bladder contraction is insufficient for normal voiding—maybe even in the absence of frank outlet obstruction. Alternatively, the relative insufficiency of bladder contraction may reflect decline in compensatory processes. Thus, DUA is defined as a contraction of reduced strength and/or duration, resulting in prolonged bladder emptying and/or a failure to achieve complete bladder emptying within a normal time span. The variables of outlet obstruction severity, detrusor contraction strength and contraction duration lead to varied

T. Renninson, M.B.Ch.B.
Department of Medicine, Frenchay Hospital,
Bristol, Avon, UK

M.J. Drake, M.A. (Cantab),
D.M. (Oxon.), F.R.C.S. (Urol.)
University of Bristol and Bristol Urological Institute,
Bristol, UK

B.A. Parsons, B.Sc., M.B.Ch.B., M.R.C.S. (✉)
Department of Urology, Cheltenham General Hospital,
Cheltenham, Gloucestershire GL53 7AN, UK
e-mail: brianaparsons@hotmail.com

A.J. Wein et al. (eds.), *Bladder Dysfunction in the Adult: The Basis for Clinical Management*, Current
Clinical Urology, DOI 10.1007/978-1-4939-0853-0_4, © Springer Science+Business Media New York 2014

Table. 4.1 Symptoms seen in outlet obstruction as standardised by the International Continence Society [2], comprising voiding lower urinary tract symptoms (LUTS) (slow stream, hesitancy, straining and terminal dribble) and post-micturition LUTS (post-micturition dribble and feeling of incomplete emptying)

LUTS suggestive of BOO	A term used when a man complains predominately of voiding symptoms in the absence of infection or obvious pathology other than possible causes of outlet obstruction
Slow stream	Reported by the individual as his or her perception of reduced urine flow, usually compared to previous performance or in comparison to others
Intermittent stream (intermittency)	The term used when the individual describes urine flow which stops and starts, on one or more occasions, during micturition
Hesitancy	Used when an individual describes difficulty in initiating micturition resulting in a delay in the onset of voiding after the individual is ready to pass urine
Straining to void	Describes the muscular effort used to either initiate, maintain or improve the urinary stream
Terminal dribble	Used when an individual describes a prolonged final part of micturition, when the flow has slowed to a trickle/dribble
Post-micturition dribble	Describes the involuntary loss of urine immediately after a person has finished passing urine, usually after leaving the toilet in men or after rising from the toilet in women
Feeling of incomplete emptying	A self-explanatory term for a feeling experienced by the individual after passing urine

Table. 4.2 Key issues of outlet obstruction [2]

BOO	The generic term for obstruction during voiding, characterised by increased detrusor pressure and reduced urine flow rate. It is usually diagnosed by studying the synchronous values of flow rate and detrusor pressure
Benign prostatic hyperplasia (BPH)	A term used (and reserved) for the typical histological pattern which defines the disease
Benign prostatic enlargement (BPE)	Prostatic enlargement due to histological BPH. The term 'prostatic enlargement' should be used in the absence of prostatic histology
Benign prostatic obstruction (BPO)	A form of BOO which may be diagnosed when the cause of outlet obstruction is known to be benign prostatic enlargement, due to histological BPH
Dysfunctional voiding	Voiding characterised by an intermittent and/or fluctuating flow rate due to involuntary intermittent contractions of the periurethral striated muscle during voiding in neurologically normal individuals
Acute retention of urine	A painful, palpable or percussible bladder, when the patient is unable to pass any urine
Chronic retention of urine	A non-painful bladder, which remains palpable or percussible after the patient has passed urine. Such patients may be incontinent. *The term chronic retention excludes transient voiding difficulty, for example, after surgery for stress incontinence, and implies a significant residual urine; a minimum figure of 300 mL has been previously mentioned*
Post-void residual (PVR)	The volume of urine left in the bladder at the end of micturition

clinical features of symptom severity, symptom bother and urodynamic changes (Table 4.2).

In some patients, BOO may be asymptomatic and only become manifest on development of urinary retention, sepsis or upper tract pathology. Often however, BOO produces LUTS, but the degree of associated bother is highly variable and not predictable on the basis of the specific underlying aetiology or the severity of the obstruction. Voiding symptoms are a subset of LUTS experienced during the voiding phase of micturition and

comprise slow stream, intermittency, hesitancy, straining and terminal dribbling [2]. Although voiding LUTS and a feeling of incomplete emptying may be suggestive of obstruction, BOO commonly presents as complex array of symptoms that often includes daytime frequency, urgency, nocturia and incontinence (storage symptoms).

Using gender- and age-specific prevalence data from the EPIC study [4] and population estimates from the US Census Bureau International Database, Irwin and colleagues have attempted to estimate worldwide numbers of individuals aged 20 years and over experiencing LUTS suggestive of BOO (LUTS/BOO) [5]. The authors defined LUTS/BOO as the presence of any voiding symptom and estimated that 21.5 % of the world's population in 2008 (917 million individuals) experienced such symptoms with a greater prevalence among men than women. This is likely to be an underestimate, as some patients may have a main complaint of storage symptoms whilst others may remain asymptomatic.

Secondary Consequences of Outlet Obstruction

The generation of high-amplitude sustained contractions for voiding against a partially obstructed outlet leads to alterations in structure and physiology of the bladder wall. Localised muscle hypertrophy gives a trabeculated appearance to the bladder wall, often with small diverticula, visible endoscopically and on imaging [6]. The thickness of the detrusor is increased, and the whole bladder wall increases as a result of this and other cellular responses.

The higher contractile force impairs blood flow, leading to hypoxia [7–9]. Since neurones are very active metabolically, they may be differentially affected by hypoxia, leading potentially to partial denervation in BOO [10]. In the longer term, fibrosis within muscle bundles is evident. The fibrosis may be influenced by small leucine-rich proteoglycans [11]. At a cellular level, diverse changes have been reported. Interstitial cell numbers and interactions are altered in experimental models of BOO (e.g. in rat [12]). The bladder urothelium, a structure of considerable physiological implication [13, 14], shows cellular hypertrophy, though with limited effect on second messenger signalling [15]. Expression of cell surface receptors changes in the various cell types present in the bladder, for example, purinergic receptors on interstitial cells [16]. Increased sensitivity of detrusor muscle to acetylcholine is seen [17]. Angiotensin II receptor type 1 expression, normally present on detrusor and interstitial cells, is not seen in an animal model of outlet obstruction [18]. Increased

expression of nicotinic acetylcholine receptors is seen in sensory nerves [19], and trophic influences such as nerve growth factor [20] and basic fibroblast growth factor [21] are altered. The nature of transmitter release also changes; in normal human bladder, cholinergic transmission predominates, but increased purinergic transmission is seen in partial BOO [22].

Behaviour of the smooth muscle changes, perhaps mediated by alterations in intracellular mechanisms such as calcium handling [23] and Rho-kinase [24]. Increased spontaneous activity is seen in muscle strips [25]. Enhanced coordination of muscle cell activity is seen, mediated by communication through increased numbers of intercellular gap junctions [26]. This is reflected at a gross level as altered autonomous activity in the isolated whole bladder [27], manifesting as spontaneous contractions of extensive proportions of the bladder wall (enhanced micromotions), detectable by their effect on luminal pressure.

These reports are examples of just some of the many changes seen. However, care is needed in deciding whether the changes are caused by BOO, compensate for BOO or unrelated. Furthermore, knowledge about how the changes translate into the clinical context is limited [28].

Benign Prostate Enlargement

In ageing men the most common cause of LUTS/BOO is benign prostatic enlargement (BPE), a clinical diagnosis made on digital rectal examination. BPE develops as a result of benign prostatic hyperplasia (BPH) occurring in the transition zone and periurethral glands of the prostate [29]. BPH is a histological diagnosis made on microscopic examination of prostatic biopsies/tissue and is defined by the progressive age-related hyperplasia of glandular and stromal elements. Development of BPH requires both ageing and androgens, but specific initiating and promoting factors remain elusive.

BPH is a histological diagnosis of little clinical significance unless enlargement impairs bladder outlet calibre or configuration, leading to partial BOO. BPH becomes increasingly prevalent with age, giving bothersome LUTS through benign prostatic obstruction in 30–50 %. The presence of other conditions which may present in similar fashion [30–32] needs to be considered. The incidence of bothersome symptoms increases with advancing age, regardless of ethnic origin [33].

There is no strong correlation between prostate size, symptoms and urinary flow rates in large studies on male LUTS and BPH. Nonetheless, men with larger glands and higher serum PSA values are more likely to experience clinical progression, worsening of LUTS and maximum urinary flow rates and risk of progression to prostate surgery or acute urinary retention [34, 35]. In men with no evidence of prostate cancer, serum PSA level correlates with total prostate volume [34, 36].

The relationship between BPH and LUTS is complex as histologically identifiable BPH is present at autopsy in 50 % of men aged 51–60 and increases to 90 % for men over 80 years of age and yet bothersome LUTS only occurs in 30 % of men aged 65 years and over [37]. The terms BPH and BPE must therefore be distinguished from benign prostatic obstruction (BPO), a diagnosis made after pressure-flow studies have demonstrated BOO secondary to a benign feeling prostate. Symptoms alone cannot be used for diagnosis of BOO, due to the similar nature of symptoms resulting from the disparate processes of obstruction and DUA. Instead additional tests are employed comprising noninvasive urodynamic tests and voiding cystometry, as detailed below.

Our understanding of the pathophysiology of BPE and BPO continues to develop. It has traditionally been thought that the clinical manifestations attributed to BPO are the result of dynamic and static mechanisms. The dynamic component is mediated by prostatic smooth muscle tension and is under sympathetic noradrenergic control via α-adrenoceptors. The observation by Shapiro and colleagues that 40 % of the area density of BPH is smooth muscle provides evidence for its importance in the development of clinically significant BPH [38]. The static component is attributed to the physical obstruction resulting from the presence of an enlarged prostate. This is dependent on androgen stimulation as castrated men do not develop histological BPH or

its clinical manifestations [39]. An inflammatory component to BPH pathogenesis is increasingly recognised and is evidenced by the large proportion of BPH surgical specimens that have a demonstrable inflammatory infiltrate. There is also growing interest in the role that the metabolic syndrome, cell signalling and genetics may play in the development of BPH and BPO [40].

Free Flow Rate Testing

Free flow rate (FFR) tests are a fundamental tool in assessment of voiding LUTS. They require a representative void measured with a flow rate metre, yielding information on pattern of flow and maximum flow rate (Q_{max}) (Fig. 4.1). At the time of voiding, initial bladder volume has to be adequate, since detrusor contractility is reduced if the bladder is underfilled. Repeated measurements are more accurately representative of an individual's voiding than a single FFR [41].

Uroflowmetry nomograms based on the Q_{max} are in clinical use [42–44]. However, correlation with symptoms may be weak [41], and FFR alone cannot ascertain the basis of reduction in flow, whether it be BOO or impaired detrusor contractility [45]. BOO is present in 90 % of men in the age groups at risk of BPE who have a $Q_{max} < 10$ mL/s, but it is also present in a significant proportion of men with $Q_{max} > 15$ [46].

Voiding Cystometry

Invasive urodynamic testing uses simultaneous measurement of bladder and abdominal pressure, with concurrent computed subtraction to derive the detrusor pressure throughout voiding (see also Chap. 9). When bladder pressure is at its lowest point during the peak of the flow rate, the outlet can be presumed to have reached its maximum calibre. At this point, the relationship of pressure to flow can be used as a measure of BOO. Nomograms have been used to categorise BPE patients as obstructed, equivocal or unobstructed [47, 48], derived from observing outcomes of people undergoing surgery; the nomograms are

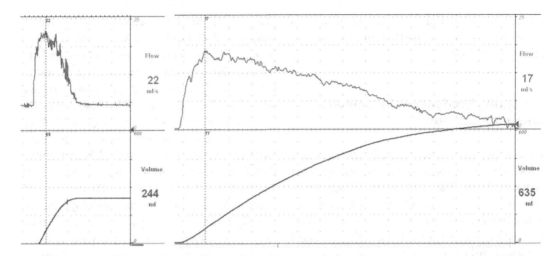

Fig. 4.1 Flow rate tests. A normal flow pattern (*left*), contrasting with that from a man with benign prostate enlargement who was subsequently shown to have bladder outlet obstruction (BOO) using invasive urodynamics (*right*). The patterns are characteristic—the relatively good maximum flow rate in the man with prostate enlargement illustrates the importance of filling volume on free flow rate (FFR), and the fact that maximum flow rate alone is not adequate as a diagnostic test for outlet obstruction

not applicable in other forms of BOO, such as urethral strictures in men or BOO in women. The most widely used is the ICS nomogram, which determines the bladder outlet obstruction index (BOOI) from maximum flow rate (Q_{max}) and the associated detrusor pressure ($P_{det}Q_{max}$) using the equation $BOOI = P_{det}Q_{max} - 2Q_{max}$. An evaluation of bladder contractility can be derived using the same parameters (bladder contractility index $= P_{det}Q_{max} + 5Q_{max}$). A third parameter, the bladder voiding efficiency (BVE) relates the degree of bladder emptying to the bladder capacity, expressed as a percentage; BVE = (voided volume/total bladder capacity) × 100 [49].

Confirmation of a BOOI > 40 (the threshold of definite obstruction) in a man with voiding LUTS is a logical basis for recommendation for surgery to relieve BOO. If BCI is >100, the threshold of normal contractility, it is reassuring that voiding LUTS are unlikely to persist postoperatively as a consequence of impaired bladder contractility. For certain groups, estimation of BOO and bladder contractility is crucial in view of potential for DUA as the basis for voiding LUTS, notably men older than 80 or younger than 50 years of age. Between these ages, clinicians may choose to use invasive urodynamic testing selectively.

Ultrasound-Based Methods

An anatomic assessment of prostate parameters can be derived using ultrasound. Prostate volume measurement using transrectal ultrasound is a simple parameter, but prostate volume correlates relatively poorly with symptoms or urodynamic parameters [50]. Transition zone volume or transition zone index has also been evaluated. Whilst they show a better correspondence with symptoms, they do not correspond reliably with findings of urodynamic testing [51, 52]. Other parameters under evaluation include the presumed prostate circle area ratio (PCAR) [53] and intravesical prostatic protrusion [54, 55].

Secondary consequences of BOO, including hypertrophy within the bladder wall, can also be measured with ultrasonography. Bladder wall thickness [56], detrusor wall thickness [57] and transabdominal ultrasound estimated bladder weight [58] are affected by BOO and have been investigated as approaches for diagnosis of BOO. A BWT cut-off of 5 mm at a volume of 150 mL has been proposed for diagnosis of BOO [56]. However, no significant difference in BWT in BOO was observed elsewhere [59]. Dynamic ultrasound parameters have also been evaluated;

for example, arterial vascular resistance is increased in BOO and partly returns to normal after surgery [60].

Measuring Urodynamic Parameters Without a Catheter

Urine flow patterns after penile compression and release (PCR) are a possible means for diagnosing BOO and DUA. The penile cuff technique interrupts voiding intermittently by rapid cycles of cuff inflation and deflation to assess isovolumetric bladder pressure [61]. A specially developed nomogram [62] can be used to classify patients as obstructed or non-obstructed. The results can anticipate clinical outcome from TURP [63]. The condom method also measures bladder pressure, but a separate FFR measurement is needed to establish whether BOO is present [64].

Urethral Stricture and Contracture

Urethral stricture disease is one of the oldest maladies known to urology, with references made about the disease and its treatment dating back to the times of the Egyptians and Greeks [65]. The male urethra can be divided into two parts: the posterior urethra including the membranous and prostatic part and the anterior urethra comprising the navicular fossa, penile and bulbar urethra. A urethral stricture is a scar of the subepithelial tissue of the corpus spongiosum that constricts the lumen [66]. The term stricture therefore applies to constrictions of the anterior urethra as this is the part that is surrounded by corpus spongiosum soft tissue [67]. A similar constricting narrowing of the urethra elsewhere is conventionally termed a stenosis or contracture. Penile urethra strictures are idiopathic in 15 %, iatrogenic in 40 %, inflammatory in 40 % or traumatic in 5 % [66]. For bulbar strictures, the figures are idiopathic 40 %, iatrogenic 35 %, inflammatory 10 % and traumatic 15 %. Most strictures are iatrogenic or idiopathic [68, 69]. Iatrogenic causes include urethral catheterisation, urinary tract endoscopy and surgery for hypospadias. Infection-related strictures appear to coincide with the location of the urethral

glands [70]. Meatal strictures may be due to ammoniacal dermatitis (i.e. skin changes caused by repeated contact with urine), lichen sclerosus (or balanitis xerotica obliterans [71]) or instrumentation. The estimated prevalence is age dependent [72, 73], and 40/100,000 may be affected by the time they reach the age of 65 years.

Urethral strictures are a common problem. Hospital episode statistics in the UK and similar data from the USA suggest an incidence of 1 in 10,000 men aged 25 and 1 in 1,000 men aged 65 years and over [74]. Stricture aetiology can be broadly divided into idiopathic, iatrogenic, traumatic and inflammatory. In the past, sexually transmitted infections were the major cause of urethral strictures, with urethritis accounting for 40 % of cases in a review of the literature published in 1981 [75]. In the developed world, the incidence of infective strictures has dramatically decreased as a result of prevention campaigns against sexually transmitted diseases and the development of effective antibiotic therapy. Consequently, most strictures are now idiopathic or iatrogenic in origin [68, 69], with lichen sclerosus (balanitis xerotica obliterans) an important 'inflammatory' cause (see Table 4.3). Iatrogenic strictures develop as a result of urinary tract instrumentation, catheterisation or previous surgery, such as transurethral resection in the older patient or hypospadias surgery in younger individuals. Instrumentation-related strictures tend to occur at the external meatus, fossa navicularis, penoscrotal junction and in the region of the urethral sphincter [89]. Idiopathic strictures have no apparent cause, but several explanations have been proposed to explain their occurrence. They are thought by some to be a delayed manifestation of unrecognised (childhood) trauma [90]. Given that idiopathic strictures are more prevalent in the bulbar urethra, the site where the part of the urethra derived from the urogenital sinus joins the part derived from the urogenital folds, it has also been suggested that these strictures may be due to incomplete canalisation during development.

In developing countries, urethritis remains an important cause of urethral strictures, accounting for up to two thirds of cases [91–95]. In these areas, there is also a higher incidence of traumatic strictures compared to the developed world

Table. 4.3 Review of the literature on anterior urethral stricture aetiology

Study authors	Stricture number (n)	Cause (n) Idiopathic	Iatrogenic	Inflammatory	Traumatic
Lumen and colleagues [69]	228	80 (35 %)	111 (49 %)	27 (12 %)	10 (4 %)
Barbagli and colleagues [76]	375	247 (66 %)	83 (22 %)	7 (2 %)	38 (10 %)
Fenton and colleagues [68]	194	65 (34 %)	63 (32 %)	38 (20 %)	28 (14 %)
Andrich and colleagues [77]	185	55 (30 %)	88 (48 %)	25 (13 %)	17 (9 %)
Elliott and colleagues [78]	60	37 (61 %)	9 (15 %)	7 (12 %)	7 (12 %)
Santucci and colleagues [79]	168	64 (38 %)	24 (14 %)	12 (7 %)	68 (41 %)
Arlen and colleagues [80]	24	12 (50 %)	5 (21 %)	1 (4 %)	6 (25 %)
O'Riordan and colleagues [81]	52	29 (55 %)	13 (25 %)	7 (14 %)	3 (6 %)
Elliott and colleagues [82]	38	6 (16 %)	18 (47 %)	8 (21 %)	6 (16 %)
Berglund and Angermeier [83]	18	4 (22 %)	8 (44 %)	3 (17 %)	3 (17 %)
Santucci and colleagues [84]	68	30 (44 %)	23 (34 %)	5 (7 %)	10 (15 %)
Barbagli and colleagues [85]	153	96 (62 %)	38 (25 %)	1 (1 %)	18 (12 %)
Kellner and colleagues [86]	23	9 (39 %)	11 (48 %)	2 (9 %)	1 (4 %)
Pansadoro and colleagues [87]	65	12 (18 %)	21 (32 %)	27 (41 %)	5 (8 %)
Meneghini and colleagues [88]	20	11 (55 %)	5 (25 %)	4 (20 %)	0 (0 %)
Total	1,296	510 (39 %)	437 (34 %)	167 (13 %)	182 (14 %)

because of the poor vehicular conditions and traffic regulations [69, 92].

It is clear that external trauma may cause partial or complete disruption of the normal urethra, leading to fibrosis and stricturing as part of the healing process. In contrast, the pathogenesis of non-traumatic stricture disease has yet to be conclusively established with multiple aetiological factors having been proposed. There is general agreement that extravasation of urine is probably the most important pathophysiological mechanism [66]. This may result from urethral injury or leakage of urine into the subepithelial tissues through fissures and ulcers. Extravasation of urine sets up an inflammatory response which ultimately leads to fibrosis of the corpus spongiosum deep to the urethral epithelium. Areas of fibrosis then coalesce over time to form a circumferential ring around the urethra. Ischaemia is another common underlying factor predisposing to stricture disease and is important in the pathogenesis of catheter-related strictures.

Stricture-related fibrosis is associated with marked changes in extracellular matrix features with a decrease in elastic fibres, changes in nitric oxide synthase metabolism and an increased proportion of type 1 collagen [96, 97]. This contrasts with wound healing in other parts of the body, where there is a lower type 1 to type 3 collagen ratio [98]. The pathology of lichen sclerosus is different

in that it is atrophic rather than proliferative with features suggestive of an autoimmune aetiology, although an infective component has not been discounted [71, 99]. Lichen sclerosus is generally confined to the prepuce and glans but can spread proximally to involve the navicular fossa, the penile urethra and rarely the bulbar urethra.

Most patients present with worsening symptoms of LUTS obstruction, haematuria and/or urinary tract infection. Strictures may be complicated by urinary retention, prostatitis, epididymo-orchitis, stone formation and upper urinary tract obstruction. If left untreated, periurethral abscess formation will occur, and eventual fistulation through the skin may result in the so-called watering-can perineum. The length and severity of the stricture seem to correlate with the risk of complications [68].

Diagnosis and management

A clinical diagnosis is largely based on the history, as physical examination is generally unrewarding unless there is a history of disease or surgery. Hesitancy, a poor stream and terminal dribbling are a common complaint, but a sensation of incomplete emptying has the strongest association with stricture disease [66]. Symptomatic assessment is best formalised using a standardised questionnaire such as the American Urological Association symptom index, but it has been shown that up to 10 % of men may be asymptomatic [100]. A urinary flow rate study may be characteristic, with a protracted low flow with a plateau appearance on the trace (Fig. 4.2) and incomplete emptying on assessment of the post-void residual. If symptoms and uroflowmetry suggest a stricture, then cystoscopy can be used to confirm the presence of a stricture. For short, mild strictures, this may provide sufficient information, but a tight stricture prevents passage of the endoscope, and visualisation above the distal limit of the stricture is restricted. A urethrogram is a radiological test, requiring retrograde instillation of contrast to map the distal limit of the stricture and screening during voiding of contrast (antegrade) to show the proximal extent (Fig. 4.3). Only a urethrogram (with retrograde and antegrade phases) is able to provide information about the exact position and length of the stricture [66]. If renal function is deranged on biochemical testing, then the upper urinary tracts should be assessed with ultrasound.

Management of Strictures

In the absence of complications, treatment should be aimed at symptom relief rather than be guided by the results of flow rate studies or imaging. Urethral strictures have traditionally been treated with dilatations or more recently by direct vision internal urethrotomy (DVIU), although there is no evidence that DVIU is better than dilatation [91]. DVIU and dilatation are potentially curative in about 50 % of cases when used in the first time

treatment of short (<1 cm) bulbar strictures [66]. However, when performed repeatedly or used to treat strictures at other sites, then these procedures are unlikely to result in cure and may exacerbate the fibrosis, thereby increasing stricture length and severity and complicating subsequent reconstruction [101]. In the presence of severe co-morbidities, palliation of symptoms by urethral dilatation or DVIU may be acceptable.

Both urethral dilatation and DVIU should be covered by prophylactic antibiotics, and limited evidence suggests that keeping a catheter for 3 days after urethrotomy reduces the risk of early postoperative urine extravasation and infective complications [102]. Urethroplasty is the only curative option currently available for the treatment of recurrent bulbar strictures and for all other anterior urethral strictures [66]. Short bulbar urethra strictures are generally amenable to complete excision with primary end-to-end anastomosis. Long bulbar strictures and penile strictures of any length are best treated by stricturotomy and a urethral substitution procedure incorporating a graft or flap to augment the stenotic segment [101].

Bladder Neck contracture and Posterior Urethra Stenosis

Bladder neck contracture can be an iatrogenic consequence of urethral instrumentation or surgery [89]. This can arise after radical treatment of prostate cancer and thus is increasingly important due to more widespread cancer diagnosis and intervention in modern practice. Incidence of bladder neck contracture after radical retropubic prostatectomy is 20–30 % [103, 104]. Incidence

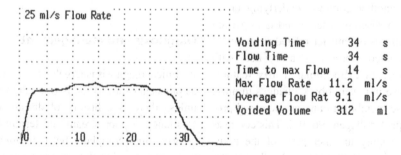

Fig. 2 An FFR test from a man with a urethral stricture, illustrating the characteristic 'plateau' pattern

Fig. 4.3 Antegrade urethrogram done by instilling contrast direct into the bladder through a suprapubic catheter and asking him to attempt voiding. In this young male, there is complete occlusion in the bulbar urethra. A retrograde urethrogram would additionally be needed to map the full extent of the stricture

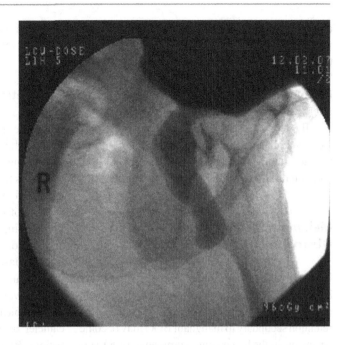

may be less using laparoscopic or robotic prostatectomy [105, 106]. Bladder neck contracture and prostatic urethral stenosis after primary radiotherapy, cryotherapy and HIFU tend to be more extensive and severe [107–110], and treatment and recovery can be problematic [89]. The incidence of iatrogenic stenoses and bladder neck contractures is more difficult to determine as they are often poorly defined due to the distortion of urethral anatomic landmarks following treatment [89]. The diagnosis is suspected on the basis of recurrent voiding symptoms and uroflowmetry data and confirmed on cystoscopy. There is often a lag phase to diagnosis which is dependent in part on the severity of the stenosis and patient tolerance of symptoms. Treatment of symptomatic patients requires a bladder neck incision.

Bladder neck contractures following radical prostatectomy occur in 0.4–32 % of cases, with a lower incidence reported after laparoscopic and robotic approaches [111–113]. A prior TURP is a preoperative risk factor as is postoperative bleeding and haematoma formation as the latter could put tension on the anastomosis. Less severe contractures can be treated endoscopically with urethral dilatation or DVIU with a single procedure being successful in 25–73 % of patients [89, 114, 115]. The patient may subsequently be taught intermittent self-catheterisation to maintain urethral patency. There is a recognised association with sphincter weakness incontinence, and after successful contracture treatment, an artificial sphincter may be needed to treat worsening incontinence [114]. For patients with more fibrotic contractures or contractures that are refractory to endoscopic treatment, a revision of the vesicourethral anastomosis may be considered. This can be performed abdominoperineally or transperineally, but only small series have been reported [89, 116, 117]. Contractures associated with external beam radiotherapy, brachytherapy, HIFU and cryotherapy are much more difficult to treat with less satisfactory outcomes. Stenosis may be amenable to an anastomotic repair or a flap repair for longer more obliterative narrowings [89]. A long-term suprapubic catheter or a supravesical diversion may be the last resort.

Other Causes of Bladder Outlet Obstruction in Men

Rarely, the outlet can be 'plugged'—for example, by a foreign body in the lumen [118], a bladder diverticulum [119] or a congenital abnormality, such as a sliding ureterocoele [120]. Posterior urethral valves (PUV) are an anatomic abnormality which can cause severe BOO, presenting in early boyhood with renal failure or detected antenatally due to hydronephrosis. There are various classifications and theories underlying the underlying embryology (reviewed in [121]). The consequences on urodynamic function can be profound, though not invariably so, and persist after treatment. Another congenital abnormality, usually less severely obstructing than PUV, is Cobb's collar—a membranous stricture of the bulbar urethra, which can lead to partial BOO and potentially to acute urinary retention [122].

Malignant Bladder Outlet Obstruction

For men with advanced prostate cancer that is not amenable to radical treatment with curative intent or those with recurrent disease, LUTS and urinary retention secondary to malignant BOO may become an increasingly bothersome complaint. BOO surgery in the context of cancer is associated with poorer outcomes than for benign disease, and consequently hormonal manipulation is the preferred first-line treatment, especially as such patients are often at a higher anaesthetic risk [123]. It has been reported that in up to two thirds of patients with urinary retention due to prostate cancer, orchidectomy alone will lead to relief of outlet obstruction within 60 days of treatment [124]. In patients with persistent symptoms, those who develop urinary retention despite endocrine therapy and in symptomatic patients with castrate-resistant disease, a palliative (or channel) TURP is an alternative to the placement of chronic indwelling catheter.

Few published studies have addressed the efficacy and morbidity of TURP in patients with locally advanced prostate cancer. The limited available data suggests that the outcomes of palliative surgery are not as good as those of TURP for benign disease, as evidenced by the smaller decrease in the IPSS of prostate cancer patients, the higher incontinence rate, the increased chance of failing a trial without catheter and the greater likelihood of needing further interventions or long-term catheterisation [125–127]. This is especially true for patients with castrate-resistant disease or men who have had prior radiotherapy [128, 129]. A channel TURP can be offered to symptomatic patients after failed hormonal manipulation but only after appropriate counselling has been given about the increased risk of complications.

Traumatic Posterior Urethral Injury

An acute posterior urethral distraction injury results when the pubis is fractured and displaced and the puboprostatic ligaments remain intact, as this leads to a shearing force across the membranous and bulbar urethra [130]. Approximately 4–14 % of pelvic fractures will cause a posterior urethral injury [131] and are more commonly associated with straddle fractures (including sacroiliac diastasis and bilateral pubic rami fractures) than other more simple pelvic fractures.

Following a pelvic fracture, a posterior urethral injury typically causes difficulty inserting a Foley catheter or an inability to void by the conscious patient. Blood at the urethral meatus is noted in about 50 % of cases and a high riding prostate due to a pelvic haematoma in 34 % of urethral distraction injuries [130]. In the emergency setting, one careful attempt at catheter placement should be made, but if this fails, then a retrograde urethrogram should be performed. If a urethral injury is confirmed, then urinary diversion with a suprapubic catheter is recommended for 3–6 months before attempting formal open reconstruction. In the absence of an intraperitoneal bladder rupture, a suprapubic catheter should be inserted percutaneously, but otherwise an open cystotomy and catheter placement would be recommended. Urinary diversion allows time for scar maturation, resorption of pelvic hematomas and relative restoration of anatomic fascial layers. Definitive treatment would then involve excision of the scarred segment of the urethra via a perineal approach with a primary anastomotic repair [130]. Substitution urethroplasty is almost never required for the repair of a posterior urethral distraction injury.

Conclusions

Anatomic causes of outlet obstruction are a common health issue in the ageing male as a consequence of two key conditions, BPE and urethral stricture. Rare causes of outlet obstruction also need to be considered, but similarity of symptoms means that DUA is one of the main issues to be considered in the differential diagnosis. Diagnostic approaches use noninvasive (particularly FFR and post-void residual assessment) and invasive urodynamic methods and endoscopic examination, as appropriate for the particular circumstances.

References

1. Wein AJ. Classification of neurogenic voiding dysfunction. J Urol. 1981;125:605–9.
2. Abrams P, Cardozo L, Fall M, et al. The standardisation of terminology of lower urinary tract function: report from the Standardisation Sub-committee of the International Continence Society. Neurourol Urodyn. 2002;21:167–78.
3. Abrams P. New words for old: lower urinary tract symptoms for "prostatism". BMJ. 1994;308:929–30.
4. Irwin DE, Milsom I, Hunskaar S, et al. Population-based survey of urinary incontinence, overactive bladder, and other lower urinary tract symptoms in five countries: results of the EPIC study. Eur Urol. 2006;50:1306–14; discussion 14–5.
5. Irwin DE, Kopp ZS, Agatep B, Milsom I, Abrams P. Worldwide prevalence estimates of lower urinary tract symptoms, overactive bladder, urinary incontinence and bladder outlet obstruction. BJU Int. 2011;108:1132–8.
6. Galosi AB, Mazzaferro D, Lacetera V, Muzzonigro G, Martino P, Tucci G. Modifications of the bladder wall (organ damage) in patients with bladder outlet obstruction: ultrasound parameters. Arch Ital Urol Androl. 2012;84:263–7.
7. Drzewiecki BA, Anumanthan G, Penn HA, et al. Modulation of the hypoxic response following partial bladder outlet obstruction. J Urol. 2012;188:1549–54.
8. Greenland JE, Brading AF. The effect of bladder outflow obstruction on detrusor blood flow changes during the voiding cycle in conscious pigs. J Urol. 2001;165:245–8.
9. Greenland JE, Hvistendahl JJ, Andersen H, et al. The effect of bladder outlet obstruction on tissue oxygen tension and blood flow in the pig bladder. BJU Int. 2000;85:1109–14.
10. Brading AF, Turner WH. The unstable bladder: towards a common mechanism. Br J Urol. 1994;73:3–8.
11. Maciejewski CC, Honardoust D, Tredget EE, Metcalfe PD. Differential expression of class I small leucine-rich proteoglycans in an animal model of partial bladder outlet obstruction. J Urol. 2012;188:1543–8.
12. Kim SO, Oh BS, Chang IY, et al. Distribution of interstitial cells of Cajal and expression of nitric oxide synthase after experimental bladder outlet obstruction in a rat model of bladder overactivity. Neurourol Urodyn. 2011;30:1639–45.
13. Birder LA. Involvement of the urinary bladder urothelium in signaling in the lower urinary tract. Proc West Pharmacol Soc. 2001;44:85–6.
14. Birder LA. Urothelial signaling. Auton Neurosci. 2010;153:33–40.
15. Bschleipfer T, Weidner W, Kummer W, Lips KS. Does bladder outlet obstruction alter the non-neuronal cholinergic system of the human urothelium? Life Sci. 2012;91:1082–6.
16. Li Y, Xue L, Miao Q, et al. Expression and electrophysiological characteristics of P2X3 receptors in interstitial cells of Cajal in rats with partial bladder outlet obstruction. BJU Int. 2013;111:843–51.
17. Sibley GN. The physiological response of the detrusor muscle to experimental bladder outflow obstruction in the pig. Br J Urol. 1987;60:332–6.
18. Tobu S, Noguchi M, Hatada T, Mori K, Matsuo M, Sakai H. Changes in angiotensin II type 1 receptor expression in the rat bladder by bladder outlet obstruction. Urol Int. 2012;89:241–5.
19. Bschleipfer T, Nandigama R, Moeller S, Illig C, Weidner W, Kummer W. Bladder outlet obstruction influences mRNA expression of cholinergic receptors on sensory neurons in mice. Life Sci. 2012; 91:1077–81.
20. Ochodnicky P, Cruz CD, Yoshimura N, Michel MC. Nerve growth factor in bladder dysfunction: contributing factor, biomarker, and therapeutic target. Neurourol Urodyn. 2011;30:1227–41.
21. Imamura M, Kanematsu A, Yamamoto S, et al. Basic fibroblast growth factor modulates proliferation and collagen expression in urinary bladder smooth muscle cells. Am J Physiol Renal Physiol. 2007; 293:F1007–17.
22. Bayliss M, Wu C, Newgreen D, Mundy AR, Fry CH. A quantitative study of atropine-resistant contractile responses in human detrusor smooth muscle, from stable, unstable and obstructed bladders. J Urol. 1999;162:1833–9.
23. Burmeister D, AbouShwareb T, D'Agostino Jr R, Andersson KE, Christ GJ. Impact of partial urethral obstruction on bladder function: time-dependent changes and functional correlates of altered expression of Ca(2)(+) signaling regulators. Am J Physiol Renal Physiol. 2012;302:F1517–28.
24. Wibberley A, Chen Z, Hu E, Hieble JP, Westfall TD. Expression and functional role of Rho-kinase in rat urinary bladder smooth muscle. Br J Pharmacol. 2003;138:757–66.
25. Brading AF. A myogenic basis for the overactive bladder. Urology. 1997;50:57–67; discussion 8–73.
26. Imamura M, Negoro H, Kanematsu A, et al. Basic fibroblast growth factor causes urinary bladder overactivity through gap junction generation in the smooth muscle. Am J Physiol Renal Physiol. 2009;297:F46–54.
27. Drake MJ, Hedlund P, Harvey IJ, Pandita RK, Andersson KE, Gillespie JI. Partial outlet obstruction enhances modular autonomous activity in the isolated rat bladder. J Urol. 2003;170:276–9.
28. Oelke M, Kirschner-Hermanns R, Thiruchelvam N, Heesakkers J. Can we identify men who will have

complications from benign prostatic obstruction (BPO)? ICI-RS 2011. Neurourol Urodyn. 2012; 31:322–6.

29. McNeal JE. Anatomy of the prostate and morphogenesis of BPH. Prog Clin Biol Res. 1984;145:27–53.

30. Girman CJ. Natural history and epidemiology of benign prostatic hyperplasia: relationship among urologic measures. Urology. 1998;51:8–12.

31. Rhodes T, Girman CJ, Jacobsen SJ, Roberts RO, Guess HA, Lieber MM. Longitudinal prostate growth rates during 5 years in randomly selected community men 40 to 79 years old. J Urol. 1999;161:1174–9.

32. Girman CJ, Jacobsen SJ, Rhodes T, Guess HA, Roberts RO, Lieber MM. Association of health-related quality of life and benign prostatic enlargement. Eur Urol. 1999;35:277–84.

33. Roehrborn CG. Male lower urinary tract symptoms (LUTS) and benign prostatic hyperplasia (BPH). Med Clin North Am. 2011;95:87–100.

34. Roehrborn CG. The utility of serum prostatic-specific antigen in the management of men with benign prostatic hyperplasia. Int J Impot Res. 2008;20 Suppl 3:S19–26.

35. Roehrborn CG. BPH progression: concept and key learning from MTOPS, ALTESS, COMBAT, and ALF-ONE. BJU Int. 2008;101 Suppl 3:17–21.

36. Bohnen AM, Groeneveld FP, Bosch JL. Serum prostate-specific antigen as a predictor of prostate volume in the community: the Krimpen study. Eur Urol. 2007;51:1645–52; discussion 52–3.

37. Berry SJ, Coffey DS, Walsh PC, Ewing LL. The development of human benign prostatic hyperplasia with age. J Urol. 1984;132:474–9.

38. Shapiro E, Hartanto V, Lepor H. Anti-desmin vs. anti-actin for quantifying the area density of prostate smooth muscle. Prostate. 1992;20:259–67.

39. Schroder FH. Medical treatment of benign prostatic hyperplasia: the effect of surgical or medical castration. Prog Clin Biol Res. 1994;386:191–6.

40. Donnell RF. Benign prostate hyperplasia: a review of the year's progress from bench to clinic. Curr Opin Urol. 2011;21:22–6.

41. Reynard JM, Yang Q, Donovan JL, et al. The ICS-'BPH' Study: uroflowmetry, lower urinary tract symptoms and bladder outlet obstruction. Br J Urol. 1998;82:619–23.

42. Siroky MB, Olsson CA, Krane RJ. The flow rate nomogram: I. Development. J Urol. 1979;122:665–8.

43. Siroky MB, Olsson CA, Krane RJ. The flow rate nomogram: II. Clinical correlation. J Urol. 1980; 123:208–10.

44. Haylen BT, Ashby D, Sutherst JR, Frazer MI, West CR. Maximum and average urine flow rates in normal male and female populations—the Liverpool nomograms. Br J Urol. 1989;64:30–8.

45. Chancellor MB, Blaivas JG, Kaplan SA, Axelrod S. Bladder outlet obstruction versus impaired detrusor contractility: the role of outflow. J Urol. 1991; 145:810–2.

46. Abrams P. Urodynamics. 3rd ed. London: Springer; 2006.

47. Abrams PH, Griffiths DJ. The assessment of prostatic obstruction from urodynamic measurements and from residual urine. Br J Urol. 1979;51:129–34.

48. Schafer W. Analysis of bladder-outlet function with the linearized passive urethral resistance relation, linPURR, and a disease-specific approach for grading obstruction: from complex to simple. World J Urol. 1995;13:47–58.

49. Abrams P. Bladder outlet obstruction index, bladder contractility index and bladder voiding efficiency: three simple indices to define bladder voiding function. BJU Int. 1999;84:14–5.

50. Bosch JL, Kranse R, van Mastrigt R, Schroder FH. Reasons for the weak correlation between prostate volume and urethral resistance parameters in patients with prostatism. J Urol. 1995;153:689–93.

51. Kaplan SA, Te AE, Pressler LB, Olsson CA. Transition zone index as a method of assessing benign prostatic hyperplasia: correlation with symptoms, urine flow and detrusor pressure. J Urol. 1995;154:1764–9.

52. Witjes WP, Aarnink RG, Ezz-el-Din K, Wijkstra H, Debruyne EM, de la Rosette JJ. The correlation between prostate volume, transition zone volume, transition zone index and clinical and urodynamic investigations in patients with lower urinary tract symptoms. Br J Urol. 1997;80:84–90.

53. Kojima M, Ochiai A, Naya Y, Ukimura O, Watanabe M, Watanabe H. Correlation of presumed circle area ratio with infravesical obstruction in men with lower urinary tract symptoms. Urology. 1997;50:548–55.

54. Chia SJ, Heng CT, Chan SP, Foo KT. Correlation of intravesical prostatic protrusion with bladder outlet obstruction. BJU Int. 2003;91:371–4.

55. Keqin Z, Zhishun X, Jing Z, Haixin W, Dongqing Z, Benkang S. Clinical significance of intravesical prostatic protrusion in patients with benign prostatic enlargement. Urology. 2007;70:1096–9.

56. Manieri C, Carter SS, Romano G, Trucchi A, Valenti M, Tubaro A. The diagnosis of bladder outlet obstruction in men by ultrasound measurement of bladder wall thickness. J Urol. 1998;159:761–5.

57. Kessler TM, Gerber R, Burkhard FC, Studer UE, Danuser H. Ultrasound assessment of detrusor thickness in men-can it predict bladder outlet obstruction and replace pressure flow study? J Urol. 2006; 175:2170–3.

58. Kojima M, Inui E, Ochiai A, Naya Y, Ukimura O, Watanabe H. Noninvasive quantitative estimation of infravesical obstruction using ultrasonic measurement of bladder weight. J Urol. 1997;157:476–9.

59. Hakenberg OW, Linne C, Manseck A, Wirth MP. Bladder wall thickness in normal adults and men with mild lower urinary tract symptoms and benign prostatic enlargement. Neurourol Urodyn. 2000; 19:585–93.

60. Wada N, Watanabe M, Kita M, Matsumoto S, Kakizaki H. Analysis of bladder vascular resistance before and after prostatic surgery in patients with lower urinary tract symptoms suggestive of benign prostatic obstruction. Neurourol Urodyn. 2012;31:659–63.

61. McIntosh SL, Drinnan MJ, Griffiths CJ, Robson WA, Ramsden PD, Pickard RS. Noninvasive assessment of bladder contractility in men. J Urol. 2004;172:1394–8.

62. Griffiths CJ, Harding C, Blake C, et al. A nomogram to classify men with lower urinary tract symptoms using urine flow and noninvasive measurement of bladder pressure. J Urol. 2005;174:1323–6; discussion 6; author reply 6.

63. Harding C, Robson W, Drinnan M, et al. Predicting the outcome of prostatectomy using noninvasive bladder pressure and urine flow measurements. Eur Urol. 2007;52:186–92.

64. Pel JJ, van Mastrigt R. Non-invasive measurement of bladder pressure using an external catheter. Neurourol Urodyn. 1999;18:455–69; discussion 69–75.

65. Chiou RK, Matamoros A, Anderson JC, Taylor RJ. Changing concepts of urethral stricture management. I: Assessment of urethral stricture disease. Nebr Med J. 1996;81:282–6.

66. Mundy AR, Andrich DE. Urethral strictures. BJU Int. 2011;107(1):6–26.

67. Chapple C, Barbagli G, Jordan G, et al. Consensus statement on urethral trauma. BJU Int. 2004;93: 1195–202.

68. Fenton AS, Morey AF, Aviles R, Garcia CR. Anterior urethral strictures: etiology and characteristics. Urology. 2005;65:1055–8.

69. Lumen N, Hoebeke P, Willemsen P, De Troyer B, Pieters R, Oosterlinck W. Etiology of urethral stricture disease in the 21st century. J Urol. 2009;182:983–7.

70. Singh M, Blandy JP. The pathology of urethral stricture. J Urol. 1976;115:673–6.

71. Das S, Tunuguntla HS. Balanitis xerotica obliterans—a review. World J Urol. 2000;18:382–7.

72. McMillan A, Pakianathan M, Mao JH, Macintyre CC. Urethral stricture and urethritis in men in Scotland. Genitourin Med. 1994;70:403–5.

73. Santucci RA, Joyce GF, Wise M. Male urethral stricture disease. J Urol. 2007;177:1667–74.

74. Mundy AR. Management of urethral strictures. Postgrad Med J. 2006;82:489–93.

75. De Sy WA, Oosterlinck W. Treatment of stricture of the male urethra. Acta Urol Belg. 1981;49:93–250.

76. Barbagli G, Guazzoni G, Lazzeri M. One-stage bulbar urethroplasty: retrospective analysis of the results in 375 patients. Eur Urol. 2008;53:828–33.

77. Andrich DE, Greenwell TJ, Mundy AR. The problems of penile urethroplasty with particular reference to 2-stage reconstructions. J Urol. 2003;170:87–9.

78. Elliott SP, Metro MJ, McAninch JW. Long-term followup of the ventrally placed buccal mucosa onlay graft in bulbar urethral reconstruction. J Urol. 2003;169:1754–7.

79. Santucci RA, Mario LA, McAninch JW. Anastomotic urethroplasty for bulbar urethral stricture: analysis of 168 patients. J Urol. 2002;167:1715–9.

80. Arlen AM, Powell CR, Hoffman HT, Kreder KJ. Buccal mucosal graft urethroplasty in the treatment of urethral strictures: experience using the two-surgeon technique. Scientific World Journal. 2010;10:74–9.

81. O'Riordan A, Narahari R, Kumar V, Pickard R. Outcome of dorsal buccal graft urethroplasty for recurrent bulbar urethral strictures. BJU Int. 2008;102:1148–51.

82. Elliott SP, Eisenberg ML, McAninch JW. First-stage urethroplasty: utility in the modern era. Urology. 2008;71:889–92.

83. Berglund RK, Angermeier KW. Combined buccal mucosa graft and genital skin flap for reconstruction of extensive anterior urethral strictures. Urology. 2006;68:707–10; discussion 10.

84. Santucci RA, McAninch JW, Mario LA, et al. Urethroplasty in patients older than 65 years: indications, results, outcomes and suggested treatment modifications. J Urol. 2004;172:201–3.

85. Barbagli G, De Angelis M, Romano G, Lazzeri M. Long-term followup of bulbar end-to-end anastomosis: a retrospective analysis of 153 patients in a single center experience. J Urol. 2007;178:2470–3.

86. Kellner DS, Fracchia JA, Armenakas NA. Ventral onlay buccal mucosal grafts for anterior urethral strictures: long-term followup. J Urol. 2004;171:726–9.

87. Pansadoro V, Emiliozzi P, Gaffi M, Scarpone P, DePaula F, Pizzo M. Buccal mucosa urethroplasty in the treatment of bulbar urethral strictures. Urology. 2003;61:1008–10.

88. Meneghini A, Cacciola A, Cavarretta L, Abatangelo G, Ferrarese P, Tasca A. Bulbar urethral stricture repair with buccal mucosa graft urethroplasty. Eur Urol. 2001;39:264–7.

89. Mundy AR, Andrich DE. Posterior urethral complications of the treatment of prostate cancer. BJU Int. 2012;110(3):304–25.

90. Baskin LS, McAninch JW. Childhood urethral injuries: perspectives on outcome and treatment. Br J Urol. 1993;72:241–6.

91. Steenkamp JW, Heyns CF, de Kock ML. Internal urethrotomy versus dilation as treatment for male urethral strictures: a prospective, randomized comparison. J Urol. 1997;157(1):98–101.

92. Ahmed A, Kalayi GD. Urethral stricture at Ahmadu Bello University Teaching Hospital, Zaria. East Afr Med J. 1998;75:582–5.

93. Fall B, Sow Y, Mansouri I, et al. Etiology and current clinical characteristics of male urethral stricture disease: experience from a public teaching hospital in Senegal. Int Urol Nephrol. 2011;43:969–74.

94. Tijani KH, Adesanya AA, Ogo CN. The new pattern of urethral stricture disease in Lagos, Nigeria. Niger Postgrad Med J. 2009;16:162–5.

95. Dubey D, Kumar A, Bansal P, et al. Substitution urethroplasty for anterior urethral strictures: a critical appraisal of various techniques. BJU Int. 2003;91:215–8.

96. Cavalcanti AG, Yucel S, Deng DY, McAninch JW, Baskin LS. The distribution of neuronal and inducible nitric oxide synthase in urethral stricture formation. J Urol. 2004;171:1943–7.

97. Cavalcanti AG, Costa WS, Baskin LS, McAninch JA, Sampaio FJ. A morphometric analysis of bulbar urethral strictures. BJU Int. 2007;100:397–402.

98. Baskin LS, Constantinescu SC, Howard PS, et al. Biochemical characterization and quantitation of the collagenous components of urethral stricture tissue. J Urol. 1993;150:642–7.

99. Meffert JJ, Davis BM, Grimwood RE. Lichen sclerosus. J Am Acad Dermatol. 1995;32:393–416; quiz 7-8.

100. Nuss GR, Granieri MA, Zhao LC, Thum DJ, Gonzalez CM. Presenting symptoms of anterior urethral stricture disease: a disease specific, patient reported questionnaire to measure outcomes. J Urol. 2012;187:559–62.

101. Waxman SW, Morey AF. Management of urethral strictures. Lancet. 2006;367(9520):1379–80.

102. Pain JA, Collier DG. Factors influencing recurrence of urethral strictures after endoscopic urethrotomy: the role of infection and peri-operative antibiotics. Br J Urol. 1984;56(2):217–9.

103. Fowler Jr FJ, Barry MJ, Lu-Yao G, Roman A, Wasson J, Wennberg JE. Patient-reported complications and follow-up treatment after radical prostatectomy. The National Medicare Experience: 1988-1990 (updated June 1993). Urology. 1993;42:622–9.

104. Hu JC, Gold KF, Pashos CL, Mehta SS, Litwin MS. Temporal trends in radical prostatectomy complications from 1991 to 1998. J Urol. 2003;169:1443–8.

105. Williams SB, Prasad SM, Weinberg AC, et al. Trends in the care of radical prostatectomy in the United States from 2003 to 2006. BJU Int. 2011;108:49–55.

106. Breyer BN, Davis CB, Cowan JE, Kane CJ, Carroll PR. Incidence of bladder neck contracture after robot-assisted laparoscopic and open radical prostatectomy. BJU Int. 2010;106:1734–8.

107. Merrick GS, Butler WM, Wallner KE. Risk factors for the development of prostate brachytherapy related urethral strictures. J Urol. 2006;175:1376–81.

108. Elliott SP, McAninch JW, Chi T, Doyle SM, Master VA. Management of severe urethral complications of prostate cancer therapy. J Urol. 2006;176:2508–13.

109. Elliott SP, Meng MV, Elkin EP, et al. Incidence of urethral stricture after primary treatment for prostate cancer: data from CaPSURE. J Urol. 2007;178:529–34.

110. Sullivan L, Williams SG, Tai KH, Foroudi F, Cleeve L, Duchesne GM. Urethral stricture following high dose rate brachytherapy for prostate cancer. Radiother Oncol. 2009;91:232–6.

111. Besarani D, Amoroso P, Kirby R. Bladder neck contracture after radical retropubic prostatectomy. BJU Int. 2004;94:1245–7.

112. Augustin H, Pummer K, Daghofer F, Habermann H, Primus G, Hubmer G. Patient self-reporting questionnaire on urological morbidity and bother after radical retropubic prostatectomy. Eur Urol. 2002;42:112–7.

113. Giannarini G, Manassero F, Mogorovich A, et al. Cold-knife incision of anastomotic strictures after radical retropubic prostatectomy with bladder neck preservation: efficacy and impact on urinary continence status. Eur Urol. 2008;54:647–56.

114. Anger JT, Raj GV, Delvecchio FC, Webster GD. Anastomotic contracture and incontinence after radical prostatectomy: a graded approach to management. J Urol. 2005;173:1143–6.

115. Borboroglu PG, Sands JP, Roberts JL, Amling CL. Risk factors for vesicourethral anastomotic stricture after radical prostatectomy. Urology. 2000;56:96–100.

116. Theodoros C, Katsifotis C, Stournaras P, Moutzouris G, Katsoulis A, Floratos D. Abdomino-perineal repair of recurrent and complex bladder neck-prostatic urethra contractures. Eur Urol. 2000;38:734–40; discusssion 40-1.

117. Simonato A, Gregori A, Lissiani A, Carmignani G. Two-stage transperineal management of posterior urethral strictures or bladder neck contractures associated with urinary incontinence after prostate surgery and endoscopic treatment failures. Eur Urol. 2007;52:1499–504.

118. Okeke LI, Takure AO, Adebayo SA, Oluyemi OY, Oyelekan AA. Urethral obstruction from dislodged bladder diverticulum stones: a case report. BMC Urol. 2012;12:31.

119. Appeadu-Mensah W, Hesse AA, Yaw MB. Giant bladder diverticulum: a rare cause of bladder outlet obstruction in children. Afr J Paediatr Surg. 2012;9:83–7.

120. Lang E, Cline K, Earhart V. Sliding ureterocele and bladder outlet obstruction. J Urol. 2005;173:601.

121. Krishnan A, de Souza A, Konijeti R, Baskin LS. The anatomy and embryology of posterior urethral valves. J Urol. 2006;175:1214–20.

122. Adorisio O, Bassani F, Silveri M. Cobb's collar: a rare cause of urinary retention. BMJ Case Rep. 2013.

123. Parsons BA, Evans S, Wright MP. Prostate cancer and urinary incontinence. Maturitas. 2009;63:323–8.

124. Fleischmann JD, Catalona WJ. Endocrine therapy for bladder outlet obstruction from carcinoma of the prostate. J Urol. 1985;134:498–500.

125. Mazur AW, Thompson IM. Efficacy and morbidity of "channel" TURP. Urology. 1991;38:526–8.

126. Crain DS, Amling CL, Kane CJ. Palliative transurethral prostate resection for bladder outlet obstruction in patients with locally advanced prostate cancer. J Urol. 2004;171:668–71.

127. Gnanapragasam VJ, Kumar V, Langton D, Pickard RS, Leung HY. Outcome of transurethral prostatectomy for the palliative management of lower urinary tract symptoms in men with prostate cancer. Int J Urol. 2006;13:711–5.

128. Kollmeier MA, Stock RG, Cesaretti J, Stone NN. Urinary morbidity and incontinence following transurethral resection of the prostate after brachytherapy. J Urol. 2005;173:808–12.

129. Fowler Jr FJ, Barry MJ, Lu-Yao G, Wasson JH, Bin L. Outcomes of external-beam radiation therapy for prostate cancer: a study of Medicare beneficiaries in three surveillance, epidemiology, and end results areas. J Clin Oncol. 1996;14:2258–65.

130. Crane C, Santucci RA. Surgical treatment of post-traumatic distraction posterior urethral strictures. Arch Esp Urol. 2011;64:219–26.

131. Colapinto V, McCallum RW. Injury to the male posterior urethra in fractured pelvis: a new classification. J Urol. 1977;118:575–80.

Thomas Renninson, Amit Mevcha, and Brian Andrew Parsons

Female voiding requires co-ordinated bladder contraction and outlet relaxation. Failure of the outlet to accommodate urine flow can occur in various circumstances in women. This chapter describes the diverse nature of the problem and its management, along with some of the limitations in the evidence base which make this a challenging clinical problem. Of these, one of the most important is the recognition that impairment of bladder contractility is common in older women [1] and this could cause overdiagnosis of bladder outlet obstruction (BOO). BOO may be asymptomatic, cause voiding LUTS, or complete obstruction resulting in inability to void (acute urinary retention—which is usually painful emergency). However, assessing the bladder contractility is difficult in women, and this hinders decision-making regarding diagnosis of BOO. Until the ability to agree definitions, and subsequently approaches to diagnosis, management of BOO in women will remain a clinical challenge.

T. Renninson, M.B.Ch.B.
Department of Medicine, Frenchay Hospital, Bristol, Avon, UK

A. Mevcha, M.B.B.S., M.R.C.S., F.R.C.S. (Urol.)
Department of Urology, Birmingham Heartlands Hospital, Birmingham, UK

B.A. Parsons, B.Sc., M.B.Ch.B., M.R.C.S. (✉)
Department of Urology, Cheltenham General Hospital, Cheltenham, Gloucestershire GL53 7AN, UK
e-mail: brianaparsons@hotmail.com

Retention in women results from a diverse set of conditions, which makes research into its epidemiology difficult. Most studies are small case series, or case reports with unusual causes. Part of the difficulty in estimating prevalence rates of obstruction relates to the fact that unlike for men, there are no universally accepted or standardised criteria for diagnosing the condition in women. Voiding symptoms have been shown to have a poor predictive value for diagnosing female voiding dysfunction, rarely exist in isolation and often occur in association with storage-related symptoms [2–4]. The true prevalence of BOO in women is unknown, but estimates from large retrospective studies range from 3 to 8 % [3–6]. A Scandinavian study revealed an incidence of AUR in women of seven per 100,000 population per year [7].

Defining Urinary Obstruction

BOO can be diagnosed on the basis of urodynamic studies, as in men (see Chap. 4). BOO has been defined as detrusor pressure of 60 cm of water (cm H_2O) or more, with a peak urine flow rate of less than 15 mL/s, though this was derived from measurements in a small number of women [8]. Another study derived criteria from evaluation of the videourodynamic studies of 261 women for non-neurogenic voiding function and defined BOO as radiographic evidence of obstruction between the bladder neck and the distal urethra in the presence of a sustained detrusor contraction of any magnitude, with reduced flow rate or delayed onset of flow [9].

Blaivas and Groutz derived a nomogram from information derived from 50 women, who were thought to be obstructed on clinical grounds [10]. Their study defined BOO by presence of maximum free flow rate (Q_{max}) of up to 12 mL/s in repeated free flow studies, combined with a sustained detrusor contraction and detrusor pressure at maximum flow ($P_{det}Q_{max}$) of at least 20 cm H_2O in a pressure flow study. Their nomogram used information from two separate voids—the Q_{max} from a free flow and the $P_{det}Q_{max}$ measured during voiding cystometry. This nomogram categorises into obstructed and non-obstructed and attempts to quantify into mild, moderate or severe BOO.

Chassange et al. compared women with anatomical outlet obstruction versus women with stress urinary incontinence (SUI) [11], defining BOO on Q_{max} 15 mL/s or less and $P_{det}Q_{max}$ of 20 cm H_2O or more. The criteria were subsequently revised [12, 13], and Q_{max} of up to 12 mL/s with a $P_{det}Q_{max}$ in excess of 25 cm H_2O may achieve the highest sensitivity and specificity for BOO in women [12].

When all the above parameters were compared in the same group of women, there were clear discrepancies between the classifications for the individual patients [14]. BOO was diagnosed with at least one diagnostic approach in 40 of the 91 study population; nine were obstructed on all the criteria, while a different nine fulfilled only one criterion.

One approach to assessing contractility is the 'stop-test', in which the urinary stream is interrupted during voiding. This normally should result in a significant rise in isovolumetric detrusor pressure ($P_{det.iso}$) during the flow interruption [15]. The test has practical problems, including the need to refill the bladder in order to assess BOO. Since there are no agreed criteria, stop tests are not commonly done.

Incomplete bladder emptying signifies the presence of a post-void residual (PVR), and it may be another manifestation of voiding dysfunction. In isolation a PVR is of limited diagnostic benefit as post-void residuals may develop as a result of either detrusor underactiv-

ity or BOO. Many women are found to have an asymptomatic PVR. While data from published studies appear to support the use of 100 mL as being a clinically significant cut-point [4], professional consensus on significant PVR has not been achieved.

Causes and Management of Female BOO

The basis of obstruction may be urethral compression, bladder neck distortion or luminal occlusion [16] and functional issues. Rarely, urinary retention might be labelled 'psychogenic' [17], but this should be used with considerable caution. CNS inflammation (sacral herpes, meningitis) [18], uterine fibroid [19], cytomegalovirus [20] and eosinophilic cystitis [21] have been described in case reports. Pelvic organ prolapse is an important consideration, as distortion of the urethra can cause partial BOO when anterior vaginal descent affects the bladder base. Table 5.1 lists recognised and rare causes of BOO in women [22].

The evaluation of women with voiding dysfunction should start with a thorough medical and surgical history to try and identify inciting events. Assessment will include an evaluation of the patient's symptoms using standardised measurements of LUTS such as the International Consultation on Incontinence Questionnaires [23] and a completed bladder diary/frequency volume chart. This information, though informative, is rarely diagnostic on its own. Instead, it helps plan further investigation and is useful in evaluating the response to any intervention. Examination of the patient needs to include an abdominal, bimanual pelvic, speculum vaginal and neurological examination. Focus should be on the examination of the pelvic organs to exclude pelvic masses and identify any evidence of prolapse. A pelvic ultrasound should be considered, especially if examination findings are inconclusive. Women complaining of difficulty in micturition should be investigated with a free flow rate and post-void residual. If abnormal, filling cystometry with a pressure flow study will help exclude detrusor underactivity as the cause. Videourodynamics will provide more information about

Table 5.1 Causes of urinary retention and bladder outlet obstruction (from [22])

Anatomical	
Extrinsic	Pelvic organ prolapse
	Gynaecological, e.g. uterine fibroid, tumour
	Poorly fitting pessary
	Post anti-incontinence procedure
Urethral	Stricture
	Meatal stenosis
	Thrombosed urethral caruncle
	Diverticulum
	Skene's gland cyst or abscess
Luminal	Stone
	Bladder/urethral tumour
	Ureterocoele
	Foreign body
Impaired detrusor contractility	Senile bladder change
	Diabetes mellitus
	Neurological disease (lower motor neurone lesions)
Functional	
Impaired co-ordination	Primary bladder neck obstruction
	Fowler's syndrome
	Pseudo-dyssynergia
	Detrusor-external sphincter dyssynergia
	Neurological disease (upper motor neurone lesions)
Peri-operative	Pain
	Analgesia or anaesthetic, e.g. epidural
Infective/inflammatory	UTI
	Acute vulvovaginitis
	Vaginal lichen planus/sclerosis
	Genital herpes
Pharmacological	Opiates
	Antipsychotics
	Antidepressants
	Antimuscarinics
	α-adrenergic agonist

the level of obstruction and the presence of urethral compression or hyperangulation due to an alteration in the relation between the bladder neck and the urethral axis. Cystoscopy can be used to assess compression and erosion of the urethra, bladder neck or bladder and will identify intraluminal bodies such as stones or tumours. Pelvic MRI provides detail of urethral anatomy and is able to identify both external compression and intrinsic pathology.

In the emergency context of AUR, expeditious catheterisation is needed to achieve bladder decompression and relieve pain. Intermittent catheterisation can be initiated, which has the advantage of gauging PVR over the following few days, and hence evaluating whether voiding is recovering [24, 25]. Reversible causes should be identified, such as severe prolapse. If urinary tract infection is present, it should be treated with appropriate antimicrobial therapy, though it should not be presumed as the causative basis without comprehensive evaluation, since it could be an incidental or unrelated issue. Presentation of previously unidentified neurological disease should be considered. Selective use of imaging and endoscopy may be informative.

If BOO is diagnosed, clinicians often recommend urethral dilatation but the rationale is not robust [26, 27]. Bladder neck incision (BNI) has been advocated [28–30], but the clinician should be extremely alert to the possibility of causing SUI. α-adrenergic antagonists may lower the resting urethral pressure [31], but do not improve outcome of trial without catheter in women [32].

BOO in Urinary Incontinence Surgery

Partial urinary retention can arise after SUI surgery, precipitated by anaesthesia, the procedure, discomfort, analgesia or haematoma formation; the mechanisms are likely to be BOO, or temporary impairment of bladder contractility and voiding reflexes. Crucially, a midurethral tape or colposuspension can cause outlet compression of distortion, leading to iatrogenic anatomical BOO (a case is illustrated in Fig. 9.4 in the chapter on Urodynamics). In colposuspension, placement of sutures close to the urethra can lead to compression or distortion [33], which was particularly evident with the Marshall-Marchetti-Krantz procedure [34]. Secondary bladder over distention injury could greatly delay recovery, so early use of catheterisation is needed as soon as it is clear that spontaneous voiding is failing to recover. Temporary intermittent catheterisation is sufficient in the majority.

A few women proceed to tape sectioning [35], but the physician responsible for the patient's care must take every step to ensure rational management; it is not appropriate simply to cut the tape in all women having difficulty recovering voiding, since there are several reversible causes of post-operative retention as listed above. Pelvic examination should identify whether the midurethral tape is overtight; it is only in this scenario that tape incision should restore voiding. Patients have to be evaluated on an individual basis, and where tape sectioning is considered appropriate, it should be undertaken in a timely manner [36]. Return of incontinence following tape sectioning is seen in a substantial proportion [37].

A compressing autologous sling can be placed with the deliberate intention of urethral compression as management of intrinsic sphincter deficiency, provided the woman has received prior training in intermittent catheterisation. This method must not be used with a midurethral tape, due to the risk of urethral erosion with overtight tapes [38].

BOO can also arise after injection of a periurethral bulking agent. This may be a short-term effect that should wear off after a couple of days. Occasionally, and generally after several treatments or administration of large volumes of injectant, patients can have symptoms which persist [39]. Diagnosis is made mainly on the history of the onset of symptoms and can be confirmed on cystoscopy. Treatment of persistent obstruction involves removal of some of the bulking material by means of a transurethral resection [40].

Fowler's Syndrome

Fowler's syndrome affects young adult women without neurological disease and is manifest as painless retention at high bladder volumes, often following an apparently unconnected precipitating event [41]. The urethral sphincter is found to be hypertrophic and overactive, as catheterisation causes spasms, and maximum urethral closure pressure may be very high. This can make intermittent catheterisation unbearable. Urethral hypertrophy can be identified with radiological imaging. A urethral sphincter EMG is diagnostic.

Management of Fowler's syndrome is specialised, comprising psychological support, reduction of medication use (especially opiates), intermittent catheterisation where possible and sacral nerve stimulation [42]. Reconstructive surgery using a continent diversion (Mitrofanoff procedure) may be necessary, so that intermittent catheterisation can be done through a non-urethral route.

Pelvic Organ Prolapse

POP is increasingly recognised as a contributing factor in the voiding dysfunction of many women. It may be the underlying aetiology of BOO in a large proportion [3]. In keeping with this, high-grade pelvic prolapse has been shown to correlate with PVR volumes of urine [43]. Using urodynamic criteria, Romanzi and colleagues prospectively evaluated 60 women with genital prolapse and diagnosed BOO in 58 % of women with high-grade anterior compartment prolapse compared with only 4 % of patients with low-grade prolapse [44]. POP may be managed conservatively with vaginal pessary placement, but severe prolapse is best managed by surgical correction. If surgery is to be undertaken, then urodynamic assessment should be considered to assess for the presence of occult SUI.

Gynaecological Masses

Pelvic masses are an uncommon cause of BOO and urinary retention. When very large, benign masses such as fibroids and pregnancy can lead to BOO by causing impaction of the enlarged uterus [45, 46]. Cervical cancer is the gynaecological malignancy most commonly associated with lower urinary tract obstruction, but vulvar carcinoma [47] and ovarian malignancy [48, 49] have been described in the literature as a cause of BOO. In addition to a full examination (including a bimanual pelvic exam), ultrasonography is indicated for the initial investigation of large pelvic masses and for the assessment of pregnant women. CT and MRI are able to yield greater detail of the relevant anatomy and the anatomical relationships of the mass. Urodynamic investigation may provide functional information. Treatment is often surgical and depends on the type of mass, its position and the patient's fitness for intervention.

Urethral Strictures

Most urethral strictures in women are iatrogenic in origin; they can occur from any previous urethral or paraurethral surgery. Other causes include recurrent infections, trauma or a congenital abnormality [50]. Urethral strictures most commonly occur in the distal urethra or at the urethral meatus. The mainstay of diagnosis is cystoscopy but strictures can be diagnosed by seeing characteristic changes on videourodynamics or on MRI [51]. Treatment is normally surgical, but there may be a role for urethral dilatation. However, evidence has shown that there is a significant recurrence rate from dilating urethral strictures and so urethral dilatation should no longer be routine [52]. Surgical treatment is cystoscopic urethrotomy making incisions at the 6 o'clock or two incisions at the 5 and 7 o'clock positions. Any patient undergoing a meatotomy or urethrotomy should be monitored post procedure as there is still significant risk of recurrence due to fibrosis [52]. More definitive specialist intervention can include reconstructive urethroplasty procedures which allow for the repair of recurrent strictures or strictures of greater length [50, 53, 54].

Luminal Obstruction

Luminal obstructions can be roughly divided into loose bodies and tumours. Loose bodies can be diagnosed and removed cystoscopically. Tumours need further investigation to define their extension outside of the lumen of the urethra. Polyps or pedunculated tumours can be removed using a cystoscope; however, larger or invasive tumours may require partial or complete urethrectomy.

References

1. Abarbanel J, Marcus EL. Impaired detrusor contractility in community-dwelling elderly presenting with lower urinary tract symptoms. Urology. 2007;69:436–40.

2. Lowenstein L, Anderson C, Kenton K, Dooley Y, Brubaker L. Obstructive voiding symptoms are not predictive of elevated postvoid residual urine volumes. Int Urogynecol J Pelvic Floor Dysfunct. 2008;19:801–4.

3. Groutz A, Blaivas JG, Chaikin DC. Bladder outlet obstruction in women: definition and characteristics. Neurourol Urodyn. 2000;19:213–20.

4. Robinson D, Staskin D, Laterza RM, Koebl H. Defining female voiding dysfunction: ICI-RS 2011. Neurourol Urodyn. 2012;31:313–6.

5. Rees DL, Whitfield HN, Islam AK, Doyle PT, Mayo ME, Wickham JE. Urodynamic findings in adult females with frequency and dysuria. Br J Urol. 1975;47:853–60.

6. Carr LK, Webster GD. Bladder outlet obstruction in women. Urol Clin North Am. 1996;23:385–91.

7. Klarskov P, Andersen JT, Asmussen CF, et al. Acute urinary retention in women: a prospective study of 18 consecutive cases. Scand J Urol Nephrol. 1987;21:29–31.

8. Diokno AC, Hollander JB, Bennett CJ. Bladder neck obstruction in women: a real entity. J Urol. 1984;132: 294–8.

9. Nitti VW, Tu LM, Gitlin J. Diagnosing bladder outlet obstruction in women. J Urol. 1999;161:1535–40.

10. Blaivas JG, Groutz A. Bladder outlet obstruction nomogram for women with lower urinary tract symptomatology. Neurourol Urodyn. 2000;19:553–64.

11. Chassagne S, Bernier PA, Haab F, Roehrborn CG, Reisch JS, Zimmern PE. Proposed cutoff values to define bladder outlet obstruction in women. Urology. 1998;51:408–11.

12. Defreitas GA, Zimmern PE, Lemack GE, Shariat SF. Refining diagnosis of anatomic female bladder outlet obstruction: comparison of pressure-flow study parameters in clinically obstructed women with those of normal controls. Urology. 2004;64:675–9; discussion 9–81.

13. Lemack GE, Zimmern PE. Pressure flow analysis may aid in identifying women with outflow obstruction. J Urol. 2000;163:1823–8.

14. Akikwala TV, Fleischman N, Nitti VW. Comparison of diagnostic criteria for female bladder outlet obstruction. J Urol. 2006;176:2093–7.

15. Tan TL, Bergmann MA, Griffiths D, Resnick NM. Which stop test is best? Measuring detrusor contractility in older females. J Urol. 2003;169:1023–7.

16. Goldman HB, Zimmern PE. The treatment of female bladder outlet obstruction. BJU Int. 2006;98 Suppl 1:17–23; discussion 4–6.

17. Sakakibara R, Uchiyama T, Awa Y, et al. Psychogenic urinary dysfunction: a uro-neurological assessment. Neurourol Urodyn. 2007;26:518–24.

18. Sakakibara R, Yamanishi T, Uchiyama T, Hattori T. Acute urinary retention due to benign inflammatory nervous diseases. J Neurol. 2006;253:1103–10.

19. Novi JM, Shaunik A, Mulvihill BH, Morgan MA. Acute urinary retention caused by a uterine leiomyoma: a case report. J Reprod Med. 2004;49:131–2.

20. Shih SL, Liu YP, Tsai JD, Tsai YS, Yang FS, Chen YF. Acute urinary retention in a 7-year-old girl: an unusual complication of cytomegalovirus cystitis. J Pediatr Surg. 2008;43:e37–9.

21. van den Ouden D, van Kaam N, Eland D. Eosinophilic cystitis presenting as urinary retention. Urol Int. 2001; 66:22–6.

22. Mevcha A, Drake MJ. Etiology and management of urinary retention in women. Indian J Urol. 2010; 26:230–5.

23. Abrams P, Avery K, Gardener N, Donovan J. The international consultation on incontinence modular questionnaire: www.iciq.net. J Urol. 2006;175:1063–6.

24. Patel MI, Watts W, Grant A. The optimal form of urinary drainage after acute retention of urine. BJU Int. 2001;88:26–9.

25. Smith NK, Morrant JD. Post-operative urinary retention in women: management by intermittent catheterization. Age Ageing. 1990;19:337–40.

26. Ramsey S, Palmer M. The management of female urinary retention. Int Urol Nephrol. 2006;38:533–5.

27. Wheeler Jr JS, Culkin DJ, Walter JS, Flanigan RC. Female urinary retention. Urology. 1990;35:428–32.

28. Blaivas JG, Flisser AJ, Tash JA. Treatment of primary bladder neck obstruction in women with transurethral resection of the bladder neck. J Urol. 2004;171: 1172–5.

29. Kumar A, Mandhani A, Gogoi S, Srivastava A. Management of functional bladder neck obstruction in women: use of alpha-blockers and pediatric resectoscope for bladder neck incision. J Urol. 1999;162: 2061–5.

30. Peng CH, Kuo HC. Transurethral incision of bladder neck in treatment of bladder neck obstruction in women. Urology. 2005;65:275–8.

31. Reitz A, Haferkamp A, Kyburz T, Knapp PA, Wefer B, Schurch B. The effect of tamsulosin on the resting tone and the contractile behaviour of the female urethra: a functional urodynamic study in healthy women. Eur Urol. 2004;46:235–40; discussion 40.

32. Hershkovitz A, Manevitz D, Beloosesky Y, Gillon G, Brill S. Medical treatment for urinary retention in rehabilitating elderly women: is it necessary? Aging Clin Exp Res. 2003;15:19–24.

33. Takacs P, Candiotti K, Medina CA. Effect of suture type on postoperative urinary retention following Burch colposuspension. Int J Gynaecol Obstet. 2008;100:193–4.

34. Zimmern PE, Hadley HR, Leach GE, Raz S. Female urethral obstruction after Marshall-Marchetti-Krantz operation. J Urol. 1987;138:517–20.

35. Hong B, Park S, Kim HS, Choo MS. Factors predictive of urinary retention after a tension-free vaginal

tape procedure for female stress urinary incontinence. J Urol. 2003;170:852–6.

36. Leng WW, Davies BJ, Tarin T, Sweeney DD, Chancellor MB. Delayed treatment of bladder outlet obstruction after sling surgery: association with irreversible bladder dysfunction. J Urol. 2004;172:1379–81.

37. Segal J, Steele A, Vassallo B, et al. Various surgical approaches to treat voiding dysfunction following anti-incontinence surgery. Int Urogynecol J Pelvic Floor Dysfunct. 2006;17:372–7.

38. Jones R, Abrams P, Hilton P, Ward K, Drake M. Risk of tape-related complications after TVT is at least 4%. Neurourol Urodyn. 2010;29:40–1.

39. Bernier PA, Zimmern PE, Saboorian MH, Chassagne S. Female outlet obstruction after repeated collagen injections. Urology. 1997;50:618–21.

40. Goldman HB, Zimmern PE. The treatment of female bladder outlet obstruction. BJU Int. 2006;98:359–66.

41. Fowler CJ, Kirby RS. Abnormal electromyographic activity (decelerating burst and complex repetitive discharges) in the striated muscle of the urethral sphincter in 5 women with persisting urinary retention. Br J Urol. 1985;57:67–70.

42. Datta SN, Chaliha C, Singh A, et al. Sacral neurostimulation for urinary retention: 10-year experience from one UK centre. BJU Int. 2008;101:192–6.

43. Gardy M, Kozminski M, DeLancey J, Elkins T, McGuire EJ. Stress incontinence and cystoceles. J Urol. 1991;145:1211–3.

44. Romanzi LJ, Chaikin DC, Blaivas JG. The effect of genital prolapse on voiding. J Urol. 1999;161:581–6.

45. Kondo A, Otani T, Takita T, Hayashi H, Kihira M, Itoh F. Urinary retention caused by impaction of enlarged uterus. Urol Int. 1982;37:87–90.

46. Silva PD, Berberich W. Retroverted impacted gravid uterus with acute urinary retention: report of two cases and a review of the literature. Obstet Gynecol. 1986;68:121–3.

47. Romero Perez P. Urinary retention caused by vulvar carcinoma. Actas Urol Esp. 1995;19:67–9.

48. Nishimoto N, Kajikawa J, Miyoshi S, Iwao N, Mizutani S, Okuyama A. Urinary retention secondary to ovarian dysgerminoma in a girl. Urology. 1985; 26:71–3.

49. Geisler JP, Perry RW, Ayres GM, Holland 3rd TF, Melton ME, Geisler HE. Ovarian cancer causing upper and lower urinary tract obstruction. Eur J Gynaecol Oncol. 1994;15:343–4.

50. Montorsi F, Salonia A, Centemero A, et al. Vestibular flap urethroplasty for strictures of the female urethra. Impact on symptoms and flow patterns. Urol Int. 2002;69:12–6.

51. Lorenzo AJ, Zimmern P, Lemack GE, Nurenberg P. Endorectal coil magnetic resonance imaging for diagnosis of urethral and periurethral pathologic findings in women. Urology. 2003;61:1129–33; discussion 33–4.

52. McCrery RJ, Appell RA. Bladder outlet obstruction in women: iatrogenic, anatomic, and neurogenic. Curr Urol Rep. 2006;7:363–9.

53. Schwender CE, Ng L, McGuire E, Gormley EA. Technique and results of urethroplasty for female stricture disease. J Urol. 2006;175:976–80; discussion 80.

54. Tanello M, Frego E, Simeone C, Cosciani Cunico S. Use of pedicle flap from the labia minora for the repair of female urethral strictures. Urol Int. 2002; 69:95–8.

Bladder Pain Syndrome

6

Marcus J. Drake

Bladder pain syndrome (BPS) is a clinical diagnosis characterised by pain in the bladder or pelvis, along with other urinary symptoms such as urgency or frequency. It overlaps with other chronic pain syndromes, such as irritable bowel syndrome, fibromyalgia and chronic fatigue syndrome. According to the European Society for the Study of Bladder Pain Syndrome (ESSIC), symptoms should have been present for at least 6 months, with sensations of pain, pressure or discomfort perceived by the patient in relation to the bladder [1]. Interstitial cystitis is a widely used term often employed interchangeably with BPS. Various organisations have put forward diagnostic parameters in addition to those of ESSIC, for example the NIDDK, in which diagnosis requires pain associated with bladder or urinary urgency, with characteristic endoscopic appearances (Hunner's ulcer or characteristic glomerulations), in patients with 9 or more months symptoms and at least eight voids per day and reduced bladder capacity (350 mL) [2]. The East Asian Guideline alludes to the fact that many patients with this type of problem do not report pain, but rather increased sensitivity [3].

The International Continence Society categorises according to location of pain [4]:

- Painful bladder syndrome is the complaint of suprapubic pain related to bladder filling, accompanied by other symptoms such as increased daytime and night-time frequency, in the absence of proven urinary infection or other obvious pathology. This term was felt to be preferable for symptom-based diagnosis to interstitial cystitis.
- Urethral pain syndrome is the occurrence of recurrent episodic urethral pain usually on voiding, with daytime frequency and nocturia, in the absence of proven infection or other obvious pathology.
- Pelvic pain syndrome is the occurrence of persistent or recurrent episodic pelvic pain associated with symptoms suggestive of lower urinary tract, sexual, bowel or gynaecological dysfunction. There is no proven infection or other obvious pathology.

Genito-urinary pain syndromes are all chronic in their nature. Pain is the major complaint but concomitant complaints are of lower urinary tract, bowel, sexual or gynaecological nature. Overall, people affected describe extremely bothersome symptoms which can be disabling for quality of life and ability to carry on daily activities. Underlying mechanisms are probably varied, explaining the difficulties achieving a universally agreed diagnosis and reliable response to treatment [5].

Epidemiology

Epidemiological studies are hampered by the difficulty achieving an agreed definition and hence diagnosis [6]. The Fifth International Consultation

6

M.J. Drake, M.A. (Cantab),
D.M. (Oxon.), F.R.C.S. (Urol.) (✉)
University of Bristol and Bristol Urological Institute,
Bristol, UK
e-mail: marcus.drake@bui.ac.uk

on Incontinence felt that it is not possible to determine an accurate estimate of the prevalence of BPS [7]. Studies done in the USA using symptom surveys suggested a high prevalence, with several million young women affected [8], while in Japan the prevalence was estimated at only 4.5 per 100,000 women [9]. This considerable range means care has to be taken interpreting the literature.

Aetiology

The Fifth International Consultation on Incontinence [7] summarised the progressive nature of aetiology, perhaps initiated by a bladder 'insult' such as cystitis, neurogenic inflammation, trauma, over distension or autoimmunity. This might then lead to impaired urothelial function causing a perpetuation of the problem and enabling urine constituents into the bladder wall. This might then set off the activation of sensory nerves, mast cells and allergic responses, giving rise to progressive bladder injury.

The urothelium has a critical role in excluding the toxic content of urine from the tissues of the bladder wall. There are numerous toxins, in particular potassium, in high concentration in the urine. The urothelium confines them to the lumen of the bladder due to the watertight nature of the cellular junctions on the luminal layers. This is supplemented by a glycosaminoglycan (GAG) layer. The GAG layer and the urothelial junctions appeared to be disrupted in people with BPS [10]. Basic science studies indicate that the potassium is a strong stimulant for both sensory nerve and muscle function. Accordingly, the potassium sensitivity test was developed to attempt to diagnose BPS, based on an overreaction to a standardised exposure to potassium [11]. While not widely employed in current practice, this is an interesting observation for understanding the condition.

Various inflammatory processes are contributory in BPS [12], and this will directly stimulate afferent nerves. The altered cytokine milieu resulting from inflammation is likely to be a factor in sensitisation of sensory nerves [13]. An important example is the activation or proliferation of mast cells leading to release of mediators such as histamine, which can be exacerbated by stress [14]. Sensory nerves from the bladder can show increased influence when they are sensitised, which can be a consequence of inflammation in other pelvic organs, particularly the large intestine [15].

No infectious organism has consistently been identified in BPS patients, even with techniques of greater sensitivity than standard urine culture [16]. However, the nature of the bladder wall alterations leads some investigators to speculate an infectious basis either for triggering or maintaining BPS. Nanobacteria have been proposed to be a factor [17].

An autoimmune process has not been ruled out, autoantibodies having been identified in various patients [18, 19]. Findings have not been consistent, but the possibility of a subgroup of BPS patients with this mechanism has to be considered.

Diagnosis

A stepwise approach is needed to evaluation, ascertaining the key aspects of the condition and excluding other diagnoses, particularly endometriosis, carcinoma in situ and urolithiasis. A separate condition which has to be considered is ketamine cystitis, caused by ingestion of ketamine as a drug of abuse [20].

1. In the clinical history, key features include the location and nature of the areas of pain and relationship to bladder filling or emptying. Relevant factors also include previous pelvic operations, urinary tract infection, urological diseases, radiation and autoimmune disease.
2. Physical examination should include any potential neurological problems. Areas of pain should be mapped by physical examination, including bimanual pelvic examination.
3. Urinalysis and screening for sexually transmitted disease should be considered. Cytology might be appropriate in certain risk groups.
4. Frequency volume charts are helpful in identifying increased daytime frequency and small voided volumes.

Fig. 6.1 Cystoscopy view of bladder after distension in a woman with bladder pain syndrome, showing small petechial 'glomerular' haemorrhages

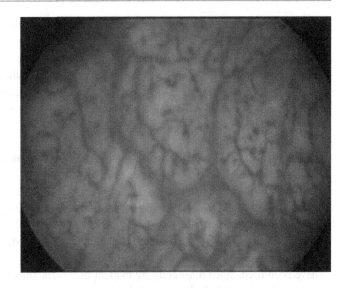

5. A symptom score should be considered. The most widely used is the O'Leary-Sant Symptom Score [21]. Pain can also be documented with a visual analogue scale.
6. Endoscopic examination under general anaesthetic can reveal two classic appearances. The first is Hunner's ulcer, in which a mild urothelial defect splits open during distension and becomes oedematous and bloody following distension. The second appearance is that of multifocal 'glomerulations', which are small bleeding points seen throughout the bladder wall (Fig. 6.1) and giving rise to bloodiness of the urine after distension. Bladder capacity is impaired. Increased autonomic reaction might be reported by the anaesthetist.
7. Biopsies might be taken, which can show denudation of the urothelium and increased mast cell numbers.
8. Other tests can be considered but are not generally undertaken as part of initial assessment. Urodynamics does not have a clear diagnostic contribution, but some aspects have been proposed to help evaluate diagnosis and prognosis [22]. Biomarkers are under investigation; while none is yet established, antiproliferative factor is showing some promise [23].

The UPOINT system is a pragmatic phenotyping scheme, which scores according to key features of urinary, psychosocial, organ specific, infection, neurological/systemic and tenderness [24]. This offers a systematic approach, which can aid diagnosis and help steer therapy appropriately.

Treatment

The area is a highly specialised one with the need for a multidisciplinary approach and access to relevant specialists such as pain experts. Support for the patient is essential for successful outcome, including easy access to information, nurse specialists and counselling. Alongside the disparate nature of pathophysiology underlying BPS, the secondary mechanisms causing pain perpetuation and dissemination, and the psychological factors, make this a difficult area. The range of treatments tried testifies to the difficult nature of the clinical problem. Indeed, placebo responses can be considerable in some of these studies. Thus, research into the area needs to be extremely well designed and has to recognise the importance of patient selection.

- *Conservative treatment.* This includes behavioural modification, physical therapy, change in diet and stress reduction. Physiotherapy aims to improve any contributory pain issues resulting from muscle spasm. Stress reduction aims to improve psychological coping mechanisms for stress, since the latter can exacerbate pain and other related symptoms. Dietary manipulation recommends avoidance of trigger substances such as acidic drinks, spices, alcohol and caffeine.

- *Oral medications.* Analgesics have to be considered. Conventional analgesics have a limited role. Gabapentin has been used to try to alter the central spinal mechanisms in handling pain. Pregabalin has also been used. Opioids have to be used if lower-level analgesics are unsuccessful. Specialist pain management should be consulted to optimise the regime and minimise potential complication. Amitriptyline is sometimes used, as it is considered beneficial in some chronic pain situations. Antihistamines have been used, since mast cells are evident in many patients with BPS. Deficient GAG layers, seen in some patients, have led to oral therapy using sodium pentosan polysulphate. It is taken three times daily and limited evidence does suggest that some patients benefit. Immuno-suppression has been tried, but in the absence of clear markers of autoimmune disease, it remains to be seen whether this is safely applicable in the general patient. Some studies have also looked at other agents such as nitric oxide donors or antibiotics.
- *Bladder instillation.* Direct instillation into the bladder through a short-term catheter is widely employed. Artificial GAG substitutes are commonly used. These include hyaluronic acid and chondroitin sulphate. Some studies have used heparin for the same reason. Historically, DMSO, a solvent agent, has been instilled into the bladder and sometimes centres still occasionally use it. Other agents have also been instilled into the bladder, such as vanilloids and BCG; however, these are felt to have significant side effects or potential serious complications and are not recommended by the International Consultation on Incontinence [7]. Botulinum A neurotoxin injections into the bladder have been used; the potential for botulinum to cause urinary retention is a significant concern since intermittent catheterisation in these patients is rarely well tolerated. Efficacy has been reported in some small studies, but caution must be employed before considering such therapy.

- *Neuromodulation.* Sacral nerve stimulation has been employed in some of these patients, with anecdotal evidence and small-scale studies giving support. General use is limited and it remains to be seen whether long-term efficacy can be anticipated.

Surgical Intervention

- *Bladder distension*: Based on the importance of sensory nerves in contributing to sensation of pain, attempts to 'denervate' the bladder and reduce stimulus transduction into the sensory nerve activity have been made. One such is bladder distension, stretching the bladder under general anaesthetic to high volume and pressure. Such attempts have produced anecdotal improvement in some patients but carry significant risk of severe complication such as bladder rupture. The evidence base is limited and long-term efficacy is uncertain.
- Transurethral resection aims to remove any ulcerated area in the hope that regrowth of urothelium would allow normal urothelium to replace the denuded area. Some patients have perceived significant improvement, specifically those with a Hunner's ulcer [25].
- Denervation techniques using various approaches to affect the sensory nerves (probably with consequent influence on motor nerves as well) have been described, but none is currently accepted as usefully or safely applicable.
- *Cystectomy and reconstruction.* Using bowel segments to augment or replace parts of the bladder has been used for many years. Cystoplasty with supratrigonal resection can be employed in selected patients with end-stage severe BPS. Subtrigonal cystectomy with cystoplasty does not carry any clear advantages and probably has a higher complication rate according to the Internal Consultation on Incontinence [7]. Urinary diversion with cystectomy and/or urethrectomy is a considerable step to take, but some patients are so severely affected that they wish for this. Sometimes, the bladder can be left in place, since diversion of the urinary stream away from the organ affected can improve symptoms without the morbidity of cystectomy.

Nonetheless, patients with bladder preservation at the time of diversion sometimes proceed to cystectomy at a later stage because of ongoing pain, or complications such as pyocystis (a mucopurulent accumulation in the bladder lumen causing offensive discharge and discomfort).

References

1. van de Merwe JP, Nordling J, Bouchelouche P, Bouchelouche K, Cervigni M, Daha LK, et al. Diagnostic criteria, classification, and nomenclature for painful bladder syndrome/interstitial cystitis: an ESSIC proposal. Eur Urol. 2008;53(1):60–7.
2. Simon LJ, Landis JR, Erickson DR, Nyberg LM. The interstitial cystitis data base study: concepts and preliminary baseline descriptive statistics. Urology. 1997;49(5A Suppl):64–75.
3. Homma Y, Ueda T, Tomoe H, Lin AT, Kuo HC, Lee MH, et al. Clinical guidelines for interstitial cystitis and hypersensitive bladder syndrome. Int J Urol. 2009;16(7):597–615.
4. Abrams P, Cardozo L, Fall M, Griffiths D, Rosier P, Ulmsten U, et al. The standardisation of terminology of lower urinary tract function: report from the standardisation sub-committee of the international continence society. Neurourol Urodyn. 2002;21(2): 167–78.
5. Hanno P, Lin A, Nordling J, Nyberg L, van Ophoven A, Ueda T, et al. Bladder pain syndrome committee of the international consultation on incontinence. Neurourol Urodyn. 2010;29(1):191–8.
6. Berry SH, Bogart LM, Pham C, Liu K, Nyberg L, Stoto M, et al. Development, validation and testing of an epidemiological case definition of interstitial cystitis/painful bladder syndrome. J Urol. 2010;183(5): 1848–52.
7. Abrams P, Cardozo L, Khoury S, Wein A, editors. Incontinence: 5th international consultation on incontinence. Paris: European Association of Urology/International Consultation on Urological Diseases; 2013.
8. Parsons CL, Tatsis V. Prevalence of interstitial cystitis in young women. Urology. 2004;64(5):866–70.
9. Ito T, Miki M, Yamada T. Interstitial cystitis in Japan. BJU Int. 2000;86(6):634–7.
10. Hauser PJ, Dozmorov MG, Bane BL, Slobodov G, Culkin DJ, Hurst RE. Abnormal expression of differentiation related proteins and proteoglycan core proteins in the urothelium of patients with interstitial cystitis. J Urol. 2008;179(2):764–9.
11. Parsons CL, Zupkas P, Parsons JK. Intravesical potassium sensitivity in patients with interstitial cystitis and urethral syndrome. Urology. 2001;57(3): 428–32; discussion 432–3.
12. Grover S, Srivastava A, Lee R, Tewari AK, Te AE. Role of inflammation in bladder function and interstitial cystitis. Ther Adv Urol. 2011;3(1):19–33.
13. Birder LA, de Groat WC. Mechanisms of disease: involvement of the urothelium in bladder dysfunction. Nat Clin Pract Urol. 2007;4(1):46–54.
14. Spanos C, Pang X, Ligris K, Letourneau R, Alferes L, Alexacos N, et al. Stress-induced bladder mast cell activation: implications for interstitial cystitis. J Urol. 1997;157(2):669–72.
15. Ustinova EE, Fraser MO, Pezzone MA. Cross-talk and sensitization of bladder afferent nerves. Neurourol Urodyn. 2010;29(1):77–81.
16. Duncan JL, Schaeffer AJ. Do infectious agents cause interstitial cystitis? Urology. 1997;49(5A Suppl):48–51.
17. Zhang QH, Shen XC, Zhou ZS, Chen ZW, Lu GS, Song B. Decreased nanobacteria levels and symptoms of nanobacteria-associated interstitial cystitis/painful bladder syndrome after tetracycline treatment. Int Urogynecol J. 2010;21(1):103–9.
18. Anderson JB, Parivar F, Lee G, Wallington TB, MacIver AG, Bradbrook RA, et al. The enigma of interstitial cystitis—an autoimmune disease? Br J Urol. 1989;63(1):58–63.
19. Jokinen EJ, Alfthan OS, Oravisto KJ. Antitissue antibodies in interstitial cystitis. Clin Exp Immunol. 1972;11(3):333–9.
20. Middela S, Pearce I. Ketamine-induced vesicopathy: a literature review. Int J Clin Pract. 2011;65(1): 27–30.
21. O'Leary MP, Sant GR, Fowler Jr FJ, Whitmore KE, Spolarich-Kroll J. The interstitial cystitis symptom index and problem index. Urology. 1997;49(5A Suppl):58–63.
22. Kuo YC, Kuo HC. The urodynamic characteristics and prognostic factors of patients with interstitial cystitis/bladder pain syndrome. Int J Clin Pract. 2013; 67(9):863–9.
23. Keay S, Warren JW, Zhang CO, Tu LM, Gordon DA, Whitmore KE. Antiproliferative activity is present in bladder but not renal pelvic urine from interstitial cystitis patients. J Urol. 1999;162(4):1487–9.
24. Nickel JC, Shoskes D, Irvine-Bird K. Clinical phenotyping of women with interstitial cystitis/painful bladder syndrome: a key to classification and potentially improved management. J Urol. 2009;182(1):155–60.
25. Peeker R, Aldenborg F, Fall M. Complete transurethral resection of ulcers in classic interstitial cystitis. Int Urogynecol J Pelvic Floor Dysfunct. 2000; 11(5):290–5.

Jonathan Williams

Overactive Bladder

Definitions

The 2002 International Continence Society definitions of lower urinary tract function included key definitions of storage dysfunction symptoms [1]. Overactive bladder (OAB) is urgency, with or without urgency incontinence, usually with increased daytime frequency and nocturia. Diagnosing OAB assumes that conflicting problems, such as urinary tract infection, are excluded. It can be categorised into OAB wet (where there is associated urgency incontinence) and OAB dry (where there is no incontinence).

The key symptom of OAB is urgency. Urgency is the complaint of a sudden compelling desire to pass urine which is difficult to defer [2]. Increased daytime frequency is the complaint by the patient who feels he/she voids too often by day. Urgency incontinence is the complaint of involuntary leakage accompanied by or immediately preceded by urgency. OAB is a symptom-based diagnosis; it differs from detrusor overactivity (DO), which is a urodynamic diagnosis, comprising bladder contractions during the filling phase, which may be spontaneous or provoked. A retrospective study

in 2006 found only 64 % of patients with OAB symptoms have DO on urodynamic investigation; conversely 30 % of those with DO did not have OAB [3].

Aetiology

The mechanisms that underlie OAB and DO are not completely understood. The pathogenesis of OAB is multifactorial, differing for different individuals and altering over time in any one person [4]. Three main theories have been proposed.

- The neurogenic hypothesis of DO [5] deals with the changes in central nervous system (CNS) pathways, leading to imbalances that tend to increase bladder excitation, reduce inhibition and increase afferent input. Damage to central inhibitory pathways or sensitisation of peripheral afferent terminals in the bladder can unmask primitive voiding reflexes that trigger bladder overactivity.
- The myogenic hypothesis [6] suggests that partial denervation of the detrusor causes an alteration of the properties of the smooth muscle ('denervation supersensitivity'), leading to increased spontaneous excitability. In addition, propagation of excitation over abnormal large distances allows spread of spontaneous excitation to affect a greater proportion of the bladder. Alterations in the functional properties of detrusor myocytes is seen in DO [7].
- The peripheral autonomous (integrative) hypothesis [8] suggests that interactions

J. Williams, M.B.B.S., B.Sc. (✉)
Department of Urology, Southmead Hospital,
Southmead, Bristol BS10 5NB, UK
e-mail: jonwilliams1981@gmail.com

A.J. Wein et al. (eds.), *Bladder Dysfunction in the Adult: The Basis for Clinical Management*, Current
Clinical Urology, DOI 10.1007/978-1-4939-0853-0_7, © Springer Science+Business Media New York 2014

between various cell types in the bladder wall determine the organ's functional properties and that any change in the integration will alter function. Thus, properties of each major cell type (detrusor, urothelium, interstitial cells, neurons) and their intercommunications determine normal function and propensity to dysfunction.

- Altered sensory function; increased afferent activity may increase sensation and predispose to reflex dysfunction.

Key Considerations

The NOBLE study suggests around 16 % of adults aged 18 and over in North America suffer from OAB [9]. Prevalence is similar in men and women, although OAB dry is more common in men and OAB wet more common in women. Prevalence increases with age in both sexes [10]. Urgency with at least one other symptom is essential for the diagnosis of OAB [11]. OAB symptoms have been shown in numerous studies to have a significant negative impact on the health-related quality of life, emotional wellbeing and work productivity of affected individuals [12]. Urgency incontinence may be due to increased filling sensation or an involuntary detrusor contraction. Due to the short warning time before having to get to the toilet, urgency incontinence is associated with an increase in falls and fractures in the elderly population [13]. Frequency in those with DO may in part be a coping mechanism in order to suppress urgency.

Diagnosis

It is important to exclude urinary tract infection and pelvic malignancy as a cause. An abdominal and pelvic examination should be done to rule out any masses and also to evaluate prostatic enlargement or malignancy in male patients. Neurological examination should be done. A urine dipstick analysis is needed to rule out infection and look for blood or glucose, which may represent other underlying pathologies. Frequency volume charts [14] are a way of objectively evaluating frequency and nocturia [14]. In a bladder diary, the patient can also document other facets, such as fluid intake. There are also a number of validated symptoms tools (e.g. the International Consultation on Incontinence Questionnaires—ICIQ) to measure severity and bother of LUTS.

Invasive urodynamics is discussed in the relevant chapter.

Management

This is discussed in more detail in the relevant chapters. Most patients can be managed with conservative management or drug therapy, without the need for specialist involvement. The principles of treatment are to reduce urinary urgency so as to decrease the number of episodes of incontinence and improve urinary frequency, nocturia and voided volumes [15]. Behavioural and lifestyle techniques involve fluid intake advice, bladder training and timed voiding. Pelvic floor exercises can be used to suppress involuntary detrusor contractions [16].

The mainstay of treatment for OAB symptoms is antimuscarinic medications. Beta-3 adrenergic agonists have recently been introduced. Neuromodulation can be used in those whose quality of life is significantly impaired by their symptoms and does not respond to more conservative measures. Sacral, paraurethral, pudendal nerve and tibial nerve stimulation have been used [17]. Surgical interventions which have been seen to be beneficial in those with refractory OAB include intravesical botulinum toxin injection [18], bladder augmentation [19] and urinary diversion [20]; however, these procedures carry a significant risk of morbidity and not all patients with OAB will be suitable for surgery.

Bladder Underactivity

Definition

The International Continence Society (2002) definition of detrusor underactivity (DUA) is a contraction of reduced strength and/or duration resulting in prolonged bladder emptying and/or failure to achieve complete bladder emptying within a normal time span [2]. DUA is a urodynamic diagnosis based on pressure flow and characterised by low pressure, poorly sustained detrusor contraction in combination with poor urinary flow [21].

Aetio-pathophysiology

The cause of DUA is likely to be multifactorial. Although detrusor contractility diminishes with age, a minority develop clinically relevant DUA [28].

Patients with DUA may experience a greater decline in detrusor contractility than normal individuals. Studies have shown a decrease in the muscle to collagen ratio [22], widened spaces between muscle cells [23], age-related increases in circulating norepinephrine [24] and decrease in M3-muscarinic receptor density [25]. Changes to potassium and calcium channels may also contribute to DUA. Decreased bladder sensation, resulting from vesical afferent dysfunction, is commonly associated.

Activation of the micturition response is dependent on a normal transmission of sensory information from the bladder to higher brain centres. The micturition reflex is based on spinobulbo-spinal pathways, regulated by higher CNS centres. DUA may reflect changes to the afferent or efferent limb of the micturition reflex or a defect of integrative control.

Epidemiology

Data from urodynamic investigations suggest that DUA is associated with ageing [26]. Twenty-two percent of men and 11 % or women over 60 report difficulties with bladder emptying [27], although DUA will not be the only cause for this. Bladder outlet obstruction is a common cause for difficulty voiding in older men; offering prostate surgery to men whose underlying pathology is DUA will be of little benefit and can cause harm [21]. Precise epidemiological data on the prevalence of DUA is difficult to establish, due to the relatively low proportion of patients who undergo urodynamic investigation.

DUA is common in patients with neurogenic bladder dysfunction. This includes those with diabetes mellitus, multiple sclerosis, Parkinson's disease or cerebral stroke [28]. DUA can also be iatrogenic, caused by peripheral denervation during pelvic surgery, such as radical prostatectomy, colorectal surgery or hysterectomy [29].

Other risk factors include constipation, immobility and drugs. Antimuscarinic drugs, calcium channel blockers, neuroleptics and alpha blockers may be contributory. It has been suggested that recurrent urinary infections may also play a role; however, clinical data from humans is lacking [21].

Diagnosis

Symptoms include frequency, urgency, feeling of incomplete bladder emptying, recurrent urinary infections and incontinence. These cannot be distinguished from bladder outlet obstruction based on history alone. Urodynamic multichannel cystometry can be used (see relevant chapter). There are several urodynamic algorithms for quantifying detrusor pressure during voiding. Abram's bladder contractility index [30], Griffiths' Watt factor [31] and Shafer's detrusor adjusted mean PURR factor [32] have been suggested but have only been validated in male patients.

Bladder biopsies or ultrasound studies of the bladder during storage or voiding have been suggested as alternative methods for diagnosing DUA, but are not widely used.

Management

Due to the relatively poor understandings of the mechanisms leading to detrusor underactivity, treatments are limited. Treatment is aimed at increasing detrusor strength and sensation or decreasing bladder outlet resistance [21].

Intermittent self-catheterisation, in willing and physically capable individuals, is the most commonly used management option. Some drug classes have been trialled for use in patients with DUA. Muscarinic receptor agonists or cholinesterase inhibitors have been used; however, efficacy is uncertain and they have significant side effects [33].

Neurostimulation [34] and neuromodulation [35] have been used to treat DUA. More invasive bladder reconstructions involving latissimus dorsi muscle flaps have also been used [36], but have not become established.

Detrusor Storage Overactivity with Voiding Underactivity

Particularly in the elderly, both DO and DUA can coexist [37]—a situation originally termed detrusor hyperactivity with impaired contractility (DHIC) [38]. DHIC is an important urinary dysfunction in institutionalised elderly people [39]. DHIC may be a coincidental occurrence of two common conditions with different etiological factors [40]. Alternatively, it may represent a more advanced stage in the natural history of DO, signifying decompensation [38].

DHIC can contribute to urinary retention in the elderly [41]. This is due to diminished detrusor contractile function and is associated with bladder trabeculation, a slow velocity of bladder contraction, little detrusor reserve power and a significant amount of post-void residual urine [38]. It can mimic other causes of urinary incontinence and can be misdiagnosed as stress incontinence or urethral instability [42]. It can also mimic urethral obstruction in men presenting with urgency, poor flow rate, elevated residual urine and bladder trabeculation [43].

Behavioural therapy can be used to manage DHIC. Bladder training regimes can extend the time between voids [44]. For those who are cognitively impaired, 'prompted voiding' can be used [45], where the patient is encouraged to void at regular intervals.

Anticholinergic medication can be used cautiously and can reduce the occurrence of urgency in those with DHIC [46]. Urinary retention may occur and post-void residuals and urine output should be measured. Subclinical urinary retention can develop, reducing functional bladder capacity and attenuating or reversing the drug benefit. If symptoms worsen and anticholinergic

dose is increased, post-void residual should be reassessed. If symptoms are persistent, it may be necessary to induce urinary retention and teach the patient (if feasible) to self-catheterise [41].

Bladder Neck Dysfunction

Bladder neck dysfunction is incomplete opening of the bladder neck during voiding. It has been referred to as smooth sphincter dyssynergia, proximal urethral obstruction, primary bladder neck obstruction and dysfunctional bladder neck [47]. Bladder neck dysfunction was elegantly described by Turner Warwick and associates in 1973 [48]. The dysfunction generally affects young and middle-aged men, who complain of long-standing voiding symptoms, sometimes combined with storage symptoms.

These patients have a normal prostate on rectal examination, minimal residual urine volume and a normal bladder on cystoscopy [47]. The diagnosis can be made in male patients with proven outflow obstruction on urodynamics, who do not have a urethral stricture, prostatic enlargement or striated sphincter dyssynergia. Involuntary bladder contractions or decreased bladder contractions are relatively common, affecting around 34 % [49].

The exact cause of the problem is not known. Theories have suggested abnormal arrangement of muscle fibres around the bladder neck, where the bladder neck contracts instead of relaxing in co-ordination with detrusor contraction [50] or sympathetic hyperactivity.

There is sometimes some relief with alpha adrenergic blockers. Patients with bladder neck dysfunction may be affected at an early age from a relatively small increase in prostate size. This may be because the prostate cannot expand into the bladder neck and expands into the urethra [51].

Dysfunctional Voiding (Striated Sphincter)

Sphincter dyssynergia refers to the involuntary contraction or lack of relaxation of either the striated sphincter or the smooth sphincter. Detrusor sphincter dyssynergia refers to the dyssynergia of the striated external sphincter and is commonly abbreviated as DSD or DESD [47]. DESD is caused by neurological disease affecting the CNS pathways between the brainstem pontine micturition centre and the sacral spinal cord [52]. Common causes include traumatic spinal cord injury, multiple sclerosis and transverse myelitis. Dysfunctional voiding is the appropriate phrase to describe the situation in people who have a similar symptomatic and urodynamic pattern but no evident neurological bases.

Blaivas described three types of DESD [53].

Type I—Increase in both detrusor pressure and sphincter EMG activity; at the peak of detrusor contraction, the sphincter suddenly relaxes and unobstructed voiding occurs.

Type II—Sporadic contraction of the striated sphincter occurs throughout detrusor contraction.

Type III—Crescendo-decrescendo pattern of sphincter contraction resulting in outlet obstruction throughout detrusor contraction.

Without intervention patients with DESD can develop serious complications. These are more common in men than women. Fifty percent of men with DESD can develop vesicoureteric reflux or obstruction, urosepsis, and bladder stones [54].

Type I DESD is usually managed by observation only; types II and III are usually treated. Medical therapy has had limited success [47]. The most common form of treatment is intermittent self-catheterisation; other rarely used interventions are sphincterotomy, stent placement across the sphincter, Botulinum toxin injections into the sphincter, continuous catheterisation or urinary diversion [55].

Nocturia

Nocturia is the complaint that the individual has to wake at night one or more times to void, each void being preceded and followed by sleep or the intention of sleep [56]. When voiding occurs during sleep, without waking, it is termed nocturnal enuresis [56].

Nocturia is a common condition and occurs more frequently in the elderly [57, 58]. Prevalence is around 60 % in people aged 50–59, whilst 72 % of women and 91 % of men over 80 experience nocturia [59]. Nocturia is often bothersome [60] and broken sleep patterns and reduced sleep quantity or quality are associated with a negative impact on quality of life [61]. Nocturia also significantly increases the risk of injury from falls during the night in the elderly population [62].

Aetiology

Various contributory factors are recognised;

- Diurnal polyuria signifies that a person produces excessive urine volume. Of various definitions, the one used most commonly is production of more than 40 mL of urine per Kg body weight over a 24 h period [56]. Affected individuals experience an increase in both day- and night-time urine production. Secondary polydipsia, where fluid loss leads to constant thirst, can be caused by diabetes mellitus and diabetes insipidus [63]. Central diabetes insipidus is due to a failure of production of antidiuretic hormone (ADH); nephrogenic diabetes insipidus is where the kidneys fail to respond to ADH. Primary polydipsia (excessive fluid intake in the absence of a physiological stimulus to drink) can also increase total daily urine volume [63].

- Nocturnal polyuria indicates a disproportionately high nocturnal urine volume—for the elderly, at least one third of the daily total urine production [56]. The precise volumes are age dependent as younger people produce less urine at night than older people [64]. Lifestyle factors such as alcohol or caffeine consumption and evening liquid intake can underlie nocturnal polyuria [56]. Congestive heart failure, low blood albumin, venous stasis and renal insufficiency may be associated with nocturnal polyuria [65]. Respiratory conditions such as sleep apnoea have also been found to be causative of nocturnal polyuria [66]. Taking diuretic medication, beta-blockers or xanthines in the evenings before bed can also lead to increased night-time voiding.

- Bladder storage problems. Reduction in the functional capacity of the bladder can cause nocturia, even when urine production is within normal limits. This can be physical or sensory. Patients with overactive bladder syndrome may also suffer from nocturia, as an intrinsic part of the condition. Bladder, prostate or urethral cancers may reduce functional capacity, whilst irritation from infection, interstitial cystitis or calculi can lead to storage problems [56]. Some patients perceive nocturia to be an inevitable part of ageing and so may not seek medical help [64].

Evaluation

A thorough history and examination are central to the diagnosis of nocturia. There may be a treatable underlying medical cause for the nocturia. Questions should relate to voiding behaviour, medical and neurological abnormalities and sleep disturbance, as well as information on relevant surgery or previous urinary infections. Patients frequently report complaints secondary to the sleep disturbance, for example, daytime tiredness, disturbed sleep patterns and insomnia.

A voiding diary is of primary importance in diagnosing nocturia [64]. This should include recording of fluid intake and urine output volumes as well as timing of voids and any incontinence that occurs. The impact on quality of life can be measured using questionnaires, e.g. the ICS male [67] or the DAN-PSS in men [68] and the BFLUTS in women [69], which allow an assessment of the occurrence of nocturia and the degree of bother that it causes. A simple urine test, e.g. dipstick or urine analysis, should be undertaken to exclude any relevant pathology.

Management

General lifestyle advice, e.g. reducing caffeine and alcohol intake and limiting excessive liquid/food volume intake before bedtime, can sometimes achieve a satisfactory response [70]. Advice on diuretic use and timed-release formulations of these drugs may be helpful [71]. Compression stockings and evening leg elevation can reduce fluid retention prior to retiring to bed.

Medical causes of nocturnal polyuria, such as diabetes mellitus, sleep apnoea and cardiac failure, warrant treatment optimisation. Sleep disorders and psychological disturbances may benefit from relevant specialist input.

Desmopressin acetate is a synthetic analogue of arginine vasopressin. It increases urinary osmolality and reduces total urinary volume [72]. It decreases the total number of night-time voids, increases the time to first night-time void and decreases the volume of urine voided at night. An important adverse effect of desmopressin use is hyponatraemia. Sodium concentrations should be monitored, especially in the elderly [73]. Women are at greater risk of hyponatraemia than men.

The use of antimuscarinic medication in those with OAB-associated nocturia can reduce night-time voids [74]. There are some studies which suggest a benefit of using antimuscarinics in those with nocturia not associated with OAB [75].

Often, reduction in nocturia can be marginal or negligible, and further research into mechanisms and diagnostic approaches is highly desirable to try to achieve improved symptomatic outcomes with treatment.

References

1. Abrams P, et al. The standardisation of terminology of lower urinary tract function: report from the standardisation sub-committee of the International Continence Society. Neurourol Urodyn. 2002;21(2): 167–78.
2. Abrams P, et al. The standardisation of terminology of lower urinary tract function: report from the standardisation sub-committee of the International Continence Society. Am J Obstet Gynecol. 2002; 187(1):116–26.
3. Hashim H, Abrams P. Is the bladder a reliable witness for predicting detrusor overactivity? J Urol. 2006;175(1):191–4; discussion 194–195.
4. Parsons BA, Drake MJ. Animal models in overactive bladder research. Handb Exp Pharmacol. 2011;202: 15–43.
5. de Groat WC. A neurologic basis for the overactive bladder. Urology. 1997;50(6A Suppl):36–52; discussion 53–56.

6. Brading AF, Turner WH. The unstable bladder: towards a common mechanism. Br J Urol. 1994; 73(1):3–8.
7. Brading AF. A myogenic basis for the overactive bladder. Urology. 1997;50(6A Suppl):57–67; discussion 68–73.
8. Drake MJ, Mills IW, Gillespie JI. Model of peripheral autonomous modules and a myovesical plexus in normal and overactive bladder function. Lancet. 2001;358(9279):401–3.
9. Stewart WF, Van Rooyen JB, Cundiff GW, Abrams P, Herzog AR, Corey R, et al. Prevalence and burden of overactive bladder in the United States. World J Urol. 2003;20(6):327–36.
10. Irwin DE, et al. Population-based survey of urinary incontinence, overactive bladder, and other lower urinary tract symptoms in five countries: results of the EPIC study. Eur Urol. 2006;50(6):1306–14; discussion 1314–1315.
11. Drake MJ, Abrams P. Overactive bladder. In: Alan J, Wein W, McDougal S, Kavoussi LR, Novick AC, editors. Campbell-Walsh urology. 10th ed. Philadelphia, PA: WB Saunders; 2011. Ch 66.
12. Abrams P, et al. Overactive bladder significantly affects quality of life. Am J Manag Care. 2000;6(11 suppl):S580–90.
13. Brown JS, et al. Urinary incontinence: does it increase risk for falls and fractures? Study of Osteoporotic Fractures Research Group. J Am Geriatr Soc. 2000; 48(7):721–5.
14. Abrams P, Klevmark B. Frequency volume charts: an indispensible part of lower urinary tract assessment. Scand J Urol Nephrol Suppl. 1996;179:47–53.
15. Hashim H, Abrams P. Overactive bladder: an update. Curr Opin Urol. 2007;17(4):231–6.
16. Yamaguchi O, et al. Clinical guidelines for overactive bladder. Int J Urol. 2009;16(2):126–42.
17. Gulur DM, Drake MJ. Management of overactive bladder. Nat Rev Urol. 2010;7(10):572–82. Review.
18. Sahai A, Dowson C, Khan MS, Dasgupta P. Improvement in quality of life after botulinum toxin-A injections for idiopathic detrusor overactivity: results from a randomized double-blind placebo-controlled trial. BJU Int. 2009;103(11):1509–15.
19. Bramble FJ. The clam cystoplasty. Br J Urol. 1990;66(4):337–41.
20. Singh G, Wilkinson JM, Thomas DG. Supravesical diversion for incontinence: a long-term follow-up. Br J Urol. 1997;79(3):348–53.
21. Thomas AW, et al. The natural history of lower urinary tract dysfunction in men: the influence of detrusor underactivity on the outcome after transurethral resection of the prostate within a minimum 10 year urodynamic follow up. BJU Int. 2004;93:745–50.
22. Lluel P, et al. Increased adrenergic contractility and decreased mRNA expression of NOSIII in ageing rat bladders. Fundam Clin Pharmacol. 2003;17:633–41.
23. Elbadwi A, Yalla SV, Resnick NM. Structural basis of geriatric voiding dysfunction II. Aging detrusor: normal vs impaired contractility. J Urol. 1993;150:1657–67.
24. Kuchel GA. Hazzard's principals of geriatric medicine and gerontology. 6th ed. New York: McGraw-Hill; 2009. p. 621–30.
25. Schneider T, et al. A role for muscarinic receptors or rho-kinase in hypertension associated rat bladder dysfunction? J Urol. 2005;173:2178–81.
26. Malone-Lee J, Wahenda I. Characterisation of detrusor contractile function in relation to old age. Br J Urol. 1993;72:966–7.
27. Diokno AC, et al. Prevalence of urinary incontinence in the non-institutionalised elderly. J Urol. 1986;136: 1022–5.
28. van Koeveringe GA, et al. Detrusor underactivity: a plea for new approaches to a common bladder dysfunction. Neurourol Urodyn. 2011;30:723–8.
29. FitzGerald MP, Brubaker L. The etiology of urinary retention after surgery for genuine stress incontinence. Neurourol Urodyn. 2001;20:13–21.
30. Abrams P. Bladder outlet obstruction index, bladder contractility index and bladder voiding efficiency: three simple indices to define bladder voiding function. BJU Int. 1999;84(1):14–5.
31. Griffiths DJ, van Mastrigt R, Bosch R. Quantification of urethral resistance and bladder function during voiding, with special reference to the effects of prostate size reduction on urethral obstruction due to benign prostatic hyperplasia. Neurourol Urodyn. 1989;8:29–52.
32. Schafer W. Analysis of bladder-outlet function with the linearized passive urethral resistance relation, lin-PURR, and a disease-specific approach for grading obstruction: from complex to simple. World J Urol. 1995;13:47–58.
33. Anderson K-E, et al. Pharmacological treatment of urinary incontinence. In: Abrahms P, Khoury S, Wein A, editors. Incontinence 3rd international consultation on incontinence. Plymouth: Plymouth Distributors Ltd; 2005. p. 811.
34. Katona F, Eckstein HB. Treatment of neuropathic bladder by transurethral electrical stimulation. Lancet. 1974;1:780–1.
35. Everaert K, et al. The urodynamic evaluation of neuromodulation in patients with voiding dysfunction. Br J Urol. 1997;79:702–7.
36. Stenzl A, et al. Restoration of voluntary emptying of the bladder by transportation of innervated free skeletal muscle. Lancet. 1998;351:1483–5.
37. Elbadawi A, Yalla SV, Resnick NM. Structural basis of geriatric voiding dysfunction I-III. Detrusor overactivity. J Urol. 1993;150:1650–80.
38. Resnick NM, Yalla SV, Laurino E. The pathophysiology and clinical correlates of established urinary incontinence in frail elderly. N Engl J Med. 1989; 320:1–7.
39. Resnick NM, Yalla SV. Detrusor hyperactivity with impaired contractility; an unrecognized but common cause of incontinence in elderly patients. JAMA. 1987;257:3076–81.
40. Griffiths DJ, McCracken PN, Harrison GM, Ann Gormley E, Moore KN. Urge incontinence and

impaired detrusor contractility in the elderly. Neurourol Urodyn. 2002;21:126–31.

41. Resnick NM, Yalla SV. Geriatric incontinence and voiding dysfunction. In: Walsh P, Retik A, Vaughan Jr ED, Wein AJ, editors. Campbell's urology, vol. 2. 8th ed. Philadelphia, PA: WB Saunders; 2002. p. 1222–3. Ch 36.

42. Resnick NM, et al. Misdiagnosis of urinary incontinence in nursing home women: prevalence and proposed solution. Neurourol Urodyn. 1996;15:599–618.

43. Brandeis GH, Yalla SV, Resnick NM. Detrusor hyperactivity with impaired contractility (DHIC): the great mimic. J Urol. 1990;143:223A.

44. Payne CK. Behavioural therapy for overactive bladder. Urology. 2000;55(5A):3–6.

45. Fantl JA, Newman DK, Colling J. Urinary incontinence in adults: acute and chronic management. (Clinical practice guideline, Mo.2, 1996 Update, AHCPR Publication No. 96-0682). Rockville, MD: U.S. Department of health and human services, Public health service, Agency for health care policy and research; 1996.

46. Miller KL, et al. Dose titration key to oxybutynin efficacy for geriatric incontinence, even for DHIC. Neurourol Urodyn. 2000;19:538–9 (Abstract).

47. Wein AJ. Neuromuscular dysfunction of the lower urinary tract and its management. In: Walsh PC, Retik AB, Darracot Vaughan Jr E, Wein AJ, editors. Campell's urology, vol. 2. 8th ed. Philadelphia, PA: WB Saunders; 2002. p. 957–8.

48. Turner-Warwick RT, et al. A urodynamic view if the clinical problems associated with bladder neck dysfunction and its treatment by endoscopic incision and trans-trigonal posterior prostatectomy. Br J Urol. 1973;44:45–9.

49. Trockman BA, et al. Primary bladder neck dysfunction: urodynamic finding and treatment results in 26 men. J Urol. 1996;156:1418–20.

50. Bates CP, Arnold EP, Griffiths DJ. The nature of the abnormality in bladder neck obstruction. Br J Urol. 1975;47:651–5.

51. Turner-Warwick RT. Bladder outflow obstruction in the male. In: Mundy AR, Stephenson TP, Wein AJ, editors. Urodynamic principles, practice and application. London: Churchill Livingstone; 1984. p. 183–204.

52. Wein AJ, Rovner ES. Adult voiding dysfunction secondary to neurologic disease or injury. AUA Update series, vol 18, lesson 6. Houston: American Urological Association, Inc.; 1999. pp. 42–7.

53. Blavias JG, Sinha HP, Zayed AA, et al. Detrusor sphincter dyssynergia. J Urol. 1981;125:541–5.

54. Chancellor MB, Rivas DA. Current management of detrusor-sphincter dyssynergia. In: McGuire E, editor. Advances in urology. St. Louis: CV Mosby; 1995. p. 291–324.

55. Nambirajan T, et al. Urethral stents for urethral sphincter dyssynergia. BJU Int. 2005;95:350–3.

56. Van Kerrebroek P. The standardization of terminology in nocturia: report from the standardization subcommittee of the International Continence Society. BJU Int. 2002;90 Suppl 3:11–5.

57. Malmsten UG, et al. Urinary incontinence and lower urinary tract symptoms: an epidemiological study of men aged 45 to 99. J Urol. 1997;158:1733–7.

58. Swithenbank LV, et al. Female urinary symptoms: age prevalence in a community dwelling population using a validated questionnaire. Neurourol Urodyn. 1998;16:432–4.

59. Middlekoop HA, et al. Subjective sleep characteristics of 1485 males and females aged 50-93: effects of sex and age, and factors related to self-evaluated quality of sleep. J Gerontol A Biol Sci Med Sci. 1996;51:108–15.

60. Jolleys JV, Donovan JL, Nanchahal K, Peters TJ, Abrams P. Urinary symptoms in the community: how bothersome are they? Br J Urol. 1994;74(5):551–5.

61. Kobelt G, Borgstrom F, Mattiasson A. Productivity, vitality and utility in a group of healthy professionally active individuals with nocturia. BJU Int. 2003;91(3):190–5.

62. Stewart RB, Moore MT, May FE, et al. Nocturia: a risk for falls in the elderly. J Am Geriatr Soc. 1992; 40:1217–20.

63. Weiss JP, Blaivas JG. Nocturnal polyuria versus overactive bladder in nocturia. Urology. 2002;60:28–32; discussion 32.

64. Appell RA, Sand PK. Nocturia: etiology, diagnosis and treatment. Neurourol Urodyn. 2008;27:34–9.

65. Weiss JP, Blaivas JG. Nocturia. J Urol. 2000;163: 5–12.

66. Krieger JN, et al. Nocturnal polyuria is a symptom of obstructive sleep apnoea. Urol Int. 1993;50:93–7.

67. Donovan JL, Abrams P, Peters TJ, et al. The ICS-'BPH' study. The psychometric validity and reliability of the ICS male questionnaire. Br J Urol. 1996; 77:554–62.

68. Hald T, Nordling J, Andersen JT, Bilde T, Meyhoff HH, Walter S. A patient weighted symptom score system in the evaluation of uncomplicated benign prostatic hyperplasia. Scand J Urol Nephrol Suppl. 1991;138:59–62.

69. Jackson S, Donovan J, Brookes S, Eckford S, Swithinbank L, Abrams P. The Bristol female lower urinary tract symptoms questionnaire: development and psychometric testing. Br J Urol. 1996;77: 805–12.

70. Soda T, Masui K, Okuno H, et al. Efficacy of nondrug lifestyle measures for the treatment of nocturia. J Urol. 2010;184(3):1000–4.

71. Pederson PA, Johansen PB. Prophylactic treatment of adult nocturia with bumetanide. Br J Urol. 1988;62:145–7.

72. Lose G, et al. Efficacy of desmopressin (Minirin) in the treatment of nocturia: a double blind placebo-controlled study in women. Am J Obstet Gynecol. 2003;189:1106–13.
73. Rembratt A, Riis A, Norgaard JP. Desmopressin treatment on nocturia; an analysis of risk factors for hyponatraemia. Neurourol Urodyn. 2006;25:105–9.
74. Abrams P, Swift S. Solifenacin is effective for the treatment of OAB dry patients: a pooled analysis. Eur Urol. 2005;48:483–7.
75. Kaplan SA, Walmsley K, Te AE. Tolterodine extended release attenuates lower urinary tract symptoms in men with benign prostatic hyperplasia. J Urol. 2005;174:2273–5.

Part III

Evaluation

Evaluation: History and Physical Examination, Imaging, and Endoscopy

8

Alan J. Wein

The assessment of the patient with lower urinary tract symptoms (LUTS) can include any or all of the elements of the "neurourologic evaluation" (Table 8.1). The initial assessment should, where possible:

1. Establish a differential diagnosis(es).
2. Assess the level of bother, interference with quality of life (QoL), and the patient desire for intervention and tolerance for discomfort and risk.
3. Decide whether "empiric" therapy is reasonable and safe without further complex testing and, if not, what further complex testing is desirable.

History

Symptomatology is valuable in suggesting whether a dysfunction represents an abnormality of filling/storage, emptying/voiding, or both (Table 8.2). Each of these symptoms, in turn, has a list of possible etiologies (see Table 8.3 as an example), which should be kept in mind when evaluating a patient's complaints. Specific definitions for each of the symptoms have been formulated by the International Continence Society

(ICS) and the International Urogynecological Association (IUGA) [1, 2].

Symptoms suggestion of filling/storage abnormalities include:

Urinary incontinence is the complaint of involuntary loss of urine.

Stress incontinence (SUI) is the complaint of involuntary loss of urine during coughing, sneezing, or physical exertion.

Urgency incontinence (UUI) is the complaint of involuntary loss of urine associated with urgency.

Mixed urine incontinence is the complaint of involuntary loss of urine during coughing, sneezing, or physical exertion (SUI) and with urgency (UUI).

Postural incontinence is the complaint of involuntary loss of urine associated with change in body position.

Nocturnal enuresis is the complaint of involuntary loss of urine during sleep.

Continuous incontinence is the complaint of continuous involuntary loss of urine.

Insensible incontinence is the complaint of urine loss without awareness.

Coital incontinence is the complaint of involuntary loss of urine with intercourse.

Daytime urinary *frequency* is the complaint of more frequent micturition than previously considered normal.

Nocturia is the complaint of interruption of sleep one or more times due to the need to void.

A.J. Wein, M.D., Ph.D. (Hon.), F.A.C.S. (✉)
Perelman School of Medicine, University of
Pennsylvania Health System, Philadelphia,
PA 19104, USA
e-mail: alan.wein@uphs.upenn.edu

A.J. Wein et al. (eds.), *Bladder Dysfunction in the Adult: The Basis for Clinical Management*, Current
Clinical Urology, DOI 10.1007/978-1-4939-0853-0_8, © Springer Science+Business Media New York 2014

Table 8.1 Neurourologic evaluation

History, including bladder diary and/or frequency volume chart
Quality of life assessment
Physical examination
Neurologic examination
Urine bacteriologic studies
Renal function studies
Radiologic evaluation
Upper tract
Lower tract
Urodynamic/videourodynamic study
Endoscopic examination

Table 8.2 Urinary symptoms suggestive of LUT dysfunction

Filling/storage	Emptying/voiding
Urgency	Hesitancy
Frequency	Straining to void
Nocturia	Poor stream
Incontinence	Intermittency
Bladder/urethral pain	Dysuria
Increased sensation	Feeling of incomplete emptying
Decreased/absent sensation	Double voiding
	Position-dependent micturition
	Urinary retention

Table 8.3 Classification of incontinence

I. Extraurethral
  A. Fistula (vesicovaginal, ureterovaginal, urethrovaginal)
  B. Ectopic ureter
II. Urethral
  A. Functional
    1. Because of physical disability
    2. Due to lack of awareness or concern
  B. Bladder abnormalities
    1. Overactivity
      a. Involuntary contractions
      b. Decreased compliance
      c. Hypersensitivity with incontinence
      d. Combination
    2. Underactivity (overflow incontinence)
  C. Outlet abnormalities
    1. Stress urinary incontinence (SUI)
    2. Intrinsic sphincter deficiency (ISD)
    3. Combination (SUI+ISD)
    4. Urethral instability
    5. Post-void dribbling
      a. Urethral diverticulum
      b. Vaginal or urethral pooling of urine

Urgency is the complaint of a sudden, compelling, desire to void which is difficult to defer. Previously, and in the opinion of many, more appropriately, the definition included "for fear of leaking."

The *overactive bladder (OAB) symptom syndrome* is defined as the combination of urinary urgency, usually with frequency and nocturia, with or without urinary UUI, in the absence of urinary tract infection or other obvious pathology.

Increased bladder sensation is the complaint of the desire to void at an earlier time point or smaller bladder volume than previously experienced.

Dysuria is the complaint of burning or discomfort during voiding.

Bladder pain is the complaint of suprapubic or retropubic pain, pressure, or discomfort, related to the bladder, and usually increasing with bladder filling. It may persist or be relieved with bladder emptying. This is generally not a part of the OAB symptom complex. This and increased bladder sensation may be a result of the bladder pain syndrome/interstitial cystitis (BPS/IC).

Incontinence is generally a primary symptom of filling and storage failure and may be bladder or outlet related; however, it can also result from ureteral ectopia and congenital or acquired urinary fistulas. Leakage that is associated only with increases in intra-abdominal pressure implies *SUI*, but no outlet-related incontinence can occur without at least an element of *intrinsic sphincter deficiency (ISD)*. Gravitational urethral incontinence that worsens on straining implies ISD. *Precipitous incontinence* with a more sustained type of leakage similar to voiding is characteristic of *involuntary bladder contractions* (detrusor overactivity). It can occur with sensation (*urgency*) or without urgency in the absence of sensation. Incontinence is not always, however, a primary symptom of filling and storage failure. *Overflow, or paradoxical incontinence*, can develop in a patient with insidious detrusor decompensation with emptying failure. The leakage in this case is generally most prominently associated with changes in the position or sudden increases in intra-abdominal pressure and can mimic SUI.

An *increase in daytime urinary frequency* can be psychogenic, represent a response to pain or low-volume bladder distention (usually indicative of inflammatory disease), be due to detrusor overactivity (DO), or simply be due to increased fluid intake. Increased frequency can also result from emptying failure with a substantial residual urine volume and therefore a decreased functional bladder capacity. It can also exist in association with outlet obstruction-induced DO. *Nocturia* usually accompanies nonpsychogenic urinary frequency and can be associated, on the same basis as increased daytime frequency, with either storage or emptying failure. It is commonly associated with an increased nocturnal urine output (nocturnal polyuria).

The symptom of *pressure* defies exact definition. It is not quite the urge to void but rather a feeling that the bladder is full or that the urge to void will occur shortly. There is often no discernible urodynamic dysfunction in patients who complain of this, except perhaps for hypersensitivity during filling; however, such dysfunction can be due to an elevated detrusor pressure during filling but one that is below the level necessary to elicit the sensation of distention or urgency. This symptom also may be representative of an accurate perception of inadequate emptying with a modest or large residual urine volume.

Symptoms suggestive of emptying/voiding abnormalities include:

Urinary *hesitancy* is the complaint of a delay in initiating the urinary system.

Decreased *force or urinary stream* or poor flow is the complaint of a slower stream than previously appreciated or a slower stream than peers.

Intermittency is the complaint of urinary flow that stops and starts one or more time during the voiding phase.

Straining to void is the complaint of needing to exert effort by Valsalva, suprapubic pressure, or other means of increasing abdominal pressure in order to initiate or maintain the urinary stream.

Position-dependent micturition is the complaint of having to contort one's body into a specific position in order to improve the force of urinary stream or bladder emptying.

Double voiding or the need to immediately re-void is the complaint that further micturition is needed soon after voiding.

Past void dribbling is the complaint of involuntary urinary leakage immediately after voiding.

Urinary retention is the complaint of the persistent inability to pass urine.

Hesitancy, straining to void and poor or interrupted stream generally may reflect a *failure to empty adequately, but they can occur in an individual with frequency and urgency who, on toileting, simply has difficulty initiating a voluntary bladder contraction with a small intravesical urine content.*

Chronicling the history by charting is valuable in establishing a diagnoses or possible diagnoses and in assessing whether improvement has occurred. Three types of charts are described, each useful under specific circumstances [3–5]:

1. Micturition time chart: records only the times of micturition, day and night
2. Frequency-volume chart: records the volumes voided as well as the times of each void, day and night
3. Bladder diary: records the times of each void, voided volumes, incontinence episodes (including the degree of incontinence, pad usage, and associated symptoms or actions), degree of urgency, and the fluid intake

Certain patterns can be described and suggest specific pathologies. Such recordings over as long a period as possible are obviously desirable, but practicality limits are generally 2–7 days. The diary also allows an accurate estimate of the true functional capacity of the bladder, which is useful in evaluating filling volumes for urodynamics and endoscopy.

Pad Testing [6] The object of pad testing is to quantify the volume of urine lost into a perineal pad before and during some type of leakage provocation. A pad weight gain of >1 g is considered positive for a 1 h test, >4 g for a 24 h test. For tests involving exercises, these are generally done with a full bladder or with a known volume of saline instilled into the bladder. At the time of this writing, the Urodynamics Committee of the ICS is working on a standardization of pad testing.

A complete history should include, in addition to current symptomatology and bother:

1. Time of onset and duration of symptoms, precipitating (seemingly) events
2. History of neurologic disease or symptoms, diabetes, prior congenital abnormalities, and prior surgery
3. Current medications
4. Relevant general health issues
5. Prior treatment(s) and result(s)
6. Sexual function
7. Bowel function
8. For women, obstetrics and menstrual history

These are a number of questionnaires and symptom scores designed to assess various sets of lower urinary tract and pelvic symptoms and their effects on quality of life. These are also useful in assessing, over time, outcomes of interventions. The last (5th) edition of the International Consultation of Incontinence text [7] lists 21 International Consultation Modular Questionnaires (ICIQ) assessing the severity of various sets of "core symptoms" and the effect(s) on Quality of Life (QoL). An additional 74 health-related QoL measures for LUTS are chronicled in that text. Obviously, the selected use of these requires a well-thought out choice or choices for a particular purpose.

Physical Examination [3, 4, 6, 8]

To begin with, the *mental status, mobility, and dexterity* of the patient must be assessed, as these could influence and be related to the symptomatology and affect the strategy of management. Findings from a general physical examination are usually nonspecific. A *focused physical examination* should include the lower abdomen, genitalia, and rectum in both sexes and a neurologic examination.

Abdominal examination may reveal scars from prior forgotten surgeries, obesity should be noted, body mass index should be calculated, and suprapubic palpation and pressure should note a palpable bladder (generally >300 mL), pain, or the desire to void.

The *neurologic examination* should pay particular attention to the sacral dermatomes. In patients with known neurologic disease, a more thorough assessment should be carried out, and in spinal cord injured (SCI) patients, the level and completeness of the injury should be noted. In this regard, it must be remembered that the level of the vertebral lesion (as in SCI or disc disease) usually differs from the spinal cord segmental level. Sacral cord segments S2–S4 are generally at vertebral bone levels L1–L2. Evaluation of the *deep tendon reflexes* provides an indication of segmented spinal cord function as well as suprasegmental function. *Hypoactivity* of the deep tendon reflexes generally is associated with a lower motor neuron (LMN) lesion (in this context, meaning the anterior horn cells to the periphery), whereas hyperactivity generally indicates an upper motor neuron (UMN) lesion (between the brain and anterior horn cells of the spinal cord). *Commonly tested deep tendon reflexes* include the *biceps* (C5–C6), *triceps* (C6–C7), *quadriceps or patellar* (L2–L4), and *Achilles* (L5–S2). A pathologic toe sign (*Babinski reflex*) generally indicates a somatic UMN lesion but can be absent with a complete lesion and marked spasticity. A Babinski reflex may be present contralaterally with a unilateral lesion or may be present unilaterally with a bilateral lesion. The generic term *bulbocavernosus reflex* (BCR) describes contractions of the bulbocavernosus and ischiocavernosus muscles after penile glans or clitoral stimulation or after stimulation of the urethral or bladder mucosa by pulling an indwelling Foley catheter. These reflexes are mediated by pudendal and/or pelvic afferents and by pudendal nerve efferents and, as such, represent a local sacral spinal cord reflex. Most would agree that the BCR reflects activity in S2–S4, but some believe that this may involve segments as high as L5. Motor control of the *external anal sphincter* (EAS) is variously described as being served by sacral cord segments S2–S4 or S3–S5. A visible contraction of the EAS after pinprick of the mucocutaneous junction constitutes the *anal reflex*, and its activity usually parallel that of the BCR. *EAS tone*, when strong, indicates that activity of the conus medullaris is present, whereas absent anal sphincter tone usually indicates absent conal activity. Volitional control of the EAS indicates intact control by supraspinal centers. Patients should be able to voluntarily increase anal sphincter pressure. The *cough reflex* (contraction of the EAS with cough) is a spinal reflex that depends on volitional innervation of the abdominal musculature T6–L1. The afferent limb is apparently from muscle receptors in the abdominal wall that enter the spinal cord and ascend. As long as one of these segments remains under volitional control, the cough reflex may be positive. If a lesion above the outflow to the abdominal musculature exists, the cough reflex is generally absent.

Examination of the external genitalia and perineal and genital skin may detect penile and scrotal/testicular abnormalities in the male and vulvar and urethral meatal abnormalities in the female. Excoriation and irritation from urinary and fecal incontinence should be obvious. Digital rectal exam of the *prostate* for size, nodularity, induration, and tenderness seems prudent although the evidence for detecting prostate cancer, the occasional anal canal or rectal tumor, or estimating prostate size is weak. Likewise, the subject of *urinalysis* and the detection of infection and small amounts of microscopic hematuria is a matter of discussion. We do a dipstick urinalysis and, on positives, a microscopic exam, with a culture on those with significant pyuria or bacteriuria and a cytology and subsequent evaluation on those with significant microhematuria. The level of evidence for *renal function studies* in non-neurologic patients is weak, although many still feel that a baseline is useful. Biochemical screening for prostate cancer is a matter of local guidelines and personal conviction. The level of evidence for measurement of *post-voiding residual* in the standard male patient with LUTS is low and mainly based on expert opinion. Personal convictions for this seem stronger for patients with neurologic disease or more significant symptoms that could be due in part to a decreased functional bladder capacity.

Gynecologic exam should include *inspection of the perineal and genital regions* as well as *digital vaginal assessment of pelvic floor muscle strength*. It is otherwise important to *assess estrogen status* by looking for signs of vaginal atrophy and similar changes around the urethral meatus. *Urethral palpation* for tenderness or mass (diverticulum or the rare stone or carcinoma) or discharge is important. The exam should ideally include a gross assessment of the *size and mobility of the uterus and the adnexal structures and the capacity and mobility of the vagina. Pelvic floor muscle strength* is qualitatively defined by the tone at rest and the strength of a voluntary or reflex contraction as normal, absent, weak, or strong or by a validated grading system. *Assessment of pelvic organ prolapse (POP) (and pelvic floor muscle strength)* should be done in accordance with the IUGA/ICS recommendations published in 2010 [2, 6]. Exams should be done with the bladder empty and in the position that best demonstrates the prolapse.

POP is defined as the descent of one or more of the anterior vaginal wall, posterior vaginal wall, uterus/cervix, or the apex of the vagina (vaginal vault or cuff scar after hysterectomy) at the level of the hymen (the fixed point of reference) or beyond. Cystocele, rectocele, vaginal vault prolapse, and enterocele are terms used interchangeably with anterior, posterior, or apical vaginal prolapse. Stage 1 prolapse indicates that the most distal portion of the prolapse is more than 1 cm above the level of the hymen. Stage 2 indicates that the most distal portion is 1 cm or less proximal to or distal to the plane of the hymen. Stage 3 indicates descent of the most distal portion of the prolapse >1 cm below the hymenal plane. Stage 4 indicates complete eversion of the total length of the lower genital tract. The *POP-Q system* represents an objective, validated, and site-specific method for quantifying POP. The POP-Q records defects relative to the hymenal remnants in centimeter gradients and further staged according to the distal—most defect. A detailed and pictorial description of this methodology can be found in Staskin et al. [6] and Haylen et al. [2]. For initial assessment of the woman with urinary incontinence, the ICI Committee on initial assessment recommends only a simple description of the relationship of the anterior, superior, and posterior vaginal wall at rest and with straining.

A *stress test* is simple and useful. This involves observation of urine loss with cough or Valsalva. This can be done in lithotomy or standing position (helpful to place 1 ft on a stool) and should be done with a comfortably full bladder. Instantaneous urine leakage is considered positive and a sign of SUI. The *Q-tip test* is a traditional way of assessing mobility of the vesicourethral junction, but the accuracy has been questioned, and other imaging techniques are supplanting this as an assessment of bladder neck mobility.

Imaging Evaluation [8]

Upper tract imaging is generally recommended only in specific situations in the adult: (1) decreased bladder compliance, (2) neurogenic LUT dysfunction, (3) severe urethral obstruction, (4) incontinence associated with significant postvoid residual, (5) coexisting loin and flank pain, (6) severe untreated POP, and (7) suspected extraurethral UI.

Some urologists still prefer contrast imaging (CT urography or intravenous urography) as the optimal screening study of the upper tracts (kidneys and ureters) in patients with significant LUT dysfunction. *Ultrasonography*, however, can give adequate information about hydronephrosis, the presence of calculi, and, occasionally, hydroureter. *Isotope studies* can be useful to evaluate renal blood flow and function and to establish the presence of renal or ureteral obstruction. Dilation of the ureters or renal collecting system, or a decrease in function, can represent significant complications of LUT dysfunction and may be indications for intervention. Cystourethrography, either alone or as a component of a videourodynamic study, may add valuable information if the basic patterns are understood. A cystogram in the erect position at rest and during straining may be useful in quantitating the degree of classical SUI (bladder neck closed at rest, open with straining, associated with hypermobility) versus classical ISD (bladder neck open at rest, more leakage with straining, no hypermobility). Voiding cysto-urethrography is useful to diagnose the site of obstruction in a patient with proven urodynamic evidence of obstruction.

There are only a few basic cystourethrographic radiologic configurations, but proper interpretation requires concomitant urodynamic study or knowledge. A *closed bladder neck* is normal in a resting individual whose bladder is undergoing either physiologic or urodynamic filling. However, it can also occur in an individual with an areflexic bladder who is straining to void and in an individual in whom a micturition reflex is occurring but whose smooth sphincter area is dysfunctional or dyssynergic. The closed appearance can sometimes be mimicked to a great degree by significant prostatic enlargement with bladder neck and urethral compression as well. An *open bladder neck* is normal during voluntarily induced bladder micturition and during most involuntary bladder contractions as well. However, this appearance during filling/storage may also be due to ISD, seen in some types of neurologic injury or disease, or to endoscopic or open surgical alteration, and opening of the bladder neck at rest may be seen normally in some women whose continence level is at the mid-urethra.

A *closed striated sphincter* is normal during physiologic or urodynamic filling and is normally seen with an attempt to stop normal urination or to abort an involuntary bladder contraction. The sphincter also normally remains closed during abdominal straining. During voluntary micturition or during micturition secondary to an involuntary bladder contraction caused by neurologic disease at or above the brain stem, the striated sphincter should open unless the patient is trying to abort the bladder contractions by voluntary sphincter contraction or true detrusor sphincter dyssynergia is present.

Endoscopic Examination [8]

Lower Urinary Tract. *Endoscopy is recommended only in specific situations in the adult with LUTS*: (1) when initial testing suggests other types of pathology (significant microscopic or gross hematuria; pain, discomfort, and persistent or severe symptoms of bladder overactivity; and suspected extraurethral incontinence); (2) in patients who have previously undergone bladder, prostate, or other pelvic surgery; and (3) in men with incontinence. Some feel it is valuable for evaluation of the outlet and bladder in men with obstruction who are contemplating outlet reduction. Endoscopic examination does not necessarily or exclude anatomic obstruction at a particular site, as it should be recognized that not everything that appears occlusive endoscopically is obstructive urodynamically (all large prostates are not obstructive), and the lack of a visually appreciated occlusion does not exclude functional obstruction (striated or smooth sphincter dyssynergia) during bladder emptying/voiding. In describing findings on an endoscopic exam, it is better to use the term "occlusion," as "obstruction" implies urodynamic significance. The presence or absence of trabeculation (which is compatible with obstruction, involuntary bladder contractions, or neurologic decentralization) can also be determined. Bladder washings or a voided urine for cytology should be sent if symptoms suggest the possibility of neoplastic or preneoplastic changes in the bladder or urethral epithelium.

References

1. Abrams P, Cardozo L, Fall M, et al. The standardization of terminology of lower urinary tract function: report from the standardization subcommittee of the International Continence Society. Neurourol Urodyn. 2002;21:167–78.
2. Haylen BT, de Ridder D, Freeman RM, et al. An International Urogynecological Association (IUGA)/ International Continence Society (ICS) joint report on the terminology for female pelvic floor dysfunction. Neurourol Urodyn. 2010;29:4–20.
3. Abrams O, D'Ancona C, Griffiths D, et al. Lower urinary tract symptoms: etiology, partial assessment and predicting outcome from therapy. In: McConnell J, Abrams P, Denes L, Khoury S, Roehiboin C, editors. Male lower urinary tract dysfunction: evaluation and management, ICUD, SIU, EORTC-GU, editions 21. Paris: Health Publications Ltd; 2006. p. 69–142.
4. Abrams P. Urodynamics. 3rd ed. London: Springer; 2006.
5. Newman DK, Wein AJ. Managing and treating urinary incontinence. Baltimore: Health Professions Press; 2009.
6. Staskin D, Kelleher C, Bosh R, et al. Initial assessment of urinary incontinence in adult male and female patients. In: Abrams P, Cardozo L, Khoury S, Wein A, editors. Incontinence, EAU-ICUD. 5th ed. Plymouth: Health Publications Ltd; 2013. p. 361–89.
7. Kelleher C, Staskin D, Cherian P, et al. Partial-reported outcome assessment. In: Abrams P, Cardozo L, Khoury S, Wein A, editors. Incontinence, EAU-ICUD. 5th ed. Plymouth: Health Publication Ltd; 2013. p. 389–428.
8. Wein AJ, Moy AL. Voiding function and dysfunction; urinary incontinence. In: Hanno PM, Malkowicz SB, Wein AJ, editors. Plain clinical manual of urology. Philadelphia, PA: Saunders/Elsevier; 2007. p. 314–78.

Urodynamics

Marcus J. Drake

Urodynamics is a general term that covers any test that gives a dynamic evaluation of lower urinary tract (LUT) function. At its most simple, free flow rate testing with post-void residual measurement is a urodynamic test. The term is more generally applied to cystometry, which is the synchronous measurement of abdominal and bladder pressure, with flow. Its full title is multichannel cystometry, since two basic pressures are measured. The test can be further embellished by synchronous imaging (videourodynamics), ambulatory methods and more specialised tests, such as electromyography and urethral pressure profilometry.

The Basic Principles of Cystometry

The bladder is an abdominal organ, so any change in abdominal pressure should be transmitted to the bladder, confusing interpretation of whether the bladder has contracted or not. Accordingly, multichannel cystometry records both abdominal and bladder pressure, the first being subtracted from the second by continuous computer calculation to give the 'detrusor pressure'.

M.J. Drake, M.A. (Cantab),
D.M. (Oxon.), F.R.C.S. (Urol.) (✉)
University of Bristol and Bristol Urological Institute,
Bristol, UK
e-mail: marcus.drake@bui.ac.uk

Filling cystometry means the monitoring of these three basic pressures (the two measured and one calculated pressure) as the bladder is being filled, usually with body-warm saline. Bladder filling requires a second catheter into the bladder alongside the catheter used to measure bladder pressure. Often, these two bladder catheters are combined into a single catheter known as a 'double lumen line'.

As the bladder is filled, the person is asked to report any sensations that arise. The normal sensations documented are those of first awareness of filling, normal desire to void and strong desire to void [1]. A normal desire to void is best understood as the sensation that would make a person go to the toilet if they were not engaged in other activities. A strong desire to void could be viewed as the sensation which would cause somebody to interrupt an activity they are engaged in, in order to go to the toilet. Urgency is an abnormal sensation which should be distinguished from a strong desire to void—the two terms are not interchangeable. With ongoing filling, the person will feel that their bladder is full in due course, which could be at the point of a strong desire to void or a severe urgency episode. This is referred to as 'cystometric capacity'.

During filling, provocation tests are undertaken in order to reproduce the symptoms of which the patient complains. For example, a series of coughs can be used to reproduce stress incontinence. The sound of running water can sometimes elicit an urgency sensation, and this can be simply undertaken during a urodynamics test by turning on taps in a basin. The voiding phase is defined where the urodynamic investigator gives permission to the patient to pass urine. The voiding phase is a pressure-flow study, since pressures are measured whilst flow is also recorded.

Good Urodynamic Practice

The International Continence Society (ICS) defined good urodynamic practices in a standards document published in 2002 [2]. This is a detailed document by which urodynamic units are expected to run. Some of the key points are illustrated in Fig. 9.1 and include:

1. Calibration. All equipment should be calibrated according to manufacturer's instructions to ensure that flow rate recording and

pressure readings are accurate. This needs to be verified regularly.

2. Zeroing. All urodynamic machines have a 'zero button', to set the baseline relative pressure to zero. Good urodynamic practice specifies that baseline pressure should be atmospheric pressure ('zeroed to atmosphere'), since otherwise important artefacts may go undetected [3]. Assuming the transducers are zeroed to atmosphere, once they are opened to the patient's bladder or abdomen, the pressures will go up— these 'resting pressures' will be somewhere between 5 and 40 cmH$_2$O, depending on posture (supine, seated or upright). They should be similar in both bladder and abdomen, though there can be a small difference.

3. Quality of subtraction. A cough produces a short sharp rise in abdominal pressure which

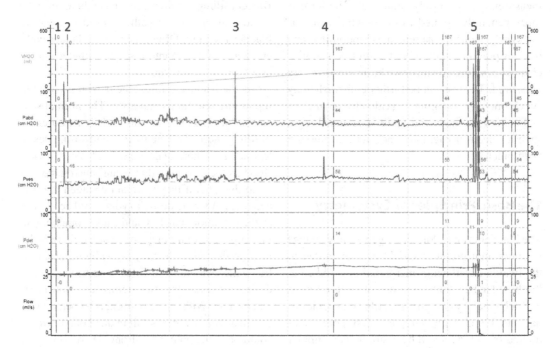

Fig. 9.1 Good urodynamic practices, illustrated using a filling phase in a man with post-prostatectomy stress incontinence. At point *1*, the transducers for measuring abdominal (P_{abd}, in *red*) and bladder (P_{ves}, in *blue*) pressure are open to the atmosphere, which is set as the baseline ('zeroed'); the transducers are then turned to record from the patient, with resting pressure seen to be about 45 cmH$_2$O (*2*). Between *1* and *2*, the patient has been asked to cough, causing a spike in pressure which is equal in height in both bladder and abdominal lines (so it is almost invisible in the detrusor line, P_{det}, in *green*, indicating 'good subtraction').

Coughs were done regularly throughout filling (*3, 4* and *5*) to check lines were still subtracting well. Bladder filling was started at *2* and stopped at *4*, shown by the *orange line* (V_{H2O}). As the bladder was filled, detrusor pressure rose, the rise halting when filling was stopped, suggesting the detrusor was not fully compliant. At *5*, a series of coughs was done to provoke stress incontinence; a small leakage happened, visible as a small amount in the flow trace (the bottom line, in *black*). The compliance, calculated from the pressure and volume at points *2* (0 mL, 1 cmH$_2$O) and *4* (167 mL, 14 cmH$_2$O), is (167−0/14−1) = 12.8 mL/cmH$_2$O should be picked up equally by both the abdominal and the bladder line. Therefore, the detrusor line should subtract both out together to give no deflection or a small biphasic artefact (i.e. small deflections of equal size above and below the line, in rapid succession). Cough testing of subtraction quality needs to be undertaken at the very start of the test, throughout filling and after the void. The latter is particularly important to ensure that pressure recorded during voiding was accurate.

4. Trace labelling. Since management decisions may be undertaken by somebody that was not present at the urodynamic test, the report should be clear and should be supported with clear labelling of any important events on the trace itself. The report should also be explicit on whether there were any problems with the test and whether the patient's day-to-day symptoms were genuinely reproduced.

Who Should Undergo Invasive Cystometry?

Patients undergoing urodynamics should have a well-defined problem. Full history and examination should have been undertaken, and ideally, a symptom score should be used to identify the severity and bother of individual lower urinary tract symptoms (LUTS), in order to direct the urodynamic methodology. A frequency volume chart is very valuable in identifying complicating factors such as polyuria. The frequency volume chart can also identify the maximum voided volume, which is a useful broad guide for the likely cystometric capacity. Based on this, a urodynamic question can be formulated to identify the issues that have to be considered. Ideally, the patient should have completed conservative management for their problem, since if conservative management alone is successful, the patient would not be seeking invasive testing and subsequent treatment. Thus, women with stress incontinence should have completed a trained, supervised regime of pelvic floor muscle exercises. Likewise, men with voiding LUTS and people with overactive bladder (OAB) should have tried behavioural

therapy and indicated medications. If a patient has comorbidity, making them inappropriate for subsequent surgical intervention, the urodynamic unit should consider whether it is genuinely worth undertaking an invasive test.

What Does Invasive Urodynamics Tell Us?

The test is aimed at achieving a clear diagnosis, so that it is possible to identify the main problem causing symptoms, additional factors that might be relevant and potential complicating factors that could increase the risk of adverse events. During the filling phase, the following diagnoses may be identified:

1. Urodynamic stress incontinence (USI) (Fig. 9.1). This is noted during filling cystometry and is defined as the involuntary leakage of urine during increased abdominal pressure, in the absence of a detrusor contraction [4]. This can occur due to urethral hypermobility, which is the commonest explanation in women with post-obstetric stress urinary incontinence (SUI). It means that the urethra is insufficiently supported, which can be identified on physical examination. Alternatively, USI can be caused by intrinsic sphincter deficiency, in which trauma to the sphincter or its innervation prevents the sphincter from functioning effectively. This is more common in people with neurological disease or who have had previous pelvic or incontinence surgery.

2. Detrusor overactivity (DO) (Fig. 9.2). Detrusor overactivity is a urodynamic observation characterised by involuntary detrusor contractions during the filling phase which may be spontaneous or provoked [4]. DO may be symptomatic, i.e. associated with urgency. Alternatively, some people have overactive detrusor contractions of which they are not aware (asymptomatic DO). DO can cause incontinence.

3. Increased filling sensation. Patients presenting with OAB symptoms most often have DO, but some instead report filling sensations at low bladder volumes or urgency in the absence of

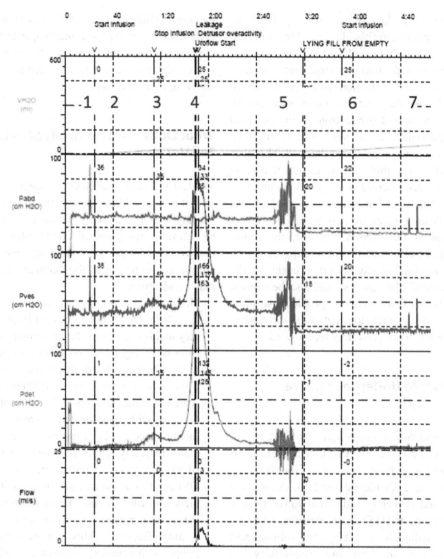

Fig. 9.2 A woman with a history of urgency and stress urinary incontinence (SUI). At *1*, resting pressures are consistent with her upright posture seated on a commode, and a cough test shows good subtraction. At *2*, filling was started. At *3*, she had a small overactive detrusor (DO) contraction. At *4*, there was a large DO contraction, causing incontinence. This confirmed the mechanism of her urgency incontinence, but did not allow assessment for urodynamic stress incontinence (for which, absence of DO is required by definition). Thus, she was asked to lie flat at *5*, since the supine position often stabilises DO; [17] it was successful for this lady, as DO settled (*6*). Thus, cough testing could be undertaken (*7*) in the absence of DO, the perineum being inspected to look for SUI (she could not be put above a flow metre when lying supine)

DO, resulting in a low cystometric capacity. It is important to consider whether stress incontinence could be causing urgency in these people—where a cough causes a small leak, which stimulates the urethral receptors and gives a sensation of desire to pass urine.

4. Reduced bladder compliance. Bladder compliance describes the relationship between change in bladder volume and change in detrusor pressure. It is calculated by dividing the volume change by the change in detrusor pressure during that change in bladder volume. The two standard points used to work out compliance are (1) the detrusor pressure at the start of bladder filling and the corresponding bladder volume (usually zero) and (2) the detrusor

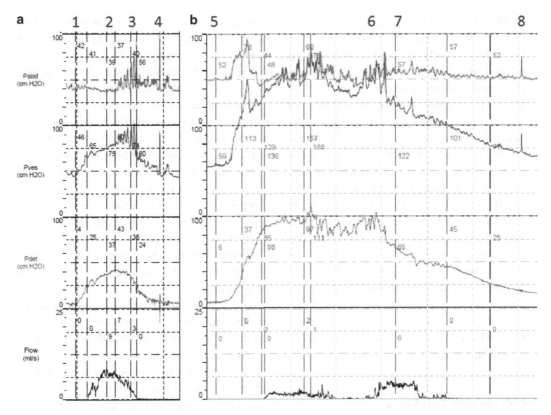

Fig. 9.3 Two men with voiding LUTS, caused by differing mechanisms: (**a**) impaired bladder contractility and (**b**) bladder outlet obstruction (BOO). (**a**); A 41-year-old man. The bladder contractility index (BCI) is calculated from the equation $BCI = P_{det}Q_{max} + 5Q_{max}$. Q_{max} was at point *2* and was 9 mL/s. The P_{det} at that moment was 37, so BCI is $37 + 45 = 82$. Any BCI value below 100 signifies impaired contractility (for men only). This man did not have BOO as the BOO index (BOOI) was 19. (**b**); A 73-year-old man. The BOOI is calculated from the equation $BOOI = P_{det}Q_{max} - 2Q_{max}$. Q_{max} was at point *7* and was 6 mL/s. The $P_{det}Q_{max}$ was 65, so BOOI is 53—any value above 40 signifying partial BOO (for men only). For both BCI and BOOI, the resting P_{det} immediately before the void (at points *1* and *6* in the illustrated examples) should be considered; it may be necessary to subtract the resting P_{det} from the $P_{det}Q_{max}$ if the BCI/BOOI is borderline or resting P_{det} is very high. In case (**b**), the BCI was close to 100; accordingly, subtracting resting P_{det} from $P_{det}Q_{max}$ reduces the latter to 59 cmH$_2$O, which gives a BCI of 89—so this man had both BOO and reduced contractility. In all cases, the post-void cough (at *4* and *8*) should be checked, as poor subtraction after the void would put the accuracy of $P_{det}Q_{max}$ recording in doubt. As is common with voiding LUTS, both men did some straining (at *3* and *6*), reflected in simultaneous transitory rises in both P_{ves} and P_{abd}

pressure (and corresponding bladder volume) at cystometric capacity or immediately before the start of any detrusor contraction that causes significant leakage (Fig. 9.1). There should overall be minimal pressure change during bladder filling. If filling causes a clear rise in pressure, it could signify potential risk to renal function in the future. The appearance of reduced compliance should prompt the urodynamicist to reduce the filling rate down to 10 mL/min [2], particularly in neuropathic patients, since a higher filling rate can cause an artefactual reduction in compliance.

Voiding Phase Diagnoses

1. Bladder outlet obstruction. Voiding at a low flow rate, but with high detrusor pressure, indicates that there is blockage at some point in the bladder outlet—in men, this is most typically caused by the prostate. For men with benign prostate enlargement, the ICS bladder outlet obstruction index (BOOI) has been derived based on the relationship between the detrusor pressure at maximum flow time and the actual maximum flow rate (Q_{max}) [5] (Fig. 9.3) to decide whether they have prostatic obstruction. For women, there is no agreed definition of

bladder outlet obstruction, though approaches to diagnosis have been attempted [6].

2. Detrusor underactivity is a contraction of reduced strength and/or duration, resulting in prolonged bladder emptying and/or a failure to achieve complete bladder emptying within a normal time span [4]. This is the alternative cause of voiding symptoms, and it is the key reason why men planning prostate surgery would undergo invasive urodynamic testing. The same parameters used in calculating BOOI, but with a modified equation, can be used to derive the bladder contractility index for men [7] (Fig. 9.3). Detrusor underactivity is more prevalent in older men and to a certain extent in younger age groups.

3. Incomplete bladder emptying. Most centres simply define a post-void residual, but the bladder voiding efficiency [7] can also be used, which relates the post-void residual to the bladder capacity.

Problems and Artefacts

Invasive urodynamics can be associated with some minor complications. There is a small rate of urinary tract infection, particularly in those people with bacteriuria before the test. Accordingly, dipstick urinalysis is usually undertaken, and cystometry deferred if nitrites are present in the urine sample. The patient may report some blood in the urine after urodynamic catheterisation. The test can be uncomfortable, so the catheters do have to be placed with care. Finally, it is an embarrassment for most people, given that the urethra and anus have to be catheterised. These aspects do have to be respected by the urodynamics unit, and consideration should be used at all times.

Patient factors are important. The patients will often be nervous before attending the test. Likewise, they might struggle to pass urine in the setting of a urodynamic unit ('bashful bladder'). Most importantly, sometimes the symptoms are not fully reproduced, or the findings might be unrepresentative of the patient's day-to-day urinary function. If the patient says that the problem

of which they are most bothered was not evident during the test, the final urodynamic report should state this clearly, so that any person making a decision based on the urodynamic test does not come to a wrong conclusion.

Technical factors are important, as described in the ICS Good Urodynamic Practices recommendations [2]. Important considerations include:

- The need to ensure equipment is appropriately maintained and calibrated.
- The importance of checking that both recorded pressures (P_{abd} and P_{ves}) are equal in size during coughs done throughout the filling phase and after the void.
- Transducers must be connected with watertight connections, and there should be no air in the system.

Artefacts tend to have characteristic features that an experienced urodynamicist can identify, and these have been categorised and described [8]. Nonetheless, even for an experienced unit, it can be difficult to maintain ideal recordings in practice. For example, sometimes, it can be difficult to ensure the lines to stay in place in the lumen of the organ, particularly in neuropathic patients or women with severe pelvic floor dysfunction.

Videourodynamics

Instead of filling the bladder with body-warm saline, X-ray contrast is used; with an image intensifier, it is then possible to look for key anatomical and functional aspects (Fig. 9.4). Typically, the X-ray source is placed behind the patient, and the image intensifier in front of the patient, so the radiation passes in the posteroanterior (PA) direction during the filling phase. The PA direction is also used during the voiding phase in women, but in men this would cause the urethra to be foreshortened and superimposed on itself on the screen. Thus, an oblique angle of about 45° is used in men to view the voiding urethrogram. Screening duration is kept as short as possible to minimise X-ray dose to the patient, and measures are taken to shield staff and others who might come into the vicinity, particularly

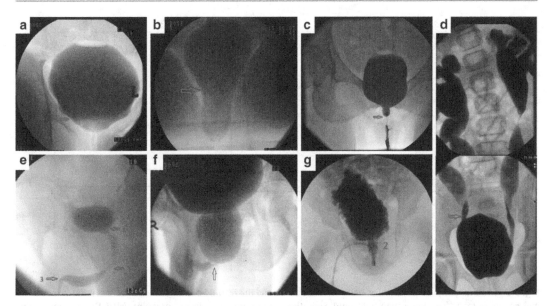

Fig. 9.4 Examples of representative images from videourodynamic studies. (**a**) Normal female cystogram. The base of the bladder lies level with the pubic symphysis (*arrow* indicates superior margin of symphysis). (**b**) Woman with pelvic organ prolapse. The base of the bladder extends below the vaginal vestibule (*arrow* indicates level of inferior margin of pubic symphysis). (**c**) Voiding phase in a woman who has previously had mid-urethral tape placement (*arrow* indicates mid-urethral point), showing obvious change in urethral calibre at the tape location. (**d**) Child (male) with bilateral grade 5 reflux (*arrow* indicates distal end of right ureter). (**e**) Normal male urethrogram (oblique projection); *1* indicates bladder neck, *2* the lower distal limit of the sphincter complex and *3* the start of the penile pendulous urethra. Between *1* and *2* is the prostatic urethra, and between *2* and *3* is the bulbar urethra. (**f**) Oblique projection of male urethra in an adolescent, showing posterior urethral valves (*arrow*). The prostatic urethra proximal to the valves is grossly distended. (**g**) Child (male, PA projection) with neurological disease, showing trabeculated and diverticulated bladder (*1*) and open bladder neck (*2*)

screens and aprons made of lead. It should be confirmed that female patients are not pregnant.

Examples of abnormalities visible with this approach include:

- Vesicoureteric reflux.
- Alterations in the bladder shape, such as trabeculation or diverticula.
- Quality of pelvic floor support; a poorly supported pelvic floor can bulge downwards at rest or during a rise in abdominal pressure.
- Incontinence.
- The location of outlet obstruction.
- Incomplete bladder emptying.

It is not necessary to use videourodynamics where the pathophysiology is predictable (best exemplified for women with post-obstetric SUI or men in the age range of benign prostate enlargement presenting with voiding symptoms). For other groups, videourodynamics provides additional information of benefit, particularly neuropathic patients or people who have previously had surgery.

Special Tests

Urethral Pressure Profilometry

This is a test in which a small catheter, continuously perfused at a rate of 2 mL per minute, is drawn along the urethra. The pressure needed to maintain the perfusion at the same rate is proportionate to the squeeze at each point along the urethra [9]. Accordingly, the squeeze can be plotted at distance, allowing identification of the external sphincter, as this is the point of maximum urethral closure pressure (MUCP) (Fig. 9.5). In men, there is often a smaller elevation in closure pressure at

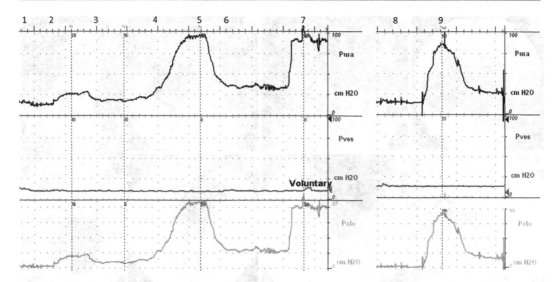

Fig. 9.5 Urethral pressure profiles for two men—a normal continent man (*left*) and a man with mild SUI after radical prostatectomy (*right*). The *black line* plots the profile, and the *blue* plots the bladder pressure. The *yellow line* is a calculated pressure subtracting the bladder pressure from the profile to give 'closure pressure' (the extent to which the outlet pressure is greater than bladder pressure at all points along its length). At point *1*, the urethral transducer is in the bladder and is gradually withdrawn, reaching the bladder neck at point *2*, the prostatic urethra at *3*, the start of the sphincter complex at *4* and the bulbar urethra at *6*. Point *5* is the maximum pressure in the outlet, and the reading of the *yellow line* at this point is the maximum urethral closure pressure (MUCP). At point *7*, the catheter had been returned to the sphincter region, and the man was asked to do a pelvic floor contraction—only a small, short-lasting contraction was achieved. For the man with mild post-prostatectomy incontinence, the bladder pressure is shown at *8* and the MUCP at *9*; consistent with his surgical history, there is no evident bladder neck and prostatic urethra. The MUCP is lower than for the continent man, and the functional length of the sphincter complex is shorter, but the differences are not substantial, which explains why symptom severity is mild

the bladder neck. MUCP is lower in people with stress incontinence, and very low values are seen in people with intrinsic sphincter deficiency. Thus, profilometry can deliver information that might help decide on subsequent treatment [10]. However, it is not widely used, and the evidence to support the treatment selection based on urethral closure pressure is limited.

Ambulatory Urodynamics

For those patients in whom prior conventional urodynamics failed to reproduce symptoms, ambulatory urodynamics is a more sensitive technique [11], perhaps because it enables more representative circumstances and more realistic provocation testing. Pressures are measured using a smaller device that can be worn by the patient, enabling them to undertake activities that might reproduce their symptoms [12]. It is a more intensive test and more demanding of resources, so it is not widely available.

Non-invasive Testing

Measurement of bladder pressure can be undertaken in men using a cuff around the penis [13]. This compresses the penile urethra, interrupting urine flow. Multiple cycles of rapid filling and emptying of the cuff cause an interrupted stream but enable the estimation of bladder pressure at maximum flow rate. Algorithms have been derived to enable the calculation of an outlet obstruction index [14], and it can anticipate response to surgery [15]. Other methods attempting to derive key urodynamic information noninvasively have been attempted but remain experimental [16].

References

1. Wyndaele JJ, De Wachter S. Cystometrical sensory data from a normal population: comparison of two groups of young healthy volunteers examined with 5 years interval. Eur Urol. 2002;42(1):34–8.
2. Schafer W, Abrams P, Liao L, Mattiasson A, Pesce F, Spangberg A, et al. Good urodynamic practices: uroflowmetry, filling cystometry, and pressure-flow studies. Neurourol Urodyn. 2002;21(3):261–74.
3. Gammie A, Drake M, Swithinbank L, Abrams P. Absolute versus relative pressure. Neurourol Urodyn. 2009;28(5):468.
4. Abrams P, Cardozo L, Fall M, Griffiths D, Rosier P, Ulmsten U, et al. The standardisation of terminology of lower urinary tract function: report from the standardisation sub-committee of the International Continence Society. Neurourol Urodyn. 2002;21(2):167–78.
5. Abrams PH, Griffiths DJ. The assessment of prostatic obstruction from urodynamic measurements and from residual urine. Br J Urol. 1979;51(2):129–34.
6. Akikwala TV, Fleischman N, Nitti VW. Comparison of diagnostic criteria for female bladder outlet obstruction. J Urol. 2006;176(5):2093–7.
7. Abrams P. Bladder outlet obstruction index, bladder contractility index and bladder voiding efficiency: three simple indices to define bladder voiding function. BJU Int. 1999;84(1):14–5.
8. Hogan S, Gammie A, Abrams P. Urodynamic features and artefacts. Neurourol Urodyn. 2012;31(7):1104–17.
9. Brown M, Wickham JEA. The urethral pressure profile. Br J Urol. 1969;41:211–7.
10. Kapoor D, White P, Housami F, Swithinbank L, Drake MJ. Maximum urethral closure pressure in women: normative data and evaluation as a diagnostic test. Int Urogynecol J. 2012;23:1613–8.
11. Heslington K, Hilton P. Ambulatory monitoring and conventional cystometry in asymptomatic female volunteers. Br J Obstet Gynaecol. 1996;103(5):434–41.
12. Swithinbank LV, James M, Shepherd A, Abrams P. Role of ambulatory urodynamic monitoring in clinical urological practice. Neurourol Urodyn. 1999;18(3):215–22.
13. Harding CK, Robson W, Drinnan MJ, Griffiths CJ, Ramsden PD, Pickard RS. An automated penile compression release maneuver as a noninvasive test for diagnosis of bladder outlet obstruction. J Urol. 2004;172(6 Pt 1):2312–5.
14. Griffiths CJ, Harding C, Blake C, McIntosh S, Drinnan MJ, Robson WA, et al. A nomogram to classify men with lower urinary tract symptoms using urine flow and noninvasive measurement of bladder pressure. J Urol. 2005;174(4 Pt 1):1323–6. discussion 1326; author reply 1326.
15. Harding C, Robson W, Drinnan M, Sajeel M, Ramsden P, Griffiths C, et al. Predicting the outcome of prostatectomy using noninvasive bladder pressure and urine flow measurements. Eur Urol. 2007;52(1):186–92.
16. Parsons BA, Bright E, Shaban AM, Whitehouse A, Drake MJ. The role of invasive and non-invasive urodynamics in male voiding lower urinary tract symptoms. World J Urol. 2011;29(2):191–7.
17. Al-Hayek S, Belal M, Abrams P. Does the patient's position influence the detection of detrusor overactivity? Neurourol Urodyn. 2008;27(4):279–86.

Special Tests

Jalesh N. Panicker and Marcus J. Drake

Where diagnostic pathways fail to establish underlying diagnosis or cause, additional tests may have a role. Particular interest is placed in radiological tests, since increasing technological and protocol development can generate useful insights. In this short chapter, we outline some current tests used in lower urinary tract dysfunction (LUTD). However, it should be recognised that the sheer scope of the field means it cannot be a comprehensive review and much of the content described will be superseded in the near future due to the pace of advances.

Magnetic Resonance Imaging

Magnetic resonance imaging (MRI) offers highly detailed imaging of anatomy, with technology to deliver reconstructions in 3 dimensions. It exploits the property of nuclear magnetic resonance (NMR) to image nuclei of atoms inside the body. The patient lies in a powerful magnetic field, which aligns the magnetization of specified

atomic nuclei, and radio frequency magnetic fields are applied to alter their alignment. Consequently, the nuclei produce a rotating magnetic field which is detectable by the scanner. The gradient of the magnetic fields affects various nuclei differently, so that spatial information can be deduced using Fourier analysis. Using gradients in different directions allows images (2D) or volumes (3D) to be obtained in any orientation. It is contraindicated in people who have certain types of metal implant or metal foreign bodies, due to the potential damage resulting from interaction of the metal with the extremely powerful magnetic field in the MRI scanner.

In functional urology, MRI can be used for circumstances where additional anatomical information is needed and where symptoms remain unexplained by standard tests. For example, urethral diverticula in women (Fig. 10.1) require careful assessment to give the best chance of successful clinical outcome and are best evaluated with MRI. Chronic pelvic pain (CPP) can result from nerve entrapment, for example, entrapment of the pudendal nerve in Alcock's canal, adjacent to the ischiopubic ramus. MRI is able to identify such patients.

MRI may also be used for the non-invasive assessment of central nervous system functions in individuals with LUTD. The science of functional brain imaging has witnessed an explosive growth over the last couple of decades. Functional MRI (fMRI) measures localised changes in cerebral blood flow related to neural activity, known as activations. This is based upon the principle that changes in neural activity are coupled with

J.N. Panicker, M.D., D.M., M.R.C.P. (UK)
Department of Uroneurology, The National Hospital for Neurology and Neurosurgery, London, UK

M.J. Drake, M.A. (Cantab.), D.M. (Oxon.), F.R.C.S. (Urol.) (✉)
University of Bristol and Bristol Urological Institute, Bristol, UK
e-mail: marcus.drake@bui.ac.uk

A.J. Wein et al. (eds.), *Bladder Dysfunction in the Adult: The Basis for Clinical Management*, Current Clinical Urology, DOI 10.1007/978-1-4939-0853-0_10, © Springer Science+Business Media New York 2014

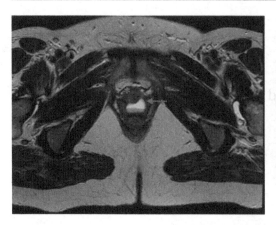

Fig. 10.1 MRI cross-sectional image at the level of the urethra in a woman, showing a urethral diverticulum (*arrowed*). Well-selected radiological scanning protocols allow a clear distinction between the diverticulum, which stands out from adjacent tissues, such as the urethra itself (*asterisk*), due to its lighter colour. There is some liquid in the diverticulum giving rise to a horizontal fluid level

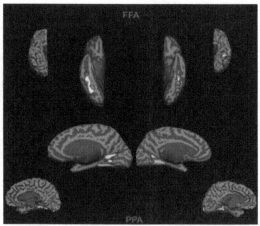

Fig. 10.2 BOLD activation from an fMRI study illustrated on three-dimensional brains. Fusiform face area (FFA) (*upper* 4) and parahippocampal place area (PPA) (*lower* 4) identified following initial 'localiser' session. FreeSurfer programme was used to inflate the brains (*central* images) to better visualise activations within folds, i.e. gyri. Courtesy Mr. Jinendra Ekanayake, Institute of Cognitive Neurosciences, Queen Square, University College London

changes in cerebral blood flow, and when a region of the brain is activated, the blood flow to that area also increases.

fMRI is potentially a useful tool for understanding the central control of lower urinary tract functions. Changes in blood-oxygen level-dependent (BOLD) contrast are studied to map neural activity in the brain during lower urinary tract-specific tasks (Fig. 10.2). Most commonly, protocols involve repeatedly filling and emptying the bladder through an indwelling catheter whilst the patient lies in the scanner. Protocols of natural bladder filling or of pelvic floor contractions have been used as well. Changes in activity have been seen in patients with idiopathic detrusor overactivity including inadequate orbitofrontal activation [1] and altered functional connectivity between the right insula, anterior cingulate gyrus and other relevant areas for bladder control [2]. Increased activation of the anterior cingulate gyrus during these studies has been interpreted as a possible correlate to the symptom of urinary urgency [3]. Examining the functional connectivity during activity or resting state may enable the creation of functional connectivity maps of temporally correlated but spatially distinct brain regions called functional networks.

fMRI is a safe and non-invasive tool, and the scanner used is available at most centres.

The procedure entails little risk to staff or patients because of the absence of radiation exposure. Moreover, the images obtained are of high spatial resolution with greater localisation of changes in brain activity, though at the expense of temporal resolution of these brain events. fMRI is therefore the imaging modality most commonly used nowadays. Only a few centres worldwide however are actively involved in brain imaging research for understanding the central control of bladder functions. Common to all brain imaging studies is the expense and level of specialist expertise required for carrying out studies. The challenge of functional imaging lies in the interpretation of data and the availability of a dedicated team comprising the clinician, medical physicist and neuroscientist. Nevertheless, fMRI has opened up a new field of investigations and is now an established tool to understand the supraspinal neural networks controlling lower urinary tract functions. The exact role of fMRI in the clinical work up and management of the patient with LUTD is still to be determined; however, it is anticipated that with further research, information obtained will contribute to diagnostics and therapeutic strategies in the coming years.

Biomarkers

A biomarker can be used to define the presence of a condition, where it is referred to as a diagnostic biomarker. Alternatively, prognostic and predictive biomarkers can be used to categorise severity, progression or likely response to treatment. Biomarkers are well recognised in many areas of medicine, and extensive research is ongoing in functional urology to identify biomarkers for syndromes such as overactive bladder (OAB) and CPP. Urinary biomarkers are a particularly attractive prospect, due to ease of collection and ready availability. However, the conditions reflect diverse pathophysiological mechanisms and varied presentations, such that no biomarkers are currently accepted. In OAB, several substances have been investigated (reviewed in Bhide et al. [4]), including nerve growth factor (NGF), brain-derived neurotrophic factor (BDNF), prostaglandins, cytokines, C-reactive protein and ATP [5]. In CPP, a similarly diverse group of substances has been studied, and the use of modern techniques for screening may yield beneficial insights [6]. Whilst no biomarkers are currently accepted, this is a rapidly advancing field; the experimental focus, improving insights and new methodology opportunities seem likely to bring new advances in the foreseeable future.

Ultrasound for Non-invasive Urodynamics

Voiding through a partially obstructed outlet causes detrusor muscle hypertrophy. Thus, ultrasound-derived measures of bladder wall thickness (BWT), detrusor wall thickness (DWT) and ultrasound-estimated bladder weight (UEBW) have been proposed as potential diagnostic tools for BOO. Transabdominal ultrasound can identify three distinct layers of the anterior bladder wall, of which the detrusor is a central hypoechoic layer, with hyperechoic layers of the mucosa and the subserosal tissue on either side. These parameters are still not accepted in routine use due to several limitations [7], for example, the potential

effect of sampling error and the considerable proportionate effect of any inaccuracy in measurement. Furthermore, mucosal thickness can be affected by differing pathologies, such as infection and carcinoma. Likewise, detrusor hypertrophy can result from OAB or outlet obstruction.

Neurophysiological Testing

Neurophysiological tests of the pelvic floor have been developed for assessing the innervation of muscles that are difficult to test clinically.

Electromyography

Pelvic floor electromyography (EMG) was first introduced as part of urodynamic studies to assess the extent of relaxation of the urethral sphincter during voiding, with the aim of recognising detrusor–sphincter dyssynergia. Another situation is in the evaluation of men with suspected dysfunctional voiding, where recording electrical silence from the urethral sphincter during voiding would exonerate the external sphincter as the cause for voiding dysfunction. However, it is now rarely recorded for several reasons. First, it is often technically difficult to obtain a good quality EMG signal from a site which is as inaccessible as the urethral sphincter, particularly in the environment in which urodynamic studies are performed. The best signal is obtained using a needle electrode, but the discomfort from the needle itself is likely to impair normal relaxation of the pelvic floor. Surface recording electrodes have been used, but they may record a considerable amount of noise which makes interpretation of the results difficult. Furthermore, in addition to the difficulties of making a meaningful recording, the value of the information the procedure provides is limited. Video screening provides more information about the outflow tract, and hence the indications for kinesiological sphincter EMG recording is now limited.

Concentric needle EMG studies of the pelvic floor performed separately from urodynamics have been useful to assess innervation in specific scenarios. EMG has been used to demonstrate

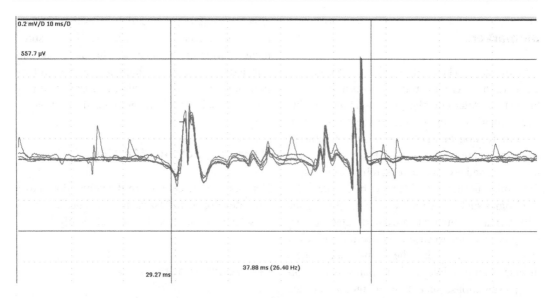

0.2 mV/D 10 ms/D

557.7 μV

29.27 ms

37.88 ms (26.40 Hz)

Fig. 10.3 Concentric needle EMG of the external anal sphincter from a 54-year-old gentleman presenting with urinary retention on the background of a recent onset Parkinsonism syndrome. Duration of the motor unit is 37.9 ms, which is prolonged and suggests chronic reinnervation. The mean duration of MUPs during the study was 19 ms (normal <10 ms), and the EMG is compatible with a diagnosis of multiple system atrophy

changes of reinnervation in the urethral or anal sphincter in a few neurogenic disorders. Well-established values exist for the normal duration and amplitude of motor units recorded from the sphincter muscles.

Some specific uses include;

1. Evaluation of suspected cauda equina lesions. Lesions of the cauda equina are an important cause for pelvic floor dysfunction and patients present with LUTD and often sexual and bowel dysfunction as well. Most often, EMG of the external anal sphincter demonstrating changes of chronic reinnervation, with a reduced interference pattern, and enlarged polyphasic motor units (>1 mV amplitude) can be found in patients with long-standing cauda equina syndrome [8]. Though EMG may demonstrate pathological spontaneous activity 3 weeks or more after injury, these changes of moderate to severe partial denervation or complete denervation often become lost in the tonically firing motor units of the sphincter.

2. Diagnosis of multiple system atrophy (MSA). Patients with a variant of Parkinson's disease known as MSA often present initially with LUTD, and, not uncommonly, they may present

to the urologist. Degenerative changes occur both in the brain and spinal cord. Neuro-pathological studies have shown that the anterior horn cells in the Onuf's nucleus are selectively lost in MSA, and this results in changes in the sphincter muscles that can be identified by EMG. The anal sphincter is once again most often studied, and changes of chronic reinnervation in MSA tend to result in prolonged duration motor units, and these changes can be detected easily (Fig. 10.3). Although the value of sphincter EMG in the differential diagnosis of Parkinsonism has been widely debated, a body of opinion exists that maintains that a highly abnormal result in a patient with mild Parkinsonism is of value in establishing a diagnosis of probable MSA [9]. This correlation is important not only for the neurologist but also for the urologist, because inappropriate surgery for a suspected prostate enlargement as the cause for bladder troubles can then be avoided.

3. Urinary retention in young women. Isolated urinary retention in young women can arise in the absence of evident cause. Neurological examination is normal, and investigations such as MRI exclude a neurological cause for void-

ing dysfunction. A characteristic abnormality, however, can be found on urethral sphincter EMG, consisting of complex repetitive discharges, akin to the 'sound of helicopters', and decelerating bursts, a signal somewhat like myotonia and akin to the 'sound of underwater recording of whales'. It has been proposed that this abnormal spontaneous activity results in impairment of relaxation of the urethral sphincter, which may cause urinary retention in some women and obstructed voiding in others. This condition, nowadays known as Fowler's syndrome, is also characterised by elevated urethral pressures.

Penilo-Cavernosus Reflex

The nomenclature of the various reflex responses that can be recorded from pelvic structures in response to electrical stimulation was recently rationalised so that the term used gives an indication as to the site of stimulation and recording. The penilo-cavernosus reflex, or 'bulbocavernosus' reflex, assesses the sacral root afferent and efferent pathways. The dorsal nerve of the penis (or clitoris) is electrically stimulated, and recordings are made from the bulbocavernosus muscle, usually with a concentric needle. It may be of value in patients with bladder dysfunction suspected to be secondary to cauda equina damage or damage to the lower motor neurone pathway. However, a normal value does not exclude the possibility of an axonal lesion.

Pudendal Nerve Terminal Motor Latency

The only test of motor conduction for the pelvic floor is the pudendal nerve terminal motor latency (PMNTL). The pudendal nerve is stimulated either per rectally or vaginally adjacent to the ischial spine using the St. Mark's electrode, a finger-mounted stimulating device with a surface EMG recording electrode 7 cm proximal located around the base of the finger. This records from the external anal sphincter. Prolongation was

initially considered evidence for pudendal nerve damage, although a prolonged latency is a poor marker of denervation. This test has not proved contributory in the investigation of patients with suspected pudendal neuralgia.

Pudendal Somatosensory Evoked Potentials

Pudendal somatosensory evoked potentials can be recorded from the scalp following electrical stimulation of the dorsal nerve of penis or clitoral nerve. Although this may be abnormal when a spinal cord lesion is the cause of sacral sensory loss or neurogenic detrusor overactivity, such pathology is usually apparent from the clinical examination. Results are compared to latencies of the tibial evoked potentials.

References

1. Griffiths D, Derbyshire S, Stenger A, Resnick N. Brain control of normal and overactive bladder. J Urol. 2005;174(5):1862–7.
2. Tadic SD, Griffiths D, Schaefer W, Resnick NM. Abnormal connections in the supraspinal bladder control network in women with urge urinary incontinence. Neuroimage. 2008;39(4):1647–53.
3. Griffiths D, Tadic SD, Schaefer W, Resnick NM. Cerebral control of the bladder in normal and urge-incontinent women. Neuroimage. 2007;37(1):1–7.
4. Bhide AA, Cartwright R, Khullar V, Digesu GA. Biomarkers in overactive bladder. Int Urogynecol J. 2013;24(7):1065–72.
5. Silva-Ramos M, Silva I, Oliveira O, Ferreira S, Reis MJ, Oliveira JC, et al. Urinary ATP may be a dynamic biomarker of detrusor overactivity in women with overactive bladder syndrome. PLoS One. 2013;8(5):e64696.
6. Blalock EM, Korrect GS, Stromberg AJ, Erickson DR. Gene expression analysis of urine sediment: evaluation for potential noninvasive markers of interstitial cystitis/bladder pain syndrome. J Urol. 2012;187(2):725–32.
7. Parsons BA, Bright E, Shaban AM, Whitehouse A, Drake MJ. The role of invasive and non-invasive urodynamics in male voiding lower urinary tract symptoms. World J Urol. 2011;29(2):191–7.
8. Podnar S, Trsinar B, Vodusek DB. Bladder dysfunction in patients with cauda equina lesions. Neurourol Urodyn. 2006;25(1):23–31.
9. Vodusek DB. Sphincter EMG, and differential diagnosis of multiple system atrophy. Mov Disord. 2001; 16(4):600–7.

Behavioral Therapy

11

Alan J. Wein and Diane K. Newman

Behavioral modification is the first treatment option included under the category of conservative management of lower urinary tract symptoms (LUTS), the latter defined as any therapy not involving surgical treatment [1]. The components of behavioral modification are seen in Fig. 11.1 and the list of potential dysfunctions to which they are potentially applicable is seen in Table 11.1. In most settings the treatment programs are administered and carried out by advanced practice professionals, who have done the bulk of evidence collection attesting to the worth of these programs. These interventions are intended to follow a simple noninvasive assessment which includes a detailed history and an assessment of pelvic floor muscle (PFM) contraction and relaxation (see sections on physical examination). The latter includes instruction, where necessary, in the identification of the musculature involved and the proper techniques for contraction and relaxation. Different methodologies for education, instruction, and following are utilized by different leaders in the field. Ours, developed by Diane Newman,

11

A.J. Wein, M.D., Ph.D (Hon.), F.A.C.S. (✉)
Perelman School of Medicine, University
of Pennsylvania Health System,
Philadelphia, PA 19104, USA
e-mail: alan.wein@uphs.upenn.edu

D.K. Newman, D.N.P., A.N.P.-.B.C., F.A.A.N.
Division of Urology, Department of Surgery,
Perelman School of Medicine, University
of Pennsylvania, Philadelphia, PA, USA

along with patient self-help reminders and charts are readily available [2]. In this chapter, we will briefly define and describe "the tools," lifestyle interventions, and "active regimens" (pelvic floor muscle utilization and bladder training).

The Tools

Scheduled voiding is a term that encompasses bladder training, timed voiding, habit training, and prompted voiding [1]. Although they share in common a toileting schedule, they differ in terms of the nature of patient involvement (active or passive) and the nature of patient–provider interaction. *Bladder training* (BT) includes a program of patient education regarding lower urinary tract function (including pelvic floor) and urine output along with a program of gradually increasing scheduled voiding intervals [4]. The underlying mechanism of how this works is unknown, but various hypotheses include improved cortical control of bladder activity and urethral closure, improved central modulation of afferent stimuli, and altered behavior because of better awareness of LUT function and the causes of urinary incontinence (UI)—all of which increase the capacity of the LUT. BT may utilize the maneuvers learned in PFM training and urgency inhibition to achieve its ends. *Timed voiding* (TV) is a fixed schedule to prevent UI by bladder emptying prior to exceeding capacity [5]. The interval is typically every 2–3 h, and TV is also intended to normalize frequency in a patient with infrequent

Fig. 11.1 Components of behavioral treatment (modified after [2], p. 246)

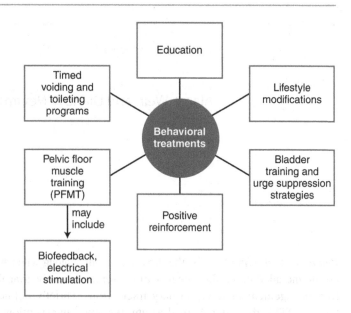

Table 11.1 Conditions for which behavioral modification has shown benefit ([2, 6])

Stress urinary incontinence
Overactive bladder ± urgency urinary incontinence
Neurogenic detrusor overactivity
Mixed urinary incontinence
Nocturia
Pelvic floor spasm (dysfunction)
Non-relaxing striated sphincter

voiding and/or diminished sensation [5]. The interval may be set permanently or gradually increased. *Habit training* refers to a toileting schedule matched to an individual voiding pattern based on their bladder diary such that the voiding interval preempts UI [7]. *Prompted voiding* is initiated by caregivers in combination with a timed voiding regimen; it is used primarily in institutionalized settings with cognitively and physically impaired older adults [8].

Pelvic floor muscle training (PFMT) involves learning how to contract and relax the PFM through instructional various types of feedback—visual, auditory, or the measurement of physiological parameters (biofeedback). Details of training regimens vary. PFMT is useful in treating both SUI and UUI and for suppressing urgency in patients with overactive bladder without urgency incontinence [1]. Active PFM contraction during activities that cause SUI has been termed "knack" and is a learned strategy [9]. Intensive PFMT is also hypothesized to reinforce structural support of the bladder neck in women and thereby facilitate the limitation of downward movement [10–12]. For the management of UUI and urgency alone, the rationale for PFMT is that detrusor contraction can be inhibited by a PFM contraction, either through electrical stimulation [13] or by voluntary contraction [14]. Repeated rapid contraction of the PFM (termed "quick flicks") with the individual remaining posturally still and waiting for the sensation to pass has proven to be a useful adjunct to BM regimen for OAB [1, 2, 5]. When PFMT is employed, the need to practice this is lifelong for the setting of both SUI and OAB.

Lifestyle modifications involve a conscious choice on the patient part to change a practice that is easily modifiable and may contribute to LUTS or bladder/pelvic pain. These include fluid intake, diet, bowel function, tobacco use, and weight control. The evidence for these will be discussed, along with the recommendations regarding each of the International Consultation on Incontinence (ICI) Committee on Conservative Management.

The Results and Conclusions

Fluid Intake and Urine Volume. Large intake volume can trigger OAB symptoms [15] and a 25 % decrease can reduce frequency, urgency, and, to a minor extent, nocturia [16]. ICI assigned a level of evidence (LOE: 3) that fluid intake may play a minor role in the pathogenesis of UI; a minor decrease by 25 % may be recommended provided baseline consumption is not <1 L/day (Grade B recommendation (R)—note—all LOE and R are from the ICI reports by Moore et al. [1] and Hanno et al. [17]). The modified Oxford system utilized is seen in Table 11.2.

Table 11.2 Oxford levels of evidence and grades of recommendation [20]

Levels of evidence

Any level of evidence may be positive (the therapy works) or negative (the therapy does not work). A level of evidence is given to each individual study

- *Level 1* evidence usually involves meta-analysis of trials (RCTs) or a good-quality randomized controlled trial, or "all-or-none" studies in which no treatment is not an option, for example, in vesicovaginal fistula

- *Level 2* evidence include "low"-quality RCT (e.g., <80 % follow-up) or meta-analysis (with homogeneity) of good-quality prospective "cohort studies." These may include a single group when individuals who develop the condition are compared with others from within the original cohort group. There can be parallel cohorts, where those with the condition in the first group are compared with those in the second group

- *Level 3* evidence includes:

  Good-quality retrospective "case–control studies" where a group of patients who have a condition are matched appropriately (e.g., for age, sex) with control individuals who do not have the condition

  Good-quality "case series" where complete group of patients, all with the same condition/disease/ therapeutic intervention, are described, without a comparison control group

- *Level 4* evidence includes expert opinion were the opinion is based not on evidence but on "first principles" (e.g., physiological or anatomical) or bench research. The Delphi process can be used to give "expert opinion" greater authority. In the Delphi process, a series of questions are posed to a panel; the answers are collected into a series of "options"; the options are serially ranked; if a 75 % agreement is reached, then a Delphi consensus statement can be made

Grades of recommendation

Any ICUD will use the four grades from the Oxford system. As with the levels of evidence, the grades of evidence may apply either positively (do the procedure) or negatively (do not do the procedure). Where there are three well-conducted RCTs indicating that Drug A was superior to placebo, but one RCT whose results show no difference, then there has to be an individual judgment as to the grade of recommendation given and the rationale explained

- *Grade A* recommendation usually depends on consistent Level 1 evidence and often means that the recommendation is effectively mandatory and placed within a clinical care pathway. However, there will be occasions where excellent evidence (Level 1) does not lead to a Grade A recommendation, for example, if therapy is prohibitively expensive, dangerous, or unethical. Grade A recommendation can follow from Level 2 evidence. However, a Grade A recommendation needs a greater body of evidence if based on anything except Level 1 evidence

- *Grade B* recommendation usually depends on consistent Level 2 and or 3 studies, or "majority evidence" from RCTs

- *Grade C* recommendation usually depends on Level 4 studies or "majority evidence" from Level 2/3 studies or Delphi processed expert opinion

- *Grade D* "No recommendation possible" would be used where the evidence is inadequate or conflicting and when expert opinion is delivered without a formal analytical process, such as by Delphi

Dietary Bladder Irritants. A large percentage of patients with bladder pain syndrome/interstitial cystitis (BPS/IC) report sensitivities to a wide variety of foods, beverages, and supplements [18]. The ICI Committee on Bladder Pain Syndrome recommended that personalized dietary manipulation be part of the therapeutic strategy for patients with BPS/IC (LOE: 2, R: B). For LUTS, a reduction in caffeine intake was recommended for those with incontinence (LOE: 2, R: B).

Bowel Function. Chronic constipation has been linked to LUTS [19] by some investigators, and the ICI concluded there is "some evidence" to suggest that chronic straining may be a risk factor for the development of UI (LOE: 3, further research recommended on the effects of resolving constipation on UI).

Smoking. Data suggest that smoking increases the risk of more severe UI (LOE: 3). Further studies were recommended to determine whether smoking cessation prevents the onset or promotes the resolution of UI. If smoking is a factor, and the reason is related to coughing and repeated increased intra-abdominal pressure, one would expect that the same association would apply to various pulmonary diseases.

Obesity and Weight Loss. Seventeen studies were reviewed by the ICI and the conclusions were that (1) obesity is an important independent risk factor for the prevalence of UI; (2) massive weight loss (15–20 BMI points) significantly decreases UI in morbidly obese women (LOE: 2); and (3) moderate weight loss may be effective in decreasing UI especially if combined with exercise (LOE: 1). A Grade A recommendation for morbidly and moderately obese women was that weight loss should be considered as a first-line treatment to reduce the prevalence of UI and that, given the high prevalence of both UI and obesity in women, the dual issues of weight loss and prevention of weight gain and exercise should be given high priority.

The ICI Committee on Conservative Therapy for sphincter- and bladder-related incontinence cited 439 articles in its well-chosen bibliography and made a number of summary statements with levels of evidence (LOE) and grades of recommendation (R), based on the modified Oxford system [1]. As a summary and conclusion, most of these are selected and reproduced here:

1. Pregnancy and birth appear to be important factors associated with the development of UI in women. Therefore, all women who have had a child or children might be considered "at risk" of developing UI at a later date.

   Continent pregnant women having their first baby who participated in a more "intensive and supervised" PFMT program than the PFMT provided as part of a usual care were less likely to experience UI from late pregnancy up to 6 months postpartum (LOE: 1). There was not sufficient evidence available to demonstrate whether this benefit persists at 12 months postpartum; results from a single trial suggest the benefit of PFMT is not maintained 8 years after treatment or with subsequent deliveries (LOE: 2). There was no evidence investigating the preventive effects of PFMT in pregnant, previously continent multiparous women.

   Continent, pregnant women having their first baby should be offered a supervised (including regular health professional contact) and intensive strengthening antepartum PFMT program to prevent postpartum UI (R: A). The usual or standard approach to PFMT for pregnancy (which is commonly verbal or written instruction without confirmation of correct contraction or supervision of training) needs to be reviewed.

   Additional trials with longer-term follow-up (greater than 12 months postnatal) are needed to determine long-term benefits of antenatal PFMT. Further large, good-quality RCTs are needed to investigate the effect of antepartum PFMT on preventing postpartum UI in multiparous women.

2. To date, only one trial has investigated the effect of PFMT for the treatment of UI in pregnant women. This was a moderate-size study that did not report allocation concealment or blinding of the assessors and did not describe the type of PFMT program employed. In the absence of any detail on the PFMT program, it is impossible to judge if the intervention had the potential to be effective.

   Postpartum women with UI who were randomized to PFMT taught and supervised by a health professional were less likely to be incontinent than controls (standard care or relaxation massage) 6–12 months following delivery (LOE: 1). Of the three trials, the one that used an extensively supervised strength training program demonstrated the greatest treatment effect. It is unclear if the benefit of PFMT is maintained over time or with subsequent deliveries (LOE: 2).

   For women who have persistent symptoms of UI at 3 months postpartum, PFMT is a more effective treatment than standard postnatal or relaxation massage; effects might be greater with supervised and intensive strengthening PFMT (with the addition of electrical stimulation).

It is not clear if the effect can be sustained over the long term; there is also no data on the effect or short periodic refresher sessions on long-term effect.

PFMT should be offered as first-line conservative therapy to women with persistent UI symptoms 3 months after delivery (R: A); an "intensive" PFMT program (in terms of supervision and exercise content) is likely to increase the treatment effect (R: B).

There is a need for at least one large, pragmatic, well-conducted, and explicitly reported trial with long-term follow-up (5+ years) of postpartum PFMT that investigates the effect of "intensive" treatment followed by periodic refresher sessions.

3. The effect of antepartum PFMT or postpartum PFMT, in groups of women where some did and some did not have prior UI symptoms, varied by study with some showing benefit on UI prevalence whereas some did not (LOE: 2). The characteristics of the three trials, all methodologically robust, that demonstrated some effects were:

   a. *For antepartum PFMT*: pregnant women having their first baby and using intensively supervised strengthening PFMT programs; PFMT reduced UI prevalence in late pregnancy and 3–6 months postpartum, but this was not evident 6 years after the index delivery.

   b. *For postpartum PFMT*: primiparous and multiparous women at potentially greater risk of postpartum UI after a large baby or forceps delivery and using a strengthening PFMT program; PFMT reduced UI prevalence at 3 months postpartum but not at 1 year.

   Health providers should carefully consider the cost/benefit of population-based approaches to health professional-taught antepartum or postpartum PFMT, that is, health professional instruction to all pregnant or postpartum women regardless of their current or prior incontinence status (R: B).

   Where a population approach is used, the "best" evidence to date suggests the following: (a) an intervention comprising a daily home PFMT and weekly physiotherapist-led exercise classes for 12 weeks, starting at 20–24 weeks of gestation for pregnant women having their first baby, and (b) an individually taught strengthening PFMT program that incorporates adherence strategies for postpartum women who have had a forceps delivery or a vaginal delivery of a large baby (4,000 g or more) (R: C).

4. PFMT is better than no treatment, a placebo drug, or an inactive control treatment for women with SUI, UUI, or MUI (LOE: 1). Women treated with PFMT were more likely to report a cure or improvement and a better quality of life; they also indicated fewer daily leakage episodes and had less urine leakage on a pad and paper towel test than those in the control group immediately after treatment and in long term. The effect of PFMT in women with SUI does not seem to decrease with increased age: in trials with older women with SUI, it appeared both primary and secondary outcome measures were comparable to those in trials focused on younger women. Moreover, the treatment effect appears to be enhanced where PFMT is based on sound muscle training principles such as specificity, overload progression, correct contraction confirmed prior to training, and use of the Knack (LOE: 4). Supervised PFMT should be offered as a first-line conservative therapy for women of all ages with SUI, urge, or MUI (R: A).

5. With regard to clinic-based biofeedback (BF), studies were inconsistent. The larger trials indicated no statistically significant differences between BF-assisted and non-BF groups for self-reported cure, cure/improvement, or leakage episodes per day or quality of life (LOE: 1). This pattern appeared to be consistent across trials that recruited women with SUI, UUI, or MUI. There were similar numbers of trials addressing the effect of home BF, but fewer data. In a single robust trial, there were no statistically significant differences between home BF and non-BF groups for self-reported cure, cure/improvement, or quality of life for women with urodynamic SUI (LOE: 2).

Clinicians should provide the most intensive health provider (HP)-led PFMT program possible within service constraints because HP-taught and HP-supervised programs are better than self-directed programs, and more HP contact is better than less (R: A). Although studies are inconsistent, this does not appear to be a clear benefit of adding clinic- (R: A) or home-based BF (R: B) to a PFMT program. Based on limited available data, it appears that PFMT with regular (e.g., weekly) supervision is better than PFMT with little or no supervision. However, the data were unclear if supervision is more effective in individual or group settings. Clinicians should provide the most intensive supervision-led PFMT program possible within service constraints because supervised PFMT programs are better than those with little or no supervision (R: A).

6. In the 11 trials that compared PFMT with vaginal cones (VCs) in women with SUI, no consistent pattern emerged in the data. Further, data on self-reported cure in eight of the trials were inconsistent and there was no difference in the pooled data from six trials for self-reported cure/improvement. Notably, there were in fact fewer daily leakage episodes with PFMT in the pooled data from three trials (LOE: 1).

PFMT and EStim in women with SUI were compared in six trials. Pooled data demonstrated that self-reported cure and cure/improvement were more likely in PFMT than in EStim groups (LOE: 1). It is worth noting that only one trial individually demonstrated a statistically significant difference in these outcomes and there was more health professional contact in the PFMT arm. There were no statistically significant differences between PFMT and EStim groups for leakage episodes or quality of life, based on a single trial on MUI (LOE: 2). In one of the trials that recruited women with SUI, UUI, or MUI, self-reported cure/improvement rates were not statistically significantly different (LOE: 2). Self-reported cure and cure/improvement rates and satisfaction were not statistically significant different in the two trials in women with UUI, although PFMT women had fewer leakage episodes per day, and women in the

EStim group had better quality of life in three of the nine domains measured on the KHQ (LOE: 2). Some women reported adverse events attributed to electrical stimulation.

A comparison of PFMT and bladder training (BT) was reported in three trials but only two included data of interest. In women with SUI, symptomatic improvement, leakage episodes, and quality of life were statistically significantly better in the PFMT group (LOE: 2). In contrast, the study that recruited women with SUI, UUI, and MUI did not find statistically significant differences between the groups (LOE: 2).

There is insufficient evidence to determine if PFMT is better than vaginal estrogens. Neither trial that compared an adrenergic agonist with PFMT in women with SUI or MUI found a difference in self-reported cure/improvement, and adrenergic side effects were bothersome (LOE: 2). One trial of PFMT versus oxybutynin in women with DO or DO with urodynamic SUI found women doing PFMT were more likely to report improvement and have fewer leakage episodes per day after treatment (LOE: 2). Many women taking oxybutynin reported drug-related side effects. One trial compared a serotonin–norepinephrine reuptake inhibitor (duloxetine) with PFMT, and while women who took the drug had fewer leakage episodes, there was no difference in terms of quality of life between the two groups, and drug side effects were sufficient to discontinue treatment in some women (LOE: 2).

Based on one trial, it seemed self-reported cure was more likely after surgery than PFMT for women with urodynamic SUI, but no statistically significant difference in the proportion of women reporting cure/improvement (LOE: 2). There was insufficient detail about the PFMT program to make a judgment about how effective it might have been.

For women with SUI:
- PFMT is better than EStim as first-line conservative therapy, particularly if PFMT is intensively supervised (R: B).
- PFMT is better than BT as first-line conservative therapy (R: B).
- PFMT and duloxetine are both effective in first-line therapy, although PFMT is better

because of the side effects experienced with the drug (R: C).

- PFMT and surgery are both effective therapies, although PFMT is better as first-line therapy because it is less invasive (R: C).

For women with SUI or MUI:

- PFMT is better than VC as first-line conservative therapy (R: B).

For women with UUI or MUI:

- PFMT and BT are effective first-line conservative therapy (R: B).
- PFMT is better than oxybutynin as first-line conservative therapy (R: B).

For women with UUI or UUI:

- PFMT and BT are effective first-line conservative therapies (R: B).
- There were few trials addressing the effect of adding PFMT to another therapy, and only five of the eight studies reported useful data. There appears to be no benefit of adding PFMT to VC or duloxetine, respectively, in women with SUI (LOE: 2). There may be benefit to adding PFMT to BT for women with urodynamic SUI or SUI with DO in the short term (3 months), but it is not clear if this benefit persists at 6 months or more (LOE: 2). There is not sufficient evidence to be sure if there is any benefit in adding PFMT to ES. There is a single trial indicating added benefit of PFMT when drug therapy is administered with the usual intensity.

For women with SUI or MUI, a combination of PFMT/BT may be better than BT alone in the short term (R: C), and a combination of PFMT/drug may be better than drug alone. IF a woman is taking duloxetine or using VC, it may not help to add PFMT (R: C). However, these recommendations are based on single trials of variable quality, and larger, good-quality trials are needed to address each of the above comparisons if these are of interest to women. Further, these studies examine the effects of combining therapies as an initial approach. Less is known about the effects of combining therapies in a stepped fashion when women do not achieve the desired outcomes with a single therapy.

8. There is no good evidence to date to suggest that "healthy" older women with UI benefit less from PFMT compared to younger women.

9. It is not clear if there are any reliable predictors of PFMT outcome. Too few trials have appropriately investigated the association between patient characteristics and outcome.

10. There is no trial evidence to suggest the more effective method or specific parameters of BT. For those undertaking BT, it is likely that more health professional contact will be better than less, based on the developing evidence for PFMT, which, like BT, requires behavioral change. The literature suggests several variables that could be investigated in future trials including the instructional approach, supervisory intensity, strategies for controlling urgency, scheduling parameters, frequency of schedule adjustments, length of treatment, and use of adjunctive treatments.

It is not clear what the most effective BT parameters are. Clinicians and researchers are advised to refer to the operant conditioning and educational literature to provide a rationale for their choice of BT parameters or approach (R: D). Clinicians should provide the most intensive BT supervision that is possible within service constraints (R: D). Most research is needed to investigate which BT parameters, supervisory intensity, and adjunctive treatments are most effective. Future trials should include outcomes that matter to patients, including the length and frequency of supervisory contact.

11. Although the few trials available were small and of variable quality, there is minimal Level 1 evidence that BT may be an effective treatment for women with UUI, SUI, and MUI (LOE: 1). BT is an appropriate first-line conservative therapy for UI in women (R: A). Additional high-quality studies are needed that examine the effect of BT versus no treatment in treatment of women with UUI, SUI, and MUI.

12. In two small trials comparing BT plus placebo drug versus BT plus drug in DO, there was a suggestion that the effect of BT might be enhanced by active drug (LOE: 2). However, both trials were small, placebo controlled, and conducted in gender-mixed sample populations, and the outcomes were

not common to both trials. Thus, there is insufficient evidence to derive a conclusion related to the effectiveness of augmenting BT with drug therapy. Direct comparisons of BT versus BT with drug are needed to address the question of whether the effect of BT can be augmented by drug therapy.

13. A single trial found that combining BT with PFMT improves short-term outcomes compared to PFMT alone, but the added benefit did not persist 3 months later. There is no evidence for an added benefit of combining brief written BT instructions with tolterodine (2 mg twice daily) compared to tolterodine alone for urge incontinence (LOE: 2), although his trial included men and women and it is not known if one gender did better than the other with respect to outcome. The use of BT with solifenacin (5/10 mg) adds benefit to symptom reduction at 8 weeks compared to solifenacin alone, mainly to symptoms of frequency (LOE: 2). This evidence is related to men and women.

    The current evidence is conflicting for the addition of written information on bladder training for women taking an antimuscarinic drug. One trial states no clinical benefit in adding brief written instruction in BT (R: B), while another suggests no significant improvements to urgency and urge incontinence but significant improvements in frequency (R: B). More research is needed using an appropriate supervised BT program combined with anticholinergic or antimuscarinic drug therapies versus drug alone.

14. There are no RCTs, or high-quality observational studies, providing evidence on the effects of timed voiding for UI in women. Based upon the data from one small uncontrolled study, it seemed a 2-h timed voiding schedule may be beneficial in treating women with mild UI, infrequent voiding patterns, and stable bladder function (LOE: 3). Timed voiding with a 2-h voiding interval may be beneficial as a sole intervention for women with mild UI infrequent voiding patterns (R: C). It may also be helpful as an adjunct to the other treatment.

15. Scheduled voiding regimens have been implemented in many forms and with a variety of intensities ranging from strict inpatient regimens to simple instruction sheets. Most research has examined BT, and most of these trials have recruited women with symptoms of UUI or OAB. The indications so far are that BT is effective for reducing UI, as well as frequency of micturition. The scant research comparing BT to drug therapy is inconsistent with some evidence for the superiority of each. It is not yet clear whether BT can enhance BT, or whether BT can enhance UI outcomes from drug therapy, although it appears that reductions in frequency of micturition may be greater with the addition of BT.

16. Overall there are still no prospective studies of lifestyle intervention to prevent prolapse. There is now further evidence that occupations involving heavy lifting/hard physical labor or being overweight may play a role in the development of POP (LOE: 3).

    Constipation is a modifiable risk factor which perhaps has potential to impact on development of prolapse symptoms. However, evidence regarding the association between constipation or straining at stool and prolapse remains conflicting. New studies were reasonably sized and adjusted for covariates. No further studies on anemia were found. A study of vitamin D found no association with self-reported bulge.

17. Currently, there is no evidence from intervention studies regarding the role of PFMT or other physical therapies in the prevention of POP; better PFM function may be associated with less risk of prolapse (LOE: 3).

18. It was concluded that PFMT can improve the symptoms of prolapse and the anatomical defects (LOE: 1).

    No further evidence is available regarding the role of PFMT as an adjunct to surgery. Pre- and postoperative PFMT may help to improve quality of life and urinary symptoms in women undergoing surgery for POP, but the findings regarding its effects on PFM strength are contradictory.

The evidence available however is based on two small trials, one of which included women undergoing surgery for UI and/or prolapse (LOE: 2).

PFMT can improve prolapse symptoms and severity (R: A). Perioperative PFMT may help improve quality of life and urinary symptoms in women undergoing surgery for prolapse (R: C). Larger trials are needed, and prolapse-specific measures should be primary outcomes in such trials. Future studies of PFMT for POP should aim to reach a consensus on the optimal intervention program prescribed and might also consider comparisons of individualized training with group training.

19. A total of ten trials were found applying a variety of pre- or postoperative PFMT-based interventions (or a combination of both). Any differences between experimental and control groups were modest and short term; differences did not appear to be sustained up to 12 months post-surgery. A particular challenge in evaluating the trials was that participant-reported outcomes in three of the studies all indicated some level of improvement in the treatment groups; however, there were no clear differences in pad test results in any of the trials. Because all the studies reviewed were generally small, varied in design, and had different outcome measures, it is difficult to interpret them as a whole. While the evidence that therapist-delivered PFMT with or without BF before or after surgery improves continence recovery after radical prostatectomy remains inconsistent, there is some suggestion that men who undergo some sort of conservative management including PFMT will achieve continence in a shorter time frame than non-treated men but that this difference is not significant at 12 months post-surgery (LOE: 2). Further discussion is needed on the outcomes of most importance. It is possible that the emphasis on quantitative outcomes is not meaningful to participants; men appear to find therapy personally helpful and value the direction provided by a therapist.

    Some preoperative or immediate postoperative instructions in PFMT for men undergoing radical prostatectomy may be helpful (R: B); whether this is in the form of "hands-on" therapy of verbal instruction and support remains unclear. Studies comparing the effectiveness of pre- versus postoperative PFMT, and the number of sessions required, are needed so that practitioners may advise men about preoperative preparation, and budget-conscious health boards can make informed decisions on program funding. In designing such studies, the natural history of UI after radical prostatectomy must be taken into account because the spontaneous recovery rate means that sample sizes must be large to detect any differences between protocols.

20. The most recent and largest trials which compared PFMT taught by digital rectal exam (DRE) or no instruction used different approaches to defining and measuring continence and showed conflicting results. In three smaller and earlier trials, in which the control groups had written or verbal instructions on PFMT, there were no statistically significant differences between groups on pad test (LOE: 2). Clinical heterogeneity makes it difficult to consider the findings from the studies as a whole.

    Some instruction in PFMT may be helpful; the objective benefit of the PFMT remains unclear. Whether PFMT taught by DRE offers any benefit over and above verbal or written instruction (R: B) is not clear. Further well-designed studies using standardized outcome measures and participant input are needed to test this hypothesis.

21. Health professional instruction in PFMT with biofeedback (BF) after radical prostatectomy when compared with control conditions seemed to reduce the amount of leakage in the early weeks of recovery (up to 3 months). However, comparisons of PFMT with clinic BF versus PFMT at home did not find similar differences. Based on the current evidence, the addition of EStim or BF does not appear to improve continence outcomes over and above PFMT (LOE: 2). However, BF may be less difficult for the therapist than DRE. It seems men who participate in PFMT

compared to no active treatment might have less leakage in the first 3 months post-operatively. To the individual, this early improvement may be important in activity, well-being, and socializing. Such concepts require further investigation.

The use of BF in clinic, over and above home PFMT, is currently a therapist/individual decision based on economics and preference (R: B).

22. Seven RCTs investigated the addition of EStim to PFMT plus or minus BF for men with post-prostatectomy incontinence. Data suggested no further benefit of EStim when added to PFMT over PFMT alone, although EStim may help achieve continence earlier in men with severe incontinence post-prostatectomy; the numbers in each trial were relatively small (LOE: 2). For men with post-prostatectomy incontinence, there does not appear to be any benefit of adding EStim to a PFMT program (R: B).

23. Based on two small studies, it seems that PFMT and urethral milking might be both effective in the control of the annoying symptom of post-micturition dribbling (PMD) (LOE: 2). Men can be offered instruction to do a strong PFM contraction immediately after voiding, or urethral massage to empty the urethra, to improve symptoms of PMD (R: C).

References

1. Moore K, Bradley C, Burgio B, et al. Adult conservative treatment. In: Abrams P, Cardozo L, Khoury S, Wein A, editors. Incontinence, EAU/ICUD. Plymouth: Health Publications Ltd; 2013. p. 1101–227.
2. Newman D, Wein A. Managing and treating urinary incontinence, Health Professions Press, Baltimore; 2009:233–244, 245–306, CD-ROM on Patient and providers Tools and Forms.
3. Wallace SA, Roe B, Williams K, Palmer M. Bladder training for urinary incontinence in adults. Cochrane Database Syst Rev. 2010:10.
4. Ostaszkiewicz J, Johnston L, Roe B. Timed voiding for the management of urinary incontinence in adults. Cochrane Database Syst Rev. 2010:11.
5. Payne CK. Conservative management of urinary incontinence. In: Wein A, Kavoussi L, Novick A, Partin A, Peters C, editors. Campbell-Walsh urology. Philadelphia: Elsevier/Saunders; 2012. p. 2003–25.
6. Newman PK, Wein AJ, Office based behavioral therapy for management of incontinence and other pelvic disorders. UROL Clinics North Am, 2013;40:613–36.
7. Ostaszkiewicz J, Chestney T, Roe B. Habit retraining for the management of urinary incontinence in adults. Cochrane Database Syst Rev. 2009:1.
8. Eustice S, Roe B, Paterson J. Prompted voiding for the management of urinary incontinence in adults. Cochrane Database Syst Rev. 2009:1.
9. Miller JM, Sampselle C, Ashton-Miller J, Hong GR, DeLancey JO. Clarification and confirmation of the Knack maneuver: the effect of volitional pelvic floor muscle contraction to preempt expected stress incontinence. Int Urogynecol J Pelvic Floor Dysfunct. 2008;19(6):773–82.
10. DeLancey JOL. Structural aspects of urethrovesical function in the female. Neurourol Urodyn. 1988;7(6):509–19.
11. Bø K. Pelvic floor muscle exercise for the treatment of stress urinary incontinence: an exercise physiology perspective. Int Urogynecol J Pelvic Floor Dysfunct. 1995;6(5):282–91.
12. Bø K. Pelvic floor muscle training is effective in treatment of female stress urinary incontinence, but how does it work? Int Urogynecol J Pelvic Floor Dysfunct. 2004;15(2):76–84.
13. Godec C, Cass AS, Ayala GF. Bladder inhibition with functional electrical stimulation. Urology. 1975;6(6):663–6.
14. Burgio KL, Whitehead WE, Engel BT. Urinary incontinence in the elderly. Bladder-sphincter biofeedback and toileting skills training. Ann Intern Med. 1985;103(4):507–15.
15. Segal S, Saks EK, Arya LA. Self-assessment of fluid intake behavior in women with urinary incontinence. J Womens Health (Larchmt). 2011;20(12):1971–21.
16. Hashim H, Abrams P. How should patients with overactive bladder manipulate their fluid intake? BJU Int. 2008;102(1):62–6.
17. Hanno P, Dinis P, Lin A, et al. Bladder pain syndrome. In: Abrams P, Cardozo L, Khoury S, Wein A, editors. Incontinence, EAU/ICUD. Plymouth: Health Publications Ltd; 2013. p. 1581–650.
18. Hanno PM. Bladder pain syndrome (interstitial Cystitis) and related disorders. In: Wein A, Kavoussi L, Novick A, Partin A, Peters C, editors. Campbell-Walsh urology. Philadelphia: Elsevier/Saunders; 2012. p. 357–401.
19. Cardozo L, Robinson D. Special considerations in premenopausal and postmenopausal women with symptoms of overactive bladder. Urology. 2002;60:64–71.
20. Abrams P, Khoury S, Grant A. Evidence based medicine—overview of the main steps for developing and grading guideline recommendation. In: Abrams P, Cardozo L, Khoury S, Wein J, editors. Incontinence, EAU/ICUD. Plymouth: Health Publications Ltd; 2013. p. 8–9.

Urinary Catheters and Other Devices

Dev Mohan Gulur and Marcus J. Drake

A urinary catheter is a device draining urine directly from the bladder. Catheter placement can employ either the urethral or suprapubic route; the latter is often necessary if urinary retention is associated with urethral stricture, or bladder neck contracture. The prevalence of long-term catheter use in the community is 0.07 % and increases to 0.5 % for people aged over 75 years [1]. A European survey reported a 23 % prevalence of long-term catheterisation (LTC) in older people in residential care [2]. Catheters can be hard to tolerate and are prone to complications. Accordingly, due consideration should be employed in deciding whether catheterisation, particularly LTC, is appropriate for management of a particular patient.

Indications

1. *Bladder outlet obstruction*: benign prostate enlargement (BPE), prostate cancer, strictures and bladder neck contractures. Retention is more common in men than women with a 13:1 ratio [3] [4]. In acute urinary retention

(AUR), which is a painful condition, a urinary catheter is used for urgent decompression of the bladder and symptom relief. AUR could be secondary to a urinary tract infection, BPE, prostate cancer, trauma and post-operatively after a general anaesthetic. Over a 4-year period, approximately 7 % of men with BPE may suffer an episode of AUR [5]. For AUR, the catheter is generally a temporary mode of decompressing the bladder in the acute setting. In high-pressure chronic retention, LTC may be needed if a patient is not suitable for definitive treatment, such as transurethral resection of the prostate.

2. *Urgency and stress urinary incontinence*: LTC is an option in an elderly, infirm patient with severe urgency incontinence resistant to behavioural modification and pharmaceutical treatment. However, the presence of a foreign body and associated bacteriuria is often poorly tolerated. Elderly patients with stress incontinence who are not medically fit for definitive surgery can be managed with LTC, as an alternative to use of containment products.

Contained incontinence is achieved with continence products like catheters in situations where a definitive surgical management is not feasible or non-existent and substantially improves the quality of life [6]. The stigma associated with incontinence is reduced if the patients are able to contain and conceal the incontinence [7].

3. *Neurological disorders*: Conditions such as spinal cord injury (SCI), spina bifida, multiple

D.M. Gulur, M.B.B.S., M.R.C.S.
Department of Urology, Aintree University Hospital NHS Foundation Trust, Liverpool, UK

M.J. Drake, M.A. (Cantab),
D.M. (Oxon.), F.R.C.S. (Urol.) (✉)
University of Bristol and Bristol Urological Institute, Bristol, UK
e-mail: marcus.drake@bui.ac.uk

A.J. Wein et al. (eds.), *Bladder Dysfunction in the Adult: The Basis for Clinical Management*, Current Clinical Urology, DOI 10.1007/978-1-4939-0853-0_12, © Springer Science+Business Media New York 2014

sclerosis, spinal tumour, prolapsed interverte-bral disc and diabetic uropathy lead to neuro-pathic lower urinary tract dysfunction. In severe cases lacking alternatives, LTC can be considered. In patients with impaired perineal sensation, particular care is needed to avoid LTC in view of potential complications such as urethral breakdown. LTC can serve to pro-tect the upper urinary tract function in severe neuropathic bladder dysfunction [8].

Types of Urinary Catheter

There are various ways by which urinary cathe-ters can be categorised, and these are set out in Table 12.1.

Indwelling Catheters

Route of access can either be urethral or suprapu-bic (SPC). SPC is generally better tolerated than urethral, with higher levels of patient comfort and satisfaction [9, 10], because of the avoidance of urethral irritation. Catheter changes are usu-ally less uncomfortable. The suprapubic route avoids potential risk of traumatic hypospadias or ischaemic urethral strictures seen with long-standing urethral catheterisation. There is evi-dence to suggest that spinal cord injury patients with long-term SPC have significantly lower incidence of UTI than those using urethral cath-eters [11]. SPC use also enables patients to retain sexual activity [12].

The insertion of an SPC may require a gen-eral anaesthetic, though insertion under local

Table 12.1 Types of urinary catheter and adaptations for specific purposes

Categorising feature	Examples
Route of access	Urethral, suprapubic, extra-anatomical
Dwell time	Indwelling, intermittent
Number of lumina	Single, double, 3-way
Retention mechanism	Balloon, malecot ("winged")
Material	Various
Coating	Various
End configuration	Angle ended, whistle tip

anaesthetic is possible with appropriate facilities and expertise [13]. Contraindications to SPC placement include haematuria of unknown ori-gin, history of bladder tumours, small-capacity bladder, presence of scars in the lower part of the abdomen, anticoagulants and presence of vascu-lar grafts (particularly femoral-femoral cross-over grafts). Bowel perforation is a recognised serious complication, especially in patients with previous lower abdominal surgery [14]. This can be prevented to a degree by using real-time ultra-sound [15, 16], but open cystotomy under general anaesthetic remains the safer option.

Intermittent Catheters

Guttman and Frankel introduced sterile intermit-tent catheterisation in spinal cord injury patients in 1947 [17]. The concept of clean intermittent self-catheterisation (CISC) was introduced by Lapides et al. in 1972 [18]. Intermittent catheterisation avoids the morbidity of an indwelling catheter and can be useful in monitoring return of voiding in potentially reversible causes, by allowing regular measurement of the postvoid residuals [19, 20]. It is preferable in spinal injury patients [21].

CISC also has an important role after endo-scopic management of urethral strictures in reduc-ing the recurrence of urethral strictures when used for sufficient duration after an optical urethrot-omy [22]. CISC may improve a patient's self-esteem relative to LTC [23], it may improve the sexual life of incontinent patients [24], and it can improve the social activities of children [25, 26].

Frequency of catheterisations for CISC is determined according to whether the patient is able to expel any urine without a catheter, what the bladder can safely hold comfortably and the overall fluid output.

Structural Catheter Adaptations

1. *Number of lumina*: Catheters can be single-lumen, 2-way or 3-way. Single-lumen cathe-ters are used for intermittent catheterisation. 2-way catheters have a second channel to inflate the balloon, along with the urine

drainage channel; this is the most commonly used variety of indwelling catheter. 3-way catheters have an additional channel used for irrigating, which is useful in haematuria and after transurethral resection of the prostate or a bladder tumour (TURP/TURBT).

2. *Configuration and retaining mechanisms*: The tip of a catheter can be open (whistle tip) or closed (for easier insertion). The end of a closed catheter can be straight or curved, for example, coude (bent), or bent and pointed (Tiemann tip). Foley catheters are held in place by an inflated balloon. A stitch is used to retain Bonanno catheters. A Malecot catheter is held in place by its retractable wings.

3. *Materials and coatings*: The most common material is latex, which can be pure latex, or latex coated with polytetrafluoroethylene (PTFE) or hydrogel. Silicone is another catheter material, which is more rigid, causes less inflammation and may be less likely to get encrusted. The nature of the material and its coatings determine the maximum duration for which a catheter can be used before it has to be changed. This is typically in the range 1–3 months. Polyvinyl chloride (PVC) catheters can be used for large-bore 3-way catheters as an alternative to silicone.

Complications and Disadvantages of Long-Term Catheters

The risk of complications of LTC may be as high as 70 % [27]. A study of 117 octogenarian incontinent medical patients given the choices of diaper, medication, scheduled toileting and catheter found that urinary catheter was their least favourite choice [28].

1. *Blockages and encrustation*: Recurrent catheter blockages due to encrustation of mineral deposits (calcium phosphate and magnesium ammonium phosphate, or struvite) occur in up to 80 % of LTC users [1, 29–31]. Precipitation of minerals in the urine is facilitated by the presence of urea-splitting organisms, like *Proteus mirabilis*, which render the urine alkaline [30, 32–34]. In vitro studies have shown that encrustation can be reduced by

increasing the fluid intake to dilute the urine and by increasing the citrate concentration of the urine by drinking orange juice and other citric fruit juices [35].

2. *Infections*: 80 % of nosocomial UTIs are in patients with indwelling catheters [36]. Risk of bacteriuria increases by 5–8 % per day after catheterisation, and all LTC patients are likely to have bacteriuria by 4 weeks [37–39], with subsequent development of catheter-associated urinary tract infection (CAUTI). Most infecting organisms are from the patient's own colonic or perineal flora or contamination from the healthcare personnel during insertion [40]. Microorganisms form a biofilm on the catheter in combination with host proteins and microbial exopolysaccharides [41, 42]; within the biofilm, bacteria are less susceptible to antibiotics [40]. A review of five randomised controlled clinical trials comparing SPC and urethral catheters after colorectal surgery found less CAUTIs with SPC, and patients reported less discomfort and pain with SPC [43]. Silver ions are bactericidal and non-toxic to humans on topical application. A Cochrane review [44] compared catheters impregnated with silver alloy or silver oxide (antiseptic catheters) and antibiotic-impregnated catheters (minocycline, rifampicin and nitrofurazone) and found that asymptomatic bacteriuria decreased in both the groups in patients catheterised for a short term (less than a week of catheterisation in hospitalised adults for antibiotic-impregnated catheters). However, a large-scale randomised Health Technology Appraisal found the clinical effectiveness for nitrofurazone-impregnated catheters was less than the pre-specified minimum, though possibly cost-effective, and found that silver alloy-coated catheters were not clinically effective or cost-effective [45].

3. *Stones*: Urinary stones can occur in 25 % of patients with LTC [46]. Incidence of bladder stones in SCI patients with LTC is between 25 and 35 % [47, 48]. The stones can cause blockage and bypassing recurrently. Encrustation and biofilm formation cause bladder stones [33, 49–51] and can occur in 45 % of patients with LTC [46].

Encrustation is due to *Proteus mirabilis* and other urease-producing bacteria [52] which render the urine alkaline and promote stone formation due to precipitation of calcium and magnesium salts. Recurrent stone formation is a problem which may warrant cystoscopic surveillance [46].

4. *Malignancy*: Squamous cell carcinoma of the bladder is a rare potential risk. It has been described in SCI patients with LTC or ISC [53, 54], and if LTC has been used for more than 10 years, the incidence of bladder SCC may be 10 % [55]. However, the exact role of the catheter needs to be ascertained, as the risk of bladder cancer in SCI patients without LTC has been reported as greater than for the general population [56]. Regular surveillance cystoscopy would be a reasonable option to monitor these patients.

5. *Urethral damage*: The urethra is a fragile structure, and placement of an indwelling catheter chronically can lead to breakdown. In men this can cause traumatic hypospadias at the urethral meatus. In women, the urethra can break down completely, resulting in expulsion of the catheter even when the retaining mechanism is functional. Consequently, the suprapubic route is preferred if long-term urinary catheter use is anticipated.

6. *Impaired quality of life (QoL)*: It can take up to a year for patients to accept an indwelling long-term catheter [57]. This may reduce if they are given information leaflets to help them understand catheters better [58]. Embarrassment and restriction of daily normal activities are problematic, particularly during catheter change, emptying of the bag or when a catheter accidentally spills or leaks in public [59, 60]. Visibility of the catheter bag has been perceived as demeaning [60, 61]. QoL questionnaires are being developed for ISC [62] and LTC [63] Catheters have a negative impact on the quality of life because of CAUTI, blockages, leakage and dislodgement. The risk of urethral trauma and bleeding is high if the catheter gets accidentally pulled with the balloon inflated. This is common in the elderly population who are not oriented to time and space, for example, as a consequence of delirium or dementia. Patients who have had catheters for a short time after an episode of acute retention have also reported a negative impact on QoL [64]. Autonomic dysreflexia (AD) is a potentially life-threatening emergency in SCI patients. This can be triggered by catheter blockages or catheter change and manifests clinically with severe headache, hypertension and sweating. Lack of awareness about AD among healthcare providers can cause significant concern to the patients [60, 65]. Pain is another factor which decreases QoL [59]. Pain and discomfort due to bladder spasms may respond to antimuscarinic drugs [66]. Other measures to prevent pain include relieving constipation, using smaller-size catheters and supporting the drainage bag to minimise inadvertent traction on the catheter.

Other Continence Products

Handheld Urinals

Female handheld urinals are made of plastic, cardboard or metal. They are designed to collect urine without spillage and are used in the standing/crouching posture or sitting on the edge of a chair, wheelchair or bed [67]. A powered urinal designed to pump urine into a reservoir has also been reported [68], which obviates the need for gravity-assisted drainage.

Male handheld urinals come in various shapes and sizes and are modified accordingly to be user-friendly for patients. For example, soft plastic urinals are easier to grip for patients with reduced manual dexterity. Urinals designed to be attached to a drainage bag have been used for men living at home with limited support [69].

Pads

Absorbent pads can either be disposable or washable. They are usually body worn but can also be used as underpads on chairs or beds.

The size of the pad depends on the degree of incontinence. Body-worn pads can be inserts (i.e. panty-liners), diapers, pull-ups (similar to toddler trainer pants) and male pouches which fit around the penis. Pads usually have three layers, with an absorbent core between an inner water-permeable coverstock and an outer waterproof layer. The absorbent layer is made of fluffy wood pulp fibre or absorbent polymer or gel.

Penile Sheaths and Mechanical Devices in Men

Close-fitting penile sheaths, also called condom catheters, uridomes or external catheters, can be attached to a drainage bag similar to indwelling catheters. The sheaths are made of various materials (latex, silicone, rubber and synthetic polymers) and come in various sizes. Some have anti-kinking and anti-blow-off features, i.e. a thickened and bulbous distal end that prevents internal walls from sticking to each other, thus minimising the risk of the sheath being dislodged at high urine flow rates. The risks associated with sheaths are skin irritation, allergy or penile compression [70]. Patients find them more comfortable than catheters, with a reduced risk of infection and pain [71]. The drainage bags can either be strapped around the leg or body worn and are made of various materials (PVC, polyvinylidene fluoride (PVDF), polyethylene, rubber or latex).

Penile clamps and peri-penile straps are available, but they have a potential to cause tissue damage and reduce cavernosal artery blood flow. They are considered appropriate only for short periods, e.g. during swimming or excursions. They are generally used as the last resort when all other methods have failed. It is imperative that the chosen patients have good cognitive function and manual dexterity [72].

Urethral Occlusion Devices and Other Mechanical Devices in Women

Devices that occlude the external meatus were reported to have varying efficacy. They are no longer generally available. Intra-urethral devices are self-inserted silicone cylinders which act by occluding the urethra or at the external urethral meatus [73]. Mechanical devices include intravaginal devices like tampons, diaphragms, pessaries and removable intravaginal silastic rings which are primarily designed to support the bladder neck, thereby helping to reduce stress incontinence.

In conclusion, there are various types of catheters and other continence products tailored to individual patients with bladder dysfunction depending on their need, tolerability, manual dexterity and mobility.

References

1. Kohler-Ockmore J, Feneley RC. Long-term catheterization of the bladder: prevalence and morbidity. Br J Urol. 1996;77(3):347–51.
2. Sorbye LW, et al. Indwelling catheter use in home care: elderly, aged 65+, in 11 different countries in Europe. Age Ageing. 2005;34(4):377–81.
3. Mevcha A, Drake MJ. Etiology and management of urinary retention in women. Indian J Urol. 2010;26(2): 230–5.
4. Klarskov P, et al. Acute urinary retention in women: a prospective study of 18 consecutive cases. Scand J Urol Nephrol. 1987;21(1):29–31.
5. McConnell JD, et al. The effect of finasteride on the risk of acute urinary retention and the need for surgical treatment among men with benign prostatic hyperplasia. Finasteride Long-Term Efficacy and Safety Study Group. N Engl J Med. 1998;338(9): 557–63.
6. Fonda D, Abrams P. Cure sometimes, help always—a "continence paradigm" for all ages and conditions. Neurourol Urodyn. 2006;25(3):290–2.
7. Paterson J. Stigma associated with postprostatectomy urinary incontinence. J Wound Ostomy Continence Nurs. 2000;27(3):168–73.
8. Drake MJ, et al. Prospective evaluation of urological effects of aging in chronic spinal cord injury by method of bladder management. Neurourol Urodyn. 2005;24(2):111–6.
9. Warren JW. Catheter-associated bacteriuria. Clin Geriatr Med. 1992;8(4):805–19.
10. Sheriff MK, et al. Long-term suprapubic catheterisation: clinical outcome and satisfaction survey. Spinal Cord. 1998;36(3):171–6.
11. Esclarin De Ruz A, Garcia Leoni E, Herruzo Cabrera R. Epidemiology and risk factors for urinary tract infection in patients with spinal cord injury. J Urol. 2000;164(4):1285–9.
12. Atkinson K. Incorporating sexual health into catheter care. Prof Nurse. 1997;13(3):146–8.

13. Khan A, Abrams P. Suprapubic catheter insertion is an outpatient procedure: cost savings resultant on closing an audit loop. BJU Int. 2009;103(5):640–4.

14. Noller KL, Pratt JH, Symmonds RE. Bowel perforation with suprapubic cystostomy report of two cases. Obstet Gynecol. 1976;48(1 Suppl):67S–9.

15. Aguilera PA, Choi T, Durham BA. Ultrasound-guided suprapubic cystostomy catheter placement in the emergency department. J Emerg Med. 2004;26(3):319–21.

16. Lee MJ, et al. Fluoroscopically guided percutaneous suprapubic cystostomy for long-term bladder drainage: an alternative to surgical cystostomy. Radiology. 1993;188(3):787–9.

17. Guttmann L, Frankel H. The value of intermittent catheterisation in the early management of traumatic paraplegia and tetraplegia. Paraplegia. 1966;4(2):63–84.

18. Lapides J, et al. Clean, intermittent self-catheterization in the treatment of urinary tract disease. J Urol. 1972;107(3):458–61.

19. Patel MI, Watts W, Grant A. The optimal form of urinary drainage after acute retention of urine. BJU Int. 2001;88(1):26–9.

20. Smith NK, Morrant JD. Post-operative urinary retention in women: management by intermittent catheterization. Age Ageing. 1990;19(5):337–40.

21. Abrams P, et al. A proposed guideline for the urological management of patients with spinal cord injury. BJU Int. 2008;101(8):989–94.

22. Harriss DR, et al. Long-term results of intermittent low-friction self-catheterization in patients with recurrent urethral strictures. Br J Urol. 1994;74(6):790–2.

23. Hill VB, Davies WE. A swing to intermittent clean self-catheterisation as a preferred mode of management of the neuropathic bladder for the dextrous spinal cord patient. Paraplegia. 1988;26(6):405–12.

24. Oakeshott P, Hunt GM. Intermittent self catheterization for patients with urinary incontinence or difficulty emptying the bladder. Br J Gen Pract. 1992;42(359):253–5.

25. Robinson RO, Cockram M, Strode M. Severe handicap in spina bifida: no bar to intermittent self catheterisation. Arch Dis Child. 1985;60(8):760–2.

26. Lapides J, et al. Further observations on self-catheterization. J Urol. 1976;116(2):169–71.

27. Kunin CM, et al. The association between the use of urinary catheters and morbidity and mortality among elderly patients in nursing homes. Am J Epidemiol. 1992;135(3):291–301.

28. Pfisterer MH, et al. Geriatric patients' preferences for treatment of urinary incontinence: a study of hospitalized, cognitively competent adults aged 80 and older. J Am Geriatr Soc. 2007;55(12):2016–22.

29. Kunin CM, Chin QF, Chambers S. Formation of encrustations on indwelling urinary catheters in the elderly: a comparison of different types of catheter materials in "blockers" and "nonblockers". J Urol. 1987;138(4):899–902.

30. Getliffe KA. The use of bladder wash-outs to reduce urinary catheter encrustation. Br J Urol. 1994;73(6):696–700.

31. Getliffe K. Managing recurrent urinary catheter blockage: problems, promises, and practicalities. J Wound Ostomy Continence Nurs. 2003;30(3):146–51.

32. Choong SK, et al. The physicochemical basis of urinary catheter encrustation. BJU Int. 1999;83(7):770–5.

33. Cox AJ, et al. Calcium phosphate in catheter encrustation. Br J Urol. 1987;59(2):159–63.

34. Stickler DJ, Zimakoff J. Complications of urinary tract infections associated with devices used for long-term bladder management. J Hosp Infect. 1994;28(3):177–94.

35. Stickler DJ, Morgan SD. Modulation of crystalline Proteus mirabilis biofilm development on urinary catheters. J Med Microbiol. 2006;55(Pt 5):489–94.

36. Edwards JR, et al. National Healthcare Safety Network (NHSN) Report, data summary for 2006, issued June 2007. Am J Infect Control. 2007;35(5):290–301.

37. Mulhall AB, Chapman RG, Crow RA. Bacteriuria during indwelling urethral catheterization. J Hosp Infect. 1988;11(3):253–62.

38. Stamm WE. Catheter-associated urinary tract infections: epidemiology, pathogenesis, and prevention. Am J Med. 1991;91(3B):65S–71.

39. Nicolle LE. The chronic indwelling catheter and urinary infection in long-term-care facility residents. Infect Control Hosp Epidemiol. 2001;22(5):316–21.

40. Maki DG, Tambyah PA. Engineering out the risk for infection with urinary catheters. Emerg Infect Dis. 2001;7(2):342–7.

41. Trautner BW, Darouiche RO. Role of biofilm in catheter-associated urinary tract infection. Am J Infect Control. 2004;32(3):177–83.

42. Nickel JC, et al. Bacterial biofilms: influence on the pathogenesis, diagnosis and treatment of urinary tract infections. J Antimicrob Chemother. 1994;33(Suppl A):31–41.

43. Branagan GW, Moran BJ. Published evidence favors the use of suprapubic catheters in pelvic colorectal surgery. Dis Colon Rectum. 2002;45(8):1104–8.

44. Schumm K, Lam TB. Types of urethral catheters for management of short-term voiding problems in hospitalised adults. Cochrane Database Syst Rev. 2008;2, CD004013.

45. Pickard R, Lam T, Maclennan G, et al. Antimicrobial catheters for reduction of symptomatic urinary tract infection in adults requiring short-term catheterisation in hospital: a multicentre randomised controlled trial. Lancet. 2012;380(9857):1927–35.

46. Khan AA, et al. Developing a strategy to reduce the high morbidity of patients with long-term urinary catheters: the BioMed catheter research clinic. BJU Int. 2007;100(6):1298–301.

47. Ord J, Lunn D, Reynard J. Bladder management and risk of bladder stone formation in spinal cord injured patients. J Urol. 2003;170(5):1734–7.

48. Linsenmeyer MA, Linsenmeyer TA. Accuracy of bladder stone detection using abdominal x-ray after spinal cord injury. J Spinal Cord Med. 2004;27(5):438–42.

49. Hedelin H, et al. Relationship between urease-producing bacteria, urinary pH and encrustation on indwelling urinary catheters. Br J Urol. 1991;67(5):527–31.

50. Morris NS, Stickler DJ, McLean RJ. The development of bacterial biofilms on indwelling urethral catheters. World J Urol. 1999;17(6):345–50.

51. Norberg B, Norberg A, Parkhede U. The spontaneous variation of catheter life in long-stay geriatric in patients with indwelling catheters. Gerontology. 1983;29(5):332–5.

52. Stickler D, et al. Proteus mirabilis biofilms and the encrustation of urethral catheters. Urol Res. 1993;21(6):407–11.

53. Esrig D, McEvoy K, Bennett CJ. Bladder cancer in the spinal cord-injured patient with long-term catheterization: a casual relationship? Semin Urol. 1992;10(2):102–8.

54. Casey RG, et al. Intermittent self-catheterization and the risk of squamous cell cancer of the bladder: an emerging clinical entity? Can Urol Assoc J. 2009;3(5): E51–4.

55. Locke JR, Hill DE, Walzer Y. Incidence of squamous cell carcinoma in patients with long-term catheter drainage. J Urol. 1985;133(6):1034–5.

56. Groah SL, et al. Excess risk of bladder cancer in spinal cord injury: evidence for an association between indwelling catheter use and bladder cancer. Arch Phys Med Rehabil. 2002;83(3):346–51.

57. Roe B. Long-term catheter care in the community. Nurs Times. 1989;85(36):43–4.

58. Roe BH. Study of the effects of education on patients' knowledge and acceptance of their indwelling urethral catheters. J Adv Nurs. 1990;15(2): 223–31.

59. Saint S, et al. Urinary catheters: what type do men and their nurses prefer? J Am Geriatr Soc. 1999;47(12): 1453–7.

60. Wilde MH. Life with an indwelling urinary catheter: the dialectic of stigma and acceptance. Qual Health Res. 2003;13(9):1189–204.

61. Fraczyk L, Godfrey H, Feneley R. A pilot study of users' experiences of urinary catheter drainage bags. Br J Community Nurs. 2003;8(3):104–11.

62. Pinder B, Lloyd AJ, Elwick H, Denys P, Marley J, Bonniaud V. Development and psychometric validation of the intermittent self-catheterization questionnaire. Clin Ther. 2012;34:2302–13.

63. Wilde MH, et al. A new urinary catheter-related quality of life instrument for adults. Neurourol Urodyn. 2010;29(7):1282–5.

64. Khoubehi B, et al. Morbidity and the impact on daily activities associated with catheter drainage after acute urinary retention. BJU Int. 2000;85(9): 1033–6.

65. Wilde MH. Understanding urinary catheter problems from the patient's point of view. Home Health Nurse. 2002;20(7):449–55.

66. Agarwal A, et al. Comparison of efficacy of oxybutynin and tolterodine for prevention of catheter related bladder discomfort: a prospective, randomized, placebo-controlled, double-blind study. Br J Anaesth. 2006;96(3):377–80.

67. Fader M, et al. The selection of female urinals: results of a multicentre evaluation. Br J Nurs. 1999;8(14): 918–20. 922-5.

68. Macaulay M, et al. A noninvasive continence management system: development and evaluation of a novel toileting device for women. J Wound Ostomy Continence Nurs. 2007;34(6):641–8.

69. Vickerman J. Selecting urinals for male patients. Nurs Times. 2006;102(19):47–8.

70. Golji H. Complications of external condom drainage. Paraplegia. 1981;19(3):189–97.

71. Saint S, et al. Condom versus indwelling urinary catheters: a randomized trial. J Am Geriatr Soc. 2006;54(7):1055–61.

72. Balmforth J, Cardozo LD. Trends toward less invasive treatment of female stress urinary incontinence. Urology. 2003;62(4 Suppl 1):52–60.

73. Moore KN, et al. Assessing comfort, safety, and patient satisfaction with three commonly used penile compression devices. Urology. 2004;63(1): 150–4.

Current Pharmacologic Treatment of Lower Urinary Tract Symptoms

Karl-Erik Andersson

Introduction

The function of the lower urinary tract (LUT)—to store and release urine—is dependent on the co-ordinated activity of smooth and striated muscles in the bladder, urethra, and pelvic floor. These structures form a functional unit, which is controlled by a complex interplay between the central and peripheral nervous systems and local regulatory factors [24, 52, 203, 277; see 46]. Malfunction at various levels may result in bladder control disorders, which roughly can be classified as disturbances of filling/storage or disturbances of voiding/emptying. Failure to store urine may lead to various forms of incontinence (mainly urgency and stress incontinence), and failure to empty can lead to urinary retention, which may result in overflow incontinence. A disturbed filling/storage function can, at least theoretically, be improved by agents decreasing detrusor activity, increasing bladder capacity, and/or increasing outlet resistance [810].

Many drugs have been tried, but the results are often disappointing, partly due to poor treatment efficacy and/or side effects. The development of pharmacologic treatment of the different forms of urinary incontinence has been slow, but several promising targets and drug principles have been identified [31, 34, 67, 133, 181].

This chapter is an update of the report from Committee 8 of the fifth International Consultation on Incontinence held in Paris, February, 2012 [40].

Pathogenesis of Bladder Control Disorders

Bladder control disorders can be divided into two general categories: disorders of filling/storage and disorders of voiding [810]. Storage problems can occur as a result of weakness or anatomical defects in the urethral outlet, causing stress urinary incontinence. Failure to store also occurs if the bladder is overactive, as in the overactive bladder syndrome (OABs). The prevalence varies with the criteria used for diagnosis, but according to Irwin et al. [392], using the International Continence Society (ICS) definition of 2002 [4], the overall prevalence of the OABs, based on computer-assisted telephone interviews (the EPIC study) was 11.8 %; rates were similar in men and women and increased with age [392]. A similar study based on a cross Canada telephone survey found the prevalence of OABs to be 13 % in men and 14.7 % in women [355]. In a Finnish study, taking into account bother, the prevalence of *clinically meaningful OABs*, was much lower than reported in these studies [786].

K.-E. Andersson, M.D., Ph.D. (✉)
Institute for Regenerative Medicine, Wake Forest University School of Medicine, Medical Center Blvd, Winston Salem, NC 27157, USA

AIAS, Aarhus Institute of Advanced Studies Aarhus University, Aarhus, Denmark
e-mail: keanders@wakehealth.edu

A.J. Wein et al. (eds.), *Bladder Dysfunction in the Adult: The Basis for Clinical Management*, Current Clinical Urology, DOI 10.1007/978-1-4939-0853-0_13, © Springer Science+Business Media New York 2014

OABs (symptomatic diagnosis) is often assumed to be caused by detrusor overactivity (DO; urodynamic diagnosis), even if this does not always seem to be the case [19, 220, 344, 382]. Only 1/3 of patients with OABs are incontinent, suggesting that the bladder may not necessarily be the source of the dysfunction, but that the problem in OABs with or without incontinence is at the level of the central nervous system (CNS), and that possible treatments for these conditions should target the micturition pathways at that level [369].

OABs/DO is multifactorial and can occur as a result of sensitization of afferent nerve terminals in the bladder or outlet region, changes of the bladder smooth muscle secondary to, e.g., denervation, or consequent upon damage to the (CNS) inhibitory pathways, as can be seen in various neurological disorders, such as multiple sclerosis, cerebrovascular disease, Parkinson's disease, brain tumors, and spinal cord injury (SCI) [48, 76, 606, 811].

Bladder Contraction

Normal bladder contraction in humans is mediated mainly through stimulation of muscarinic receptors in the detrusor muscle [32, 52]. Atropine resistance, i.e., contraction of isolated bladder muscle in response to electrical nerve stimulation after pretreatment with atropine, has been demonstrated in most animal species, but seems to be of little importance in normal human bladder muscle [24, 79]. However, atropine-resistant (non-adrenergic, non-cholinergic: NANC) contractions have been reported in normal human detrusor and may be caused mainly by adenosine triphosphate (ATP) [24, 52, 79, 440, 595]. A significant degree of atropine resistance may exist in morphologically and/or functionally changed bladders and has been reported to occur in hypertrophic bladders [703], interstitial cystitis [609], neurogenic bladders [802], in the aging bladder [834], and in females with overactive bladder [595]. The importance of the NANC component to detrusor contraction in vivo, normally, and in different micturition disorders, remains to be established [30].

Drugs Used for Treatment of Overactive Bladder Symptoms/ Detrusor Overactivity

It has been estimated that more than 50 million people in the developed world are affected by urinary incontinence, and an abundance of drugs has been used for treatment (Table 13.1). Helfand and coworkers showed that in a cohort of 7,244,501 patients over 45 years with an OABs diagnosis, 24.4 % of these were treated mainly with antimuscarinic agents; 75.6 % went untreated. Only 25.6 % of those treated were men [348]. Drugs may be efficacious in some patients, but they do have side effects, and frequently are not continued indefinitely. Hence, it would be worth considering them as an adjunct to conservative therapy.

Specific aspects of drug treatment of LUTS in the elderly can be found elsewhere [40].

Antimuscarinic (Anticholinergic) Drugs

Mechanism of Action
Antimuscarinics block, more or less selectively, muscarinic receptors irrespective of location [2, 33] (Fig. 13.1). The common view is that in OABs/DO, the drugs act by blocking the muscarinic receptors on the detrusor muscle, which are stimulated by ACh, released from activated cholinergic (parasympathetic) nerves. Thereby, they decrease the ability of the bladder to contract. However, antimuscarinic drugs act mainly during the storage phase, decreasing urgency and increasing bladder capacity, and during this phase, there is normally no parasympathetic input to the LUT [2, 33]. Furthermore, antimuscarinics are usually competitive antagonists. This implies that when there is a massive release of ACh, as during micturition, the effects of the drugs should be decreased, otherwise the reduced ability of the detrusor to contract would eventually lead to urinary retention. Undeniably, high doses of antimuscarinics can produce urinary retention in humans, but in the dose range used for beneficial effects in OABs/DO (Fig. 13.2),

Table 13.1 Drugs used in the treatment of LUTS/OABs/DO

	Level of evidence	Grade of recommendation
Antimuscarinic drugs		
Atropine, hyoscyamine	3	C
Darifenacin	1	A
Fesoterodine	1	A
Imidafenacin	1	B
Propantheline	2	B
Solifenacin	1	A
Tolterodine	1	A
Trospium	1	A
Drugs with mixed actions		
Oxybutynin	1	A
Propiverine	1	A
Flavoxate	2	D
Drugs acting on membrane channels		
Calcium antagonists	2	D
K-Channel openers	2	D
Antidepressants		
Imipramine	3	C
Duloxetine	2	C
Alpha-AR antagonists		
Alfuzosin	3	C
Doxazosin	3	C
Prazosin	3	C
Terazosin	3	C
Tamsulosin	3	C
Silodosin	3	C
Naftopidil	3	C
Beta-AR antagonists		
Terbutaline (beta 2)	3	C
Salbutamol (beta 2)	3	C
Mirabegron (beta 3)	1	B
PDE-5 inhibitors[a]		
(Sildenafil, Taladafil, Vardenafil)	1	B
COX-inhibitors		
Indomethacin	2	C
Flurbiprofen	2	C
Toxins		
Botulinum toxin (neurogenic)[b]	1	A
Botulinum toxin (idiopathic)[b]	1	B
Capsaicin (neurogenic)[c]	2	C
Resiniferatoxin (neurogenic)[c]	2	C
	Level of evidence	Grade of recommendation
Other drugs		
Baclofen[d]	3	C
Hormones		
Estrogen	2	C
Desmopressin[e]	1	A

Assessments according to the Oxford system (modified)
[a]Male LUTS/OABs
[b]Bladder wall
[c]Intravesical
[d]Intrathecal
[e]Nocturia (nocturnal polyuria), caution hyponatremia, especially in the elderly!

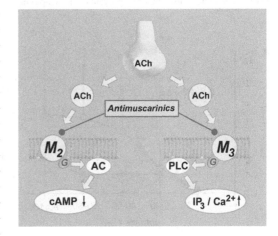

Fig. 13.1 Acetylcholine (ACh) activates all types of muscarinic receptor. The two types of muscarinic receptors dominating in the bladder contribute to bladder contraction in different ways: M3 (contraction) and M2 (inhibition of relaxation). Both subtypes of receptor are blocked by antimuscarinics

there is little evidence for a significant reduction of the voiding contraction [271]. However, there is good experimental evidence that the drugs act during the storage phase by decreasing the activity in afferent nerves (both C- and Aδ-fibers) from the bladder [206, 387] (Fig. 13.3).

Muscarinic receptors are found on bladder urothelial cells where their density can be even higher than in detrusor muscle. The role of the urothelium in bladder activation has attracted much interest [90, 91], but whether the muscarinic receptors on urothelial cells can influence micturition has not yet been established. Yoshida and colleagues [836, 838, 839] found that there is

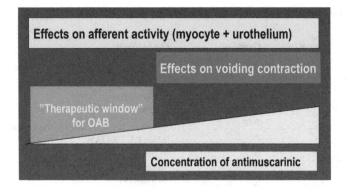

Fig. 13.2 Rationale for use of antimuscarinics for treatment of OABs/DO. Blockade of muscarinic receptors at both detrusor and nondetrusor sites may prevent OAB symptoms and DO without depressing the contraction during voiding. The "Therapeutic window for OAB" can be obtained in most patients with recommended doses of antimuscarinics

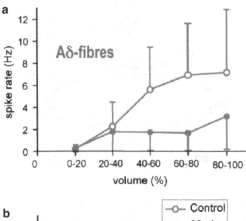

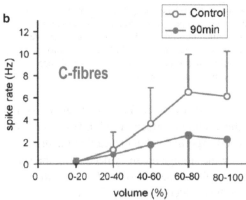

Fig. 13.3 Influence of darifenacin on volume-related nerve activity in Aδ afferents (**a**) and C afferents (**b**) in the rat pelvic nerve. From Iijima et al. Eur Urol. 2007 Sep;52(3):842

removed; thus, the released ACh was probably of non-neuronal origin and, at least partly, generated by the urothelium. There is also indirect clinical evidence for release of ACh during bladder filling. Smith and coworkers [706] found that in patients with recent spinal-cord injury, inhibition of ACh breakdown by use of cholinesterase inhibitors could increase resting tone and induce rhythmic contractions in the bladder. Yossepowitch et al. [840] inhibited ACh breakdown with edrophonium in a series of patients with disturbed voiding or urinary incontinence. They found a significant change in sensation and decreased bladder capacity, induction or amplification of involuntary detrusor contractions, or significantly decreased detrusor compliance in 78 % of the patients with the symptom pattern of overactive bladder, but in no patients without specific complaints suggesting DO. Thus, during the storage phase, ACh and ATP may be released from both neuronal and non-neuronal sources (e.g., the urothelium/suburothelium) and directly or indirectly (by increasing detrusor smooth muscle tone) excite afferent nerves in the suburothelium and within the detrusor (Fig. 13.4). These mechanisms may be important in the pathophysiology of OABs/DO and represent possible targets for antimuscarinic drugs.

Pharmacologic Properties

Generally, antimuscarinics can be divided into tertiary and quaternary amines [2, 334]. They differ

basal ACh release in human bladder. This release was resistant to tetrodotoxin and much diminished when the urothelium/suburothelium was

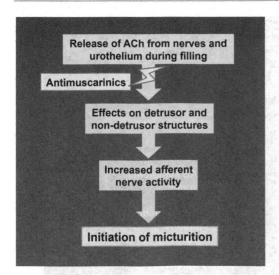

Fig. 13.4 During filling it can be assumed that acetylcholine is released from nerves and urothelium, an effect enhanced in OABs/DO. This release is reduced by antimuscarinics

with regard to lipophilicity, molecular charge, and even molecular size, tertiary compounds generally having higher lipophilicity and molecular charge than quaternary agents. Atropine, darifenacin, fesoterodine (and its active metabolite 5-hydroxy-methyl-tolterodine), oxybutynin, propiverine, solifenacin, and tolterodine are tertiary amines. They are generally well absorbed from the gastrointestinal tract and should theoretically be able to pass into the CNS, dependent on their individual physicochemical properties. High lipophilicity, small molecular size, and less charge will increase the possibilities to pass the blood brain barrier, but in some cases, such as darifenacin, that is compensated by active transport out of the CNS by the product of the MDR1 gene [112]. Quaternary ammonium compounds, like propantheline and trospium, are not well absorbed, pass into the CNS to a limited extent, and have a low incidence of CNS side effects [114, 142, 334, 796]. They still produce well-known peripheral antimuscarinic side effects, such as accommodation paralysis, constipation, increases in heart rate, and dryness of mouth.

Many antimuscarinics are metabolized by the P450 enzyme system to active and/or inactive metabolites [334]. The most commonly involved P450 enzymes are CYP2D6 and CYP3A4. The metabolic conversion creates a risk for drug–drug interactions, resulting in either reduced (enzyme induction) or increased (enzyme inhibition, substrate competition) plasma concentration/effect of the antimuscarinic and/or interacting drug. Antimuscarinics secreted by the renal tubules (e.g., trospium) may theoretically be able to interfere with the elimination of other drugs using this mechanism. Some antimuscarinics and their active metabolites are excreted in urine in amounts that may affect the mucosal muscarinic receptors from the luminal side. This has not yet been demonstrated to imply superior clinical efficacy [42].

Antimuscarinics are still the most widely used treatment for urgency and urgency incontinence [29, 39]. However, currently used drugs lack selectivity for the bladder, and effects on other organ systems (Fig. 13.5) may result in side effects, which limit their usefulness. For example, all antimuscarinic drugs are contraindicated in untreated narrow angle glaucoma.

Theoretically, drugs with selectivity for the bladder could be obtained, if the subtype(s) mediating bladder contraction, and those producing the main side effects of antimuscarinic drugs, were different. Unfortunately, this does not seem to be the case. One way of avoiding many of the antimuscarinic side effects is to administer the drugs intravesically. However, this is practical only in a limited number of patients.

Individual data on most of the antimuscarinic drugs currently used clinically are given in the "Appendix."

Clinical Use of Antimuscarinics

The clinical relevance of efficacy of antimuscarinic drugs relative to placebo has been questioned [352]. However, large meta-analyses of studies performed with the currently most widely used drugs [152–154, 161, 162, 594] clearly show that antimuscarinics are of significant clinical benefit. It was recommended that since the pharmacological profiles of each drug (see "Appendix") and dosages differ, these factors should be considered in making treatment choices.

The durability of the effects of antimuscarinics is not known and the relapse rate of symptoms after discontinuation of treatment has not been

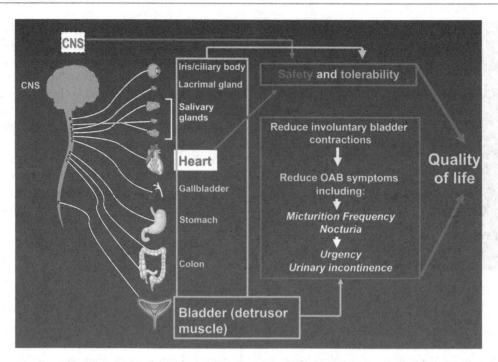

Fig. 13.5 Important sites of action of antimuscarinics. During bladder filling, there is normally no parasympathetic nervous outflow to the bladder and no release of acetylcholine (ACh). The sympathetic nervous system is active and releases noradrenaline (NA) that via β_3 adreno-ceptors stimulates adenylyl cyclase (AC) and generation of cyclic AMP (cAMP) which mediates relaxation of the bladder. In addition, β_3-adrenoceptor stimulation activates K^+ channels, stimulating outflow of K^+, which causes hyperpolarization and inhibition of Ca^{2+} inflow

systematically studies. In 173 women with OAB symptoms for >6 months, Lee et al. [480] studied in a prospective, randomized, open-label, trial what happened 3 months after the patients had been successfully treated for 1, 3, or 6-months. The relapse rate was 62 %, and the request for treatment was 65 %, indirectly suggesting an efficacy of treatment.

None of the antimuscarinic drugs in common clinical use (darifenacin, fesoterodine, imidafenacin, oxybutynin, propiverine, solifenacin, tolterodine, or trospium) is ideal as a first-line treatment for all OABs/DO patients. Optimal treatment should be individualized, implying that the patient's comorbidities and concomitant medications, and the pharmacological profiles of the different drugs, should be taken into consideration [153, 162].

To compare the effects of different antimuscarinic drugs for OAB symptoms, Madhuvrata et al. [508] analyzed 86 trials, 70 with parallel and 16 with cross-over designs (31,249 adults), drawing attention to the significance of the adverse effect of dry mouth. They concluded that when the prescribing choice is between oral immediate release oxybutynin or tolterodine, tolterodine might be preferred for reduced risk of dry mouth. Also extended release (ER) preparations of oxybutynin or tolterodine might be preferred to immediate release preparations because there is less risk of dry mouth. Comparing solifenacin and immediate release tolterodine, solifenacin might be preferred for better efficacy and less risk of dry mouth. Fesoterodine might be preferred over ER tolterodine for superior efficacy, but has higher risk of withdrawal due to adverse events in general, but in particular a higher risk of dry mouth.

Several studies have documented that the persistence with prescribed antimuscarinic therapy for overactive bladder is low [78, 436, 684, 795]. The most common causes seem to be lack of efficacy and adverse effects. However, there is some evidence suggesting that the tolerability of the different antimuscarinics may differ. Wagg et al. [795] analyzed prescription data for patients receiving antimuscarinics for treatment of the OAB syndrome over a 12-month period. At 12 months, they found that the proportions of patients still on their original treatment were: solifenacin 35 %, tolterodine ER 28 %, propiverine 27 %, oxybutynin ER 26 %, trospium 26 %, tolterodine IR 24 %, oxybutynin IR 22 %, darifenacin 17 %, and flavoxate 14 %. The longest mean persistence was reported for solifenacin (187 vs. 77–157 days for the other treatments). Gomes et al. [317] compared the persistence of oxybutynin or tolterodine therapy among older patients who were newly prescribed one of these drugs. This was a retrospective cohort study of Ontarians aged 66 years and older. Persistence with treatment was defined on the basis of refills for the drug within a grace period equal to 50 % of the prescription duration. The authors identified 31,996 patients newly treated with oxybutynin and 24,855 newly treated with tolterodine. After 2 years of follow-up, persistence on oxybutynin (9.4 %) was significantly lower than that on tolterodine (13.6 %, $p < 0.0001$). The median time to discontinuation of oxybutynin and tolterodine was 68 and 128 days, respectively. Kessler et al. [443] analyzed 69 trials enrolling 26,229 patients with OABs with the aim to compare adverse events of antimuscarinics using a network meta-analytic approach that overcomes shortcomings of conventional analyses. They found similar overall adverse event profiles for darifenacin, fesoterodine, transdermal oxybutynin, propiverine, solifenacin, tolterodine, and trospium chloride, but not for oxybutynin orally administered when currently used starting dosages were compared. They concluded that most currently used antimuscarinics seem to be equivalent first choice drugs to start the treatment of OABs, except for oral oxybutynin dosages of ≥10 mg/day, which may have more unfavorable adverse event profiles.

Even if the use of antimuscarinics is associated with many adverse effects, they are generally considered to be "safe" drugs. However, among the more serious concerns related to their use is the risk of cardiac adverse effects, particularly QT prolongation and induction of polymorphic ventricular tachycardia (torsade de pointes), and increases in heart rate (HR) [37, 47, 649]. QT prolongation and its consequences are not related to blockade of muscarinic receptors, but rather linked to inhibition of the hERG potassium channel in the heart. However, the experiences with terodiline, an antimuscarinic drug that caused torsade de pointes in patients [185, 723], have placed the whole drug class under scrutiny.

The parasympathetic actions on the heart oppose the excitatory actions of the sympathetic nervous system and slow the heart rate. An elevated resting HR has been linked to overall increased morbidity and mortality, particularly in patients with cardiovascular diseases. The prevalence of CV comorbidities was found to be significantly higher in patients with than without OABs [50]. Since mean changes in HR reported in population studies might not be applicable to an individual patient, and particularly in patients at risk of cardiac disease, even moderate increases in HR might be harmful. The potential of the different antimuscarinic agents to increase HR and/or prolong the QT time has not been extensively explored for all agents in clinical use. Differences between drugs cannot be excluded, but risk assessments based on available evidence are not possible.

Drugs Acting on Membrane Channels

Calcium Antagonists

Calcium channels play an important role in the regulation of free intracellular calcium concentrations and thereby contribute to the regulation of smooth muscle tone [86]. Two major groups of calcium channels include the voltage-gated [131] and the store-operated channels [488]. While both can contribute to the maintenance of smooth tone in general, store-operated calcium channels apparently contribute only to a limited if any extent to the regulation of bladder smooth muscle tone [675, 676]. On the other hand, various types of voltage-operated calcium channels have been implicated in the regulation of bladder smooth muscle including Q-type [286] and L-type channels [819]. The latter appears to be of particular importance as inhibitors of L-type channels have repeatedly been shown to inhibit bladder contraction in vitro with tissue from multiple mammalian species, including humans [281]. However, the relative importance of L-type channels may be somewhat less in humans than in other mammalian species [819]. In confirmation of the role of L-type calcium channels, it has been shown that knock-out mice lacking a crucial subunit of this channel exhibit a markedly impaired bladder contractility [806].

While these in vitro data suggest a possible role for calcium channel inhibitors, particularly those of L-type channels, in the treatment of DO and incontinence, only limited clinical studies are available in this regard. One urodynamic study compared the effects of intravesical installation of the calcium channel inhibitor verapamil, the muscarinic receptor antagonists oxybutynin and trospium, and placebo to patients with urgency or urgency incontinence. While the two muscarinic receptor antagonists significantly increased bladder capacity, verapamil treatment was not associated with relevant changes in bladder function [288]. In a clinical study of limited size the calcium channel inhibitor nimodipine (30 mg/day) did not significantly improve the number of incontinence episodes as compared to placebo [573]. It should be noted that despite a long-standing and widespread use of calcium channel inhibitors in the treatment of cardiovascular disease, there are no major reports on impaired bladder contractility as a side effect of such treatment. The reasons for the discrepancy between the promising in vitro and the lack of clinical data are not fully clear, but it may relate to pharmacokinetic properties of the currently used drugs which may insufficiently either reach or penetrate bladder tissue in therapeutically administered doses. At present, there is no clinical evidence to support a possible use of calcium channel inhibitors in the treatment of bladder dysfunction (Table 13.1).

Potassium Channel Openers

In a similar fashion to calcium channels, potassium channels also contribute to the membrane potential of smooth muscle cells and hence to the regulation of smooth muscle tone. Numerous types of potassium channels exist in the bladder [336, 620]. With regard to bladder function, ATP-dependent (K_{ATP}) and big calcium-activated (BK_{Ca}) channels have been studied most intensively. The BK_{Ca} channels also appear to be important physiologically as their activation can cause hyperpolarization of bladder smooth muscle cells and by this mechanism they can contribute to the relaxation of bladder smooth muscle by, e.g., β-adrenoceptor agonists [281]. Openers of both K_{ATP} [373, 375, 525] and BK_{Ca} channels [375, 691] have been shown to induce bladder smooth muscle relaxation in various mammalian species, but the density of some types of potassium channels may differ markedly between species. Some potassium channel openers have also been shown to suppress non-voiding detrusor contractions in vivo in animal models of DO [373, 525, 752] and this also includes activators of the KCNQ type of potassium channels [729]. Although potassium channel openers are believed to mainly act directly on smooth muscle cells [318, 620], they may also at least in part affect bladder function by modulating the activity of afferent neurons [752].

While the above data demonstrate the potential of potassium channel openers to inhibit non-voiding detrusor contractions, these channels are expressed not only in bladder, but also, e.g., in vascular smooth muscle. Therefore, potassium channel openers may also affect cardiovascular function, and in effective doses may considerably lower blood pressure [373, 693]. While some compounds of this class have a certain degree of selectivity for the bladder as compared to the cardiovascular system, it remains unclear whether the degree of selectivity offers a sufficiently large therapeutic window for clinical use. This consideration has led to a considerable hesitancy to study potassium channel openers in OABs patients. Nevertheless, one randomized, placebo-controlled clinical study on the K_{ATP} opener ZD0947 has been reported [159]. While

ZD0947 at the chosen dose did not lower blood pressure or cause adverse events typical for a vasodilating drug, it also failed to achieve superiority relative to placebo for the treatment of OAB symptoms. Therefore, despite promising preclinical efficacy data, potassium channel openers at present are not a therapeutic option and may never become one due to a lack of selectivity for bladder over cardiovascular tissues (Table 13.1).

Another way to use potassium channels to normalize bladder function was suggested by Christ et al. [169] in a rat model of detrusor hyperactivity. They injected "naked" hSlo/pcDNA3 (maxiK channel) into the bladder and found a significant amelioration of the hyperactivity. As to whether this principle can be therapeutically useful in man is currently under investigation.

α-Adrenoceptor (AR) Antagonists

It is well documented that α_1-AR antagonists can ameliorate lower urinary tract symptoms (LUTS) in men [28, 486, 543, 597]. Currently used α_1-AR antagonists are considered effective for treatment of both storage and voiding symptoms in men with LUTS associated with or suggestive of benign prostatic hyperplasia (BPH) [486]. However, in a study where tamsulosin was given alone, or together with tolterodine, to patients with male LUTS and OAB symptoms, monotherapy with the drug was not effective [424]. Doxazosin monotherapy resulted in only minimal effects in International Prostate Symptom Score (IPSS) storage subscore, urgency episodes, and no improvement in the patient perception of bladder condition [480]. Thus, there is no convincing evidence that α-AR antagonists, given as monotherapy, are effective in patients with storage symptoms only.

A pivotal question is if better efficacy and/or tolerability can be obtained by highly subtype selective drugs than with the commonly used alternatives. α_1-ARs include three receptor subtypes, α_{1A}, α_{1B}, and α_{1D}, which are structurally and pharmacologically distinct and have different tissue distributions [43]. α_{1A}-ARs are the predominant

subtype in the human prostate, where they mediate smooth muscle contraction. A fourth subtype, α_{1L}, also present in human prostate, is derived from the same gene as α_{1A}, but α_{1L}- and α_{1A}-receptors have different pharmacologic properties and bind some α-AR antagonists with different affinities. The precise structural relationship between the two subtypes remains to be elucidated. Selectivity for α_{1B}-AR has been considered disadvantageous from a cardiovascular point of view [682, 683]. Kojima et al. [461] studied the expression of α_1-AR in the transitional zone of prostates from 55 patients with BPH, comparing patients treated with tamsulosin presumed to block α_{1A}-ARs and naftopidil presumed to block α_{1D}-ARs. However, the selectivity of naftopidil for α_{1D}- vs. α_{1A}-ARs is modest [744] and its use as a tool to separate between α_1-AR subtypes is questionable. Nevertheless, the tamsulosin and naftopidil groups were classified as α_{1A}-AR dominant (22 and 12 patients) and α_{1D}-AR dominant (11 and 16, respectively). The efficacy of tamsulosin and naftopidil differed depending on the dominant expression of the α_1-AR subtype in the prostate. Tamsulosin was more effective in patients with dominant expression of the α_{1A}-AR subtype, whereas naftopidil was more effective in those with dominant expression of the α_{1D}-AR subtype. In another study, the same group assessed whether there was a direct correlation between the prostatic expression of α_1-AR subtype mRNA and severity of LUTS or bladder outlet obstruction [460]. They found no direct correlation between the expression of α_1-AR subtype mRNA in the prostate and severity of LUTS or BOO, although there was a significant regression of this expression with patient age. Kojima et al. [460] concluded that the expression level of α_1-AR subtype mRNA in the prostate could be a predictor of the efficacy of subtype selective α_1-AR antagonists in patients with BPH and suggested that genetic differences were responsible for the diverse responses to the drugs.

Silodosin (KD-3213), which has a high selectivity for α_{1A}-ARs [485, 753, 754, 837], had clinically good effects on both voiding and storage symptoms in men with BPH [156, 431, 522, 523, 564, 835, 837]. Chapple et al. [156] conducted a multicenter double-blind, placebo-, and active-controlled parallel group study comparing silodosin, tamsulosin, and placebo. A total of 1,228 men $\geq$50 year of age with an IPSS $\geq$13 and a urine maximum flow rate (Q_{max}) >4 and $\leq$15 mL/s were selected at 72 sites in 11 European countries. The patients were entered into a 2-week wash-out and a 4-week placebo run-in period. A total of 955 patients were randomized (2:2:1) to silodosin 8 mg ($n = 381$), tamsulosin 0.4 mg ($n = 384$), or placebo ($n = 190$) once daily for 12 week. Its overall efficacy was not inferior to tamsulosin. Only silodosin showed a significant effect on nocturia over placebo. There was no significant difference between the two α_1-AR antagonists and the placebo in terms of Q_{max}. There was also no difference between the two α-AR antagonists for the QoL parameter, whereas both were better than the placebo. Active treatments were well tolerated, and discontinuation rates due to adverse events were low in all groups (2.1 %, 1.0 %, and 1.6 % with silodosin, tamsulosin, and placebo, respectively). The most frequent adverse event with silodosin was a reduced or absent ejaculation during orgasm (14 %), a reversible effect as a consequence of the potent and selective α_{1A}-AR antagonism of the drug. The incidence was higher than that observed with tamsulosin (2 %); however, only 1.3 % of silodosin-treated patients discontinued treatment due to this adverse event. Silodosin treatment improved DO and obstruction grade by decreasing detrusor opening pressure, detrusor pressure at Q_{max}, bladder outlet obstruction index, and Schafer's obstruction class significantly [825]. In a different open, non-blinded prospective study silodosin 8 mg led to a significant increase in bladder capacity at first desire to void with no significant change in maximum cystometric capacity. In the voiding phase mean detrusor pressure at maximum flow significantly decreased, mean bladder outlet obstruction index decreased significantly, and obstruction grade as assessed by the Schaefer nomogram improved significantly [531].

It thus seems that selective blockade of α_{1A}-ARs is a clinically effective approach, and silodosin is an effective and well-tolerated treatment for the relief of both voiding and storage symptoms in male patients with LUTS, even if treatment is associated with a high incidence of ejaculatory dysfunction.

Interest has also been focused on the α_1-ARs (α_{1D}), specifically in the bladder [682, 683], assuming that these receptors were responsible for storage symptoms. However, the interrelationship between the α_{1D}-ARs in the human detrusor smooth muscle and the pathophysiology of LUTS is unclear. Naftopidil was shown to significantly improve the OAB symptom score [666] and urgency episodes [830]. Ikemoto et al. [389] gave tamsulosin and naftopidil to 96 patients with BPH for 8 weeks in a crossover study. Whereas naftopidil monotherapy decreased the I-PSS for storage symptoms, tamsulosin monotherapy decreased the I-PSS for voiding symptoms. However, this difference (which was suggested to depend on differences in affinity for α_1-AR subtypes between the drugs) could not be reproduced in a randomized head to head comparison between the drugs [319]. Based on available evidence, it therefore cannot be concluded that the α_{1D}-ARs on the detrusor smooth muscle are the main therapeutic target. However, α_{1D}-ARs may have effects on different locations in the bladder beside the detrusor smooth muscle: the detrusor vasculature, the urothelium, and the afferent and efferent nerve terminals and intramural ganglia [43]. The importance and functional role of this observation remain to be established.

In females, treatment with OABs, α_1-AR antagonists seems to be ineffective. In an RCT, comprising 364 women with OABs, no effect of tamsulosin vs. placebo could be demonstrated [640]. On the other hand, voiding symptoms in women with functional outflow obstruction, or LUTS, were treated (with modest success) with an α_1-AR antagonist [444, 500]. It should be remembered that in women, these drugs may produce stress incontinence [249].

In patients with neurogenic DO, treatment with a_1-AR antagonists was moderately successful [1].

β-Adrenoceptor Agonists

Background

The three cloned subtypes of β-ARs (β_1, β_2, and β_3) have been identified in the detrusor of most species, including humans [36, 550]. Also the

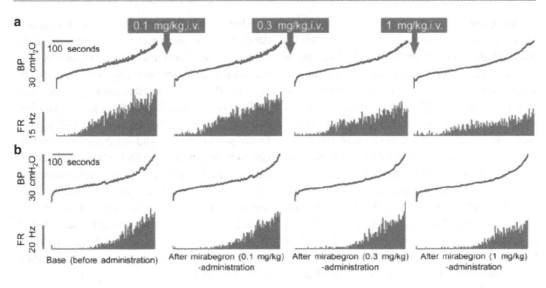

Fig. 13.6 Stimulation by highly selective β_3-adrenoceptor agonists like mirabegron inhibits afferent activity from the bladder

human urothelium contains all three receptor subtypes [605]. Studies, using real-time RT-PCR, have revealed a predominant expression of β_3-AR mRNA in human detrusor muscle [383, 550, 591] and the functional evidence for an important role in both normal and neurogenic bladders is convincing [88, 290, 383, 385, 386, 484, 550, 566, 745]. The human detrusor also contains β_2-ARs, and most probably both receptors are involved in the physiological effects (relaxation) of noradrenaline in this structure [36, 383, 550].

The generally accepted mechanism by which β-ARs induce detrusor relaxation in most species is activation of adenylyl cyclase with the subsequent formation of cAMP. However, there is evidence suggesting that in the bladder K+ channels, particularly BK_{Ca} channels, may be more important in β-AR-mediated relaxation than cAMP [280, 281, 376, 774]. Aizawa et al. [11] showed that the β_3-AR agonist, mirabegron, could inhibit filling-induced activity in both mechanosensitive Aδ-and C-fiber primary bladder afferents of the rat bladder (Fig. 13.6).

Since β-ARs are present in the urothelium, their possible role in bladder relaxation has been investigated [569, 605]. However, to what extent a urothelial signaling pathway contributes in vitro and in vivo to the relaxant effects of β-AR

agonists in general, and β_3-AR agonists specifically, remains to be elucidated.

The in vivo effects of β_3-AR agonists on bladder function have been studied in several animal models. It has been shown that compared with other agents (including antimuscarinics), β_3-AR agonists increase bladder capacity with no change in micturition pressure and the residual volume [290, 383, 412, 743, 746, 818]. For example, Hicks et al. [360] studied the effects of the selective β_3-AR agonist, GW427353, in the anesthetized dog and found that the drug evoked an increase in bladder capacity under conditions of acid-evoked bladder hyperactivity, without affecting voiding.

Clinical Use

The selective β_3-AR agonist, mirabegron, has been approved for treatment of OABs in Japan (Betanis®), USA (Myrbetriq®), and Europe (Betmiga®), and its properties and clinical effects have been extensively reviewed [45, 658]. There are proof of concept studies for other β_3-AR selective agonists such as solabegron and ritobegron [384, 600]. However, the development of ritobegron has been ceased since it failed to reach the primary efficacy endpoint in phase III studies. Other agents, e.g., TRK-380 [420], are in preclinical development for the treatment of the OAB syndrome.

Mirabegron

Pharmacokinetics. Mirabegron is rapidly absorbed after oral administration. It circulates in the plasma as the unchanged form, its glucuronic acid conjugates and other metabolites, the metabolites being inactive [747]. Of the administered dose, 55 % is excreted in urine, mainly as the unchanged form, and 34 % is recovered in feces, almost entirely as the unchanged form. Mirabegron is highly lipophilic and is metabolized in the liver via multiple pathways, mainly by cytochrome P450 3A4 and 2D6 (CYP3A4; CYP2D6) [748, 749, 779]. It may therefore be subject to clinically relevant drug–drug interactions and should therefore be used with caution in patients who are taking ketoconozole or other potent CYP3A4 inhibitors.

T_{max} in both extensive and poor metabolizers was about 2 h and the terminal elimination half-life ($t_{1/2}$) approximately 23–25 h [256, 464].

Efficacy. Several Phase II randomized controlled clinical trials (RCTs) have shown that in OABs patients mirabegron consistently improved mean number of micturitions in 24 h and number of continence episodes in 24 h [145, 149]. Mirabegron was further evaluated in three pivotal Phase III, 12-week RCTs in patients with OAB symptoms of urgency urinary incontinence, urgency, and urinary frequency [353, 446, 584]. These trials had basically similar design. Entry criteria required that patients had symptoms of overactive bladder for at least 3 months duration, at least 8 micturitions/day, and at least 3 episodes of urgency with or without incontinence over a 3-day period. The majority of patients were Caucasian (94 %) and female (72 %) with a mean age of 59 years (range 18–95 years).

In the study of Nitti et al. [584], 1,329 patients were randomized to receive placebo, or mirabegron 50 or 100 mg once daily for 12 weeks. Co-primary endpoints were change from baseline to final visit (study end) in the mean number of incontinence episodes/24 h and micturitions/24 h. At the final visit, mirabegron 50 and 100 mg showed statistically significant improvements in the co-primary efficacy endpoints and mean volume voided/micturition compared with placebo.

Khullar et al. [446] performed a similarly designed study enrolling 1,978 patients. The study included a fourth arm in which tolterodine SR 4 mg was used as a comparator. Like the study of Nitti et al. [584], it was found that mirabegron caused a statistically significant improvement from baseline compared with placebo in the number of urgency incontinence episodes and number of micturitions per 24 h. Mirabegron 50 and 100 mg was statistically superior to placebo, whereas tolterodine was not, in these two key OAB symptoms, but the study was not powered for head-to-head evaluation.

In a third phase 3 study where Herschorn et al. [353] evaluated the effects of 25 and 50 mg mirabegron, both doses were associated with significant improvements in efficacy measures of incontinence episodes and micturition frequency.

Nitti et al. [587] reported on the effects of mirabegron on maximum urinary flow rate and detrusor pressure at maximum flow rate in a urodynamic safety study on male patients with bladder outlet obstruction (BOO) and LUTS. Two hundred men with OAB symptoms and a BOO index of >20 were randomized to receive placebo, mirabegron 50 mg, or mirabegron 100 once daily for 12 weeks. Mirabegron did not adversely affect flow rate, detrusor pressure at maximum flow rate, or bladder contractile index and was well-tolerated.

Chapple et al. [151] compared the safety and efficacy of long-term administration of mirabegron 50 and 100 mg and tolterodine in a 12-month study 3-armed, parallel group study (no placebo arm). A total of 812 (50 mg) and 820 (100 mg) patients were randomized to receive mirabegron, and 812 patients received tolterodine ER 4 mg. The primary variable was incidence and severity of treatment-emergent adverse, and secondary variables were change from baseline at months 1, 3, 6, 9, and 12 in key OAB symptoms. Both mirabegron and tolterodine improved key OAB symptoms from the first measured time point of 4 week, and efficacy was maintained throughout the 12-month treatment period.

Tolerability and adverse effects. In a proof of concept study of mirabegron 100 and 150 mg

BID [145], adverse events were experienced by 45.2 % of the patients—the incidence was similar among those treated with placebo (43.2 %) and mirabegron (43.8–47.9 %). The most commonly reported adverse events considered treatment-related was gastrointestinal disorders, including constipation, dry mouth, dyspepsia, and nausea. There was no patient-reported acute retention. No significant difference in ECG parameters between the groups was demonstrated. However, a small but significant increase in mean pulse rate was observed after mirabegron 100 and 150 mg (1.6 and 4.1 beats per minute (bpm), respectively), although this was not associated with an increase in cardiovascular adverse events in this study. The overall discontinuation rate owing to adverse events was 3.2 % (placebo 3.0 % vs. mirabegron 2.4–5.3 %).

In the study of Khullar et al. [446] the incidence of adverse effects was similar across the placebo and mirabegron 50 and 100 mg groups (50.1 %, 51.6 % and 46.9 %, respectively). The most common (≥3 %) adverse effects in any treatment group were hypertension (6.6 %, 6.1 % and 4.9 %, respectively), urinary tract infection (1.8, 2.7 and 3.7 %), headache (2.0, 3.2 and 3.0 %), and nasopharyngitis (2.9, 3.4 and 2.5 %). The incidence of dry mouth was similar in the placebo and mirabegron groups (2.6 % vs. 2.8 %), and lower than observed in patients receiving tolterodine SR (10.1 %). The incidence of constipation was similar in all treatment groups (placebo 1.4 %, mirabegron 1.6 %), including tolterodine (2.0 %).

In the 12-months safety and efficacy study of mirabegron referred to previously [151], the incidence and severity of treatment-emergent and serious adverse effects (primary outcome parameters) were similar across the mirabegron 50 mg (59.7 %), mirabegron 100 mg (61.3 %), and tolterodine SR 4 mg (62.6 %) groups. The most frequent treatment-emergent adverse effects were hypertension, dry mouth, constipation, and headache, which occurred at a similar incidence across all treatment groups, while the incidence of dry mouth was more than threefold lower compared with the tolterodine SR 4 mg group [151].

One concern with the use of β₃-AR agonists has been the possibility of negative cardiovascular effects. In healthy subjects, mirabegron (50–300 mg/day for 10 days) increased *blood pressure* dose-dependently [556]. However, in the studies on OABs patients the mean increase (compared to placebo) in systolic/diastolic blood pressure after therapeutic doses of mirabegron once daily was approximately 0.5–1 mmHg and reversible upon discontinuation of treatment.

In a study on healthy volunteers, mirabegron increased *heart rate* in a dose-dependent manner. Maximum mean increases in heart rate from baseline for the 50, 100, and 200 mg dose groups compared to placebo were 6.7, 11, and 17 bpm, respectively in healthy volunteers [556]. However, in the clinical efficacy and safety studies, the change from baseline in mean pulse rate for mirabegron 50 mg was approximately 1 bpm and reversible upon discontinuation of treatment.

The cardiac safety of mirabegron was evaluated in a thorough QT/QTc (heart rate (HR)-corrected QT interval) study, including supratherapeutic dose. This was a randomized, placebo, and active-controlled (moxifloxacin 400 mg) four-treatment-arm parallel crossover study [516] and the design followed the recommendations of The International Conference on Harmonisation (ICH). Equal numbers of male and females were enrolled in each treatment group, and the pharmacokinetic and pharmacodynamic analyses comprised 333 and 317 subjects, respectively. The effect of multiple doses of mirabegron 50, 100, and 200 mg once daily on QTc interval was studied, and according to ICH E14 criteria, mirabegron did not cause QTcI prolongation at the 50-mg therapeutic and 100-mg supratherapeutic doses in either sex. Mirabegron prolonged QTcI interval at the 200-mg supratherapeutic dose (upper one-sided 95 % CI > 10 ms) in females, but not in males.

Even if the cardiovascular effects of mirabegron observed in clinical studies have been minimal and clinically not relevant, effects on heart rate and blood pressure need to be monitored when the drug is generally prescribed and patients with cardiovascular morbidities are treated.

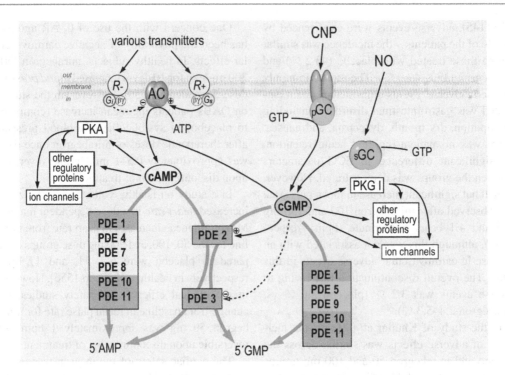

Fig. 13.7 Families of phosphodiesterases (PDE). Inhibitors of both cyclic AMP and cyclic GMP may have inhibitory effects on bladder contraction. However, so far only inhibitors of PDE5 (inhibiting degradation of cyclic GMP) have been clinically useful for treatment of lower urinary symptoms in males

Phosphodiesterase Inhibitors

Drugs stimulating the generation of cAMP are known to relax smooth muscles, including the detrusor [25, 49, 52, 309]. It is also well established that drugs acting through the NO/cGMP system can relax the smooth muscle of the bladder outflow region [36]. Use of phosphodiesterase (PDE) inhibitors to enhance the presumed cAMP- and cGMP-mediated relaxation of LUT smooth muscles (detrusor prostate, urethra) should then be a logical approach [41, 51]. There are presently 11 families of PDEs, some of which preferentially hydrolyze either cAMP or cGMP [775] (Fig. 13.7).

As a basis for PDE inhibitor treatment of LUTS, Uckert et al. [775] investigated human bladder tissue, revealing messenger RNA for PDEs 1A, 1B, 2A, 4A, 4B, 5A, 7A, 8A, and 9A; most of these PDEs preferably inhibit the breakdown of cAMP. In vitro, human detrusor muscle responded poorly to sodium nitroprusside, and to

agents acting via the cGMP system [768]. However, significant relaxation of human detrusor muscle, paralleled by increases in cyclic nucleotide levels, was induced by papaverine, vinpocetine (a low affinity inhibitor of PDE 1), and forskolin (stimulating the generation of cAMP), suggesting that the cAMP pathway and PDE 1 may be important in regulation of detrusor smooth muscle tone [769]. Significant dose-dependent relaxations were also induced by human cAMP analogs [769]. With these studies as a background, Truss et al. presented preliminary clinical data with vinpocetine in patients with urgency/urgency incontinence or low compliance bladders, and not responding to standard antimuscarinic therapy [768]. This initial open pilot study suggested a possible role for vinpocetine in the treatment of OABs. However, the results of a larger RCT in patients with DO showed that vinpocetine only showed statistically significant results for one parameter [769]. Studies with other PDE 1 inhibitors than vinpocetin (which may not be an optimal drug for elucidation of the principle) do not seem to have been performed.

PDE 4 (which also preferably hydrolyses cAMP) has been implicated in the control of bladder smooth muscle tone. PDE 4 inhibitors reduced the in vitro contractile response of guinea pig [495] and rat [413] bladder strips and also suppressed rhythmic bladder contractions of the isolated guinea pig and rat bladder [306, 307, 582]. Previous experiences with selective PDE 4 inhibitors showed emesis to be a dose-limiting effect [304]. If this side action can be avoided, PDE 4 inhibition seems to be a promising approach.

Oger and coworkers showed that PDE5-inhibitor sildenafil-induced relaxation of human detrusor smooth muscle involved cGMP-, cAMP-, and K(+) channel-dependent signaling pathways, with a minor contribution from NO [599]. In combination with the α_1-AR antagonist, doxazosin, sildenafil reduced adrenergic tone of prostatic and cavernosal smooth muscle and their combination provided a significant benefit when targeting relaxation of both tissues [598].

In vivo, several studies have indicated a role for PDE5-inhibitors in the regulation of micturition function. Systemic vardenafil reduced both non-voiding contractions and bladder afferent nerve firing in unanesthetized, decerebrate, SCI rats, indicating potential mechanisms by which PDE5-Is improve storage symptoms in SCI patients [83]. The effect of vardenafil on OAB symptoms could be related to a cGMP-dependent RhoA/ROCK signaling inhibition, as shown in spontaneously hypertensive rats (SHR) [559, 560]. Using the same animal model, bladder hypoxia was significantly reduced by acute vardenafil treatment [560]. Thus, besides relaxing muscular wall, PDE5 inhibition may positively affect urinary bladder blood perfusion. In the same respect, tadalafil was shown to increase prostate tissue oxygenation in SHR and human vesicular-deferential artery is characterized by a high expression and activity of PDE5, which was inhibited by tadalafil in vitro; these results suggest another possible mechanism through which PDE5i exert beneficial effects on LUT symptoms [561].

NO has been demonstrated to be an important inhibitory neurotransmitter in the smooth muscle of the urethra and its relaxant effect is associated with increased levels of cyclic GMP [36]. However, few investigations have addressed the cAMP- and cGMP-mediated signal transduction pathways and its key enzymes in the mammalian urethra. Morita et al. [565] examined the effects of isoproterenol, prostaglandin E_1 and E_2, and SNP on the contractile force and tissue content of cAMP and cGMP in the rabbit urethra. They concluded that both cyclic nucleotides can produce relaxation of the urethra. Werkström et al. [814] characterized the distribution of PDE 5, cGMP, and PKG1 in female pig and human urethra and evaluated the effect of pharmacological inhibition of PDE-5 in isolated smooth muscle preparations. After stimulation with the NO donor, DETA NONO-ate, the cGMP-immunoreactivity (IR) in urethral and vascular smooth muscles increased. There was a wide distribution of cGMP- and vimentin-positive interstitial cells between pig urethral smooth muscle bundles. PDE-5 IR could be demonstrated within the urethral and vascular smooth muscle cells, but also in vascular endothelial cells that expressed cGMP-IR. Nerve-induced relaxations of urethral preparations were enhanced at low concentrations of sildenafil, vardenafil, and tadalafil, whereas there were direct smooth muscle relaxant actions of the PDE-5 inhibitors at high concentrations. Fibbi et al. [269] confirmed that the highest expression and biological activity of PDE5 was found in the bladder. However, a consistent PDE5 expression and activity was also found in prostatic urethra. In contrast, the prostate gland showed the lowest PDE5 abundance and cultures derived from this tissue were less sensitive to vardenafil. Using a different animal model associated with C-fiber afferent activation, it was shown that the NO/cGMP signaling pathway is involved in the regulation of the micturition reflex, with an action that seems more predominant on the sensory rather on the motor component of the micturition reflex [128].

The observation that patients treated for erectile dysfunction with PDE5 inhibitors had an improvement of their LUTS has sparked a new interest in using these drugs also for treatment of LUTS and OABs. After the report in an open study that treatment with sildenafil appeared to improve urinary symptom scores in men with ED and LUTS [664], this observation has been confirmed in several well-designed and conducted RCTs.

To date, several RCTs have been published comparing the effect of PDE5 inhibitors alone to placebo and the combination of α_1-AR antagonists and PDE5 inhibitors vs. α_1-AR antagonists alone [80, 293, 422, 489, 542, 544, 623, 624, 644, 645, 724, 750, 772]. In these studies, different PDE5 inhibitors and different doses were administered.

PDE5-inhibitors significantly improve IPSS and IIEF scores, but not Q_{max} when compared to placebo. According to a recent meta-analysis by Gacci and coworkers, differences in IPSS score were significantly lower in older and obese patients [293]. The combination of PDE5-inhibitors and alpha-blockers led to significant improvements of the IPSS and IIEF score as well as Q_{max} when compared to the use of alpha-blockers alone. Dmochowski showed that tadalafil once daily for LUTS had no significant effect on bladder function as measured by detrusor pressure at maximum urinary flow rate or such as maximum detrusor pressure and bladder outlet obstruction index while improving IPSS [233]. PDE5-inhibitors were generally shown to be safe and well-tolerated.

The mechanism behind the beneficial effect of the PDE inhibitors on LUTS/OABs and their site(s) of action largely remains to be elucidated. If the site of action were the smooth muscles of the outflow region (and the effect relaxation), an increase in flow rate should be expected. In none of the trials referred to such an effect was found. However, there are several other structures in the LUT that may be involved, including those in the urothelial signaling pathway (urothelium, interstitial cells, and suburothelial afferent nerves). In general, it is believed that major mechanisms contributing to LUTS include reduced NO/cGMP signaling pathway, increased RhoA kinase pathway activity, autonomic overactivity, increased bladder afferent activity, and pelvic ischemia [41].

It has to be mentioned that only tadalafil has been recently approved for the treatment of LUTS due to benign prostatic obstruction (BPO); long-term experience with PDE5 inhibitors in patients with LUTS is still lacking [597]. In addition, insufficient information is available on the combination of PDE5 inhibitors with other LUTS medications such as 5-α-reductase-inhibitors.

Antidepressants

Several antidepressants have been reported to have beneficial effects in patients with DO [496, 526]. The use of antidepressants was shown to be an independent risk factor for LUTS suggestive of BPH in a community-based population of healthy aging men (Krimpen Study: [462]).

Imipramine

Imipramine is the only drug that has been widely used clinically to treat this disorder. Imipramine has complex pharmacological effects, including marked systemic antimuscarinic actions [74] and blockade of the reuptake of serotonin and noradrenaline [509], but its mode of action in DO has not been established [379]. Even if it is generally considered that imipramine is a useful drug in the treatment of DO, no good quality RCTs that can document this have been retrieved. It has been known for a long time that imipramine can have favorable effects in the treatment of nocturnal enuresis in children with a success rate of 10–70 % in controlled trials [311, 379]. It is well established that therapeutic doses of tricyclic antidepressants, including imipramine, may cause serious toxic effects on the cardiovascular system (orthostatic hypotension, ventricular arrhythmias). Imipramine prolongs QTc intervals and has an antiarrhythmic (and proarrhythmic) effect similar to that of quinidine [89, 303]. Children seem particularly sensitive to the cardiotoxic action of tricyclic antidepressants [74]. The risks and benefits of imipramine in the treatment of voiding disorders do not seem to have been assessed. Very few studies have been performed during the last decade [379, 575]. No good quality RCTs have documented that the drug is effective in the treatment DO. However, a beneficial effect has been documented in the treatment of nocturnal enuresis.

A prospective (no controls) study, the impact of the "three-drug therapy" (antimuscarinic, alpha-blocker and tricyclic antidepressants) on the treatment of refractory detrusor overactivity (DO), showed a significant increase on bladder capacity and decreases on urgency, urge-incontinence, and frequency. Objective urodynamic data as well as symptom score improved significantly with triple therapy [575].

Selective serotonin-reuptake-inhibitors (SSRIs) have been tested with regard to their effects on OAB symptoms. Milnacipran hydrochloride, a serotonin-norepinephrine reuptake inhibitor (SNRI), or paroxetine hydrochloride, a SSRI, were analyzed in a prospective open trial in neurogenic OABs patients. Milnacipran reduced daytime urinary frequency, improved the quality of life index, and increased bladder capacity as shown in urodynamic studies. No such changes were noted in the other categories of the LUTS questionnaire or urodynamic studies, or in the paroxetine group [667].

Duloxetine

Duloxetine hydrochloride is a combined norepinephrine and serotonin reuptake inhibitor, which has been shown to significantly increase sphincteric muscle activity during the filling/storage phase of micturition in the cat acetic acid model of irritated bladder function [429, 757]. Bladder capacity was also increased in this model, both effects mediated centrally through both motor efferent and sensory afferent modulation [279]. In a placebo-controlled study, the drug showed efficacy in patients with OABs [722]. The number of micturition episodes, the primary outcome, was reduced by 2 in the duloxetine arm and by 0.5 in the placebo arm. Episodes of urgency incontinence were also significantly reduced by duloxetine. These data have not been reproduced so far in another trial. However, the high withdrawal rate observed across all studies in which the drug was evaluated for SUI, affecting 20–40 %

of the patients at short-term and up to 90 % in long-term studies, do not predict clinical utility of duloxetine in OABs.

Cyclooxygenase Inhibitors

Prostanoids (prostaglandins and thromboxanes) are synthesized by cyclooxygenase (COX) from a common precursor, arachidonic acid. Prostanoids may be involved in the control of bladder function under normal and pathological conditions, including DO and OABs. Human bladder mucosa has the ability to synthesize eicosanoids [400], and these agents can be liberated from bladder muscle and mucosa in response to different types of trauma [243, 487]. Even if prostaglandins cause contraction of human bladder muscle, it is still unclear whether prostaglandins contribute to the pathogenesis of involuntary detrusor contractions. More important than direct effects on the bladder muscle may be sensitization of sensory afferent nerves, increasing the afferent input produced by a given degree of bladder filling. Involuntary bladder contractions can then be triggered at a small bladder volume. If this is an important mechanism, treatment with prostaglandin synthesis inhibitors could be expected to be effective. However, clinical evidence for this is scarce.

Cardozo et al. [127] performed a double-blind controlled study of 30 women with DO using the prostaglandin synthesis inhibitor flurbiprofen at a dosage of 50 mg three times daily. The drug was shown to have favorable effects, although it did not completely abolish DO. There was a high incidence of side effects (43 %) including nausea, vomiting, headache, and gastrointestinal symptoms. Palmer [610] studied the effects of flurbiprofen 50 mg×4 vs. placebo in a double-blind, cross-over trial in 37 patients with idiopathic DO (27 % of the patients did not complete the trial). Active treatment significantly increased maximum contractile pressure, decreased the number of voids, and decreased the number of urgent voids compared to baseline. Indomethacin

50–100 mg daily was reported to give symptomatic relief in patients with DO, compared with bromocriptine in a randomized, single-blind, cross-over study [126]. The incidence of side effects was high, occurring in 19 of 32 patients.

Although these early clinical studies with nonselective COX inhibitors showed some promise in the treatment of these disorders, the drugs were not further developed for this indication mainly due to side effects. The interest in the use of selective COX-2 inhibitors was hampered by concerns about long-term cardiovascular toxicity with these drugs.

Toxins

Intravesical pharmacological therapy for LUTS stems from the fact that circumventing systemic administration of active compounds offers two potential advantages. First, high concentrations of pharmacological agents can be given to the bladder tissue producing enhanced local effects. Second, drugs inappropriate for systemic administration due to off-target effects can be safely used. Attractive as it may be, intravesical pharmacological therapy should still be considered as a second line treatment in patients refractory to oral therapy or who do not tolerate its systemic side effects. However, this statement is based on the assumption that intervention therapy should follow oral medication. Research aiming at defining if patients' subgroups will benefit of intravesical therapy as first line is clearly necessary. Visco et al [792] performed a double-blind, double placebo-controlled, randomized trial comparing oral anticholinergic therapy and onabotulinumtoxinA by injection and found a similar reduction in the frequency of daily episodes of urgency incontinence. Patients treated with the toxin were less likely to have dry mouth, but had a higher rate of urinary retention and urinary tract infection.

Botulinum Toxin
Mechanism of Action
Botulinum toxin (BonT) is a neurotoxin produced by *Clostridium botulinum*. Of the seven subtypes of BoNT, sub-type A (BoNT-A) has the longest duration of action, making it the most relevant clinically. BoNT/A is available in three different commercial forms, with the proprietary names of Botox®, Dysport®, Xeomin®, and Prosigne. Although the toxin is the same, it is wrapped by different proteins which modify the relative potency of each brand. This was the basis for the introduction of the non-proprietary names onabotulinum toxin A (onabotA), abobotulinum toxin A (abobotA), and incobotulinum toxin A (incobotA) for Botox®, Dysport®, and Xeomin®, respectively. Prosigne is the proprietary name of a BoNT/A produced in China, which currently does not have a known non-proprietary name. Although potency of each one is usually expressed in units (U), the doses are not interchangeable. Clinical dose conversion studies for the LUT do not exist. Available information indicates that onabotA is roughly three times more potent than abobotA and equivalent to incobotA. Nevertheless, these equivalences should be approached with caution.

Most of the information available about intravesical application of BoNT/A have been derived from the use of onabotA (Botox®). However, in addition to sub-type A, some studies have investigated the effect of detrusor injection sub-type B, rimabotulinumtoxinB (proprietary names being Miobloc™ or Neurobloc™ according to countries).

BoNT consists of a heavy and a light chain linked by a disulphide bond. In the synaptic cleft the toxin binds to synaptic vesicle protein or SV2 [237] by the heavy chain before being internalized by the nerve terminal along with the recycling process of synaptic vesicles (Fig. 13.8). The two chains are then cleaved and the light chain passes into the cytosol, where it cleaves the attachment proteins involved with the mechanism of fusion of synaptic vesicles to the cytoplasmatic membrane necessary for neurotransmitter release. Attachment protein (SNARE or soluble *N*-ethylmaleimide-sensitive fusion attachment protein receptor) includes synaptosome-associated protein 25 kD (SNAP 25), synaptobrevin (vesicle-associated membrane protein—VAMP), and syntaxin. BoNT/A cleaves SNAP 25 rendering the SNARE complex inactive [138, 378]. Subtype B acts preferentially through the inactivation of VAMP [378].

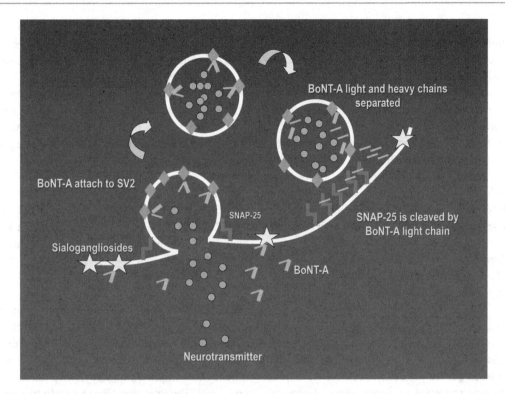

Fig. 13.8 Mechanism of action of botulinum toxin (BoNT). BoNT consists of a heavy and a light chain linked by a disulphide bond. In the synaptic cleft the toxin binds to synaptic vesicle protein or SV2 by the heavy chain before being internalized by the nerve terminal along with the recycling process of synaptic vesicles. The two chains are then cleaved and the light chain passes into the cytosol, where it cleaves the attachment proteins involved with the mechanism of fusion of synaptic vesicles to the cytoplasmatic membrane necessary for neurotransmitter release. Attachment protein (SNARE or soluble N-ethylmaleimidesensitive fusion attachment protein receptor) include synaptosome associated protein 25 kD (SNAP 25), synaptobrevin (vesicle-associated membrane protein—VAMP), and syntaxin

BonT/A application was extensively evaluated in striated muscle. In this tissue paralysis occurs by prevention of ACh release from cholinergic motor nerve endings [378]. Accumulation of neurotransmitter containing synaptic vesicles is followed by terminal axonal degeneration. Striated muscle paralysis recovers within 2–4 months time. During this time axons develop lateral sprouts and eventually regenerate completely [208].

In the human bladder SV2 and SNAP-25 expression has been demonstrated in parasympathetic, sympathetic, and sensory fibers [176–178]. Almost all parasympathetic nerves express the two proteins [177, 178]. As these nerves play a fundamental role for detrusor contraction during voiding, the blockade of ACh release is believed to play an essential role in detrusor hypo- or acontractility that follows BoNT/A injection in the bladder. In accordance with this view, it was shown that in normal or SCI animals BoNTA treatment decreased the bladder contractions evoked by electrical stimulation of spinal nerves without altering intrinsic contractions [388]. However, cholinergic axon sprouting concomitant with clinical remission could not been documented in the detrusor [340].

Bladder sensory impairment is also expected to play an important role in the final effect of BoNT/A bladder injection. BoNT/A inhibits the spinal cord release of glutamate, substance P (SP) and CGRP from sensory nerves [55, 546, 625] as well as the release of neuropeptides at the peripheral extremities [502, 629]. BoNT/A has also been shown to reduce the suburothelium immunoreactivity for TRPV1 or P2X3 [57, 60]. Morenilla-Palao et al. [563] have shown that

BonT/A impedes TRPV1 trafficking from intracellular vesicles to the neuronal membrane, a process that is also dependent on SNARE proteins. All these mechanisms may contribute to the recent observation that BonT/A reduces afferent firing from bladder afferents and antidromic release of neuropeptides [388]. Although SV2 and SNAP-25 immunoreactivity has not been detected in urothelial cells [178], urothelial function seems also compromised after BonT/A administration. BonT/A has been shown to inhibit ATP release from urothelium in animal models of SCI [445, 707]. Therefore, it is not surprising that administration of BonT/A to inflamed rat bladders reduces spinal *c-fos* counts at the L6 and S1 spinal cord segments [788].

Cleaved, inactive SNAP-25 appears rapidly after BonT/A injection. In the guinea-pig a robust expression of cleaved SNAP 25 could be detected already at 12 h and maximum intensity could be detected at 24 h with little changes afterwards. In guinea-pigs cleaved SNAP-25 expression was restricted to nerve fibers. Almost all parasympathetic fibers, either preganglionic and postganglionic, were affected while less than half of the sensory fibers express the cleaved protein [176, 177]. In the human urinary bladder cleaved SNAP 25 could be detected in NDO patients up to 11 months after BonT/A injection [681]. The longer duration of cleaved SNAP 25 in the detrusor smooth muscle, longer than in striated muscles, has no firm explanation at the moment. However, the longer persistence of the inactive form of SNAP-25 plus the involvement of pre- and post-ganglionicparasympathetic neurons may contribute to persistence of the BonT/A effect in the bladder.

Myofibroblasts form a syncytium through extensive coupling via the gap-junction protein connexin 43 and have close contacts with sensory nerves. These facts led to the hypothesis that myofibroblasts act as modulators of bladder behavior [58, 817]. However, the expression of connexin 43 is not altered by BonT/A [648]. Hence, at the moment a firm evidence for the action of BonT/A on myofibroblasts is scant.

BonT/A may decrease the levels of neurotrophic agents in the bladder tissue. Levels of nerve growth factor (NGF) [301, 302, 492] and brain-derived neurotrophic factor (BDNF) [621] have been shown to decrease in the bladder and/or urine following BonT/A injections. As both neurotrophins have paramount roles for growth, maintenance, and plasticity of peptidergic sensory nerves, these findings may point toward another mechanism whereby BonT/A acts upon the bladder.

Clinical Use

Comprehensive reviews of the clinical use of BonT/A have been produced during the last few years, covering different aspects of this treatment [158, 196, 218, 244, 245, 247, 275, 316, 427, 468–470, 521, 583, 613, 661, 762].

Efficacy. RCTs have documented the clinical effects of onabotulinumtoxinA both in neurogenic and idiopathic DO, where the drug decreases incontinence episodes, frequency, and urgency and improves quality of life [226, 518, 662, 762]. The drug was also shown to be effective in patients with OABs [585]. Successful OABs treatment with BonT/A does not appear to be related to the existence of DO. No differences in outcomes were found between those with and those without baseline DO [417, 650]. Nitti et al. [585] reported results of the first large ($N = 557$) phase 3 placebo-controlled trial of onabotulinumtoxinA in OABs patients. To be included, patients should have ≥3 urgency urinary incontinence (UI) episodes in 3 days and ≥8 micturitions/day. They were randomized 1:1 to receive intradetrusor injection of onabotulinumtoxinA 100 U or placebo (saline). Co-primary endpoints were change from baseline in UI episodes/day and proportion of patients with a positive response on the treatment benefit scale at week 12 post-treatment. Secondary endpoints included other OAB symptoms and health-related quality of life. OnabotulinumtoxinA significantly reduced the daily frequency of UI episodes vs. placebo (−2.65 vs. −0.87; $p < 0.001$) and 22.9 % vs. 6.5 % of patients became completely continent. A larger proportion of onabotulinumtoxinA-treated patients than placebo reported a positive response on the TBS (60.8 % vs. 29.2 %;

$p < 0.001$). All other OAB symptoms improved vs. placebo ($p \leq 0.05$). OnabotulinumtoxinA improved patients' health-related quality of life across multiple measures ($p < 0.001$).

The finding that onabotulinumtoxinA 100 U was consistently effective with a two to fourfold improvement over placebo in all symptoms of OABs is important: an effect of this magnitude vs. placebo does not seem to have been reported previously with antimuscarinics or β_3-AR agonists,

Adverse effects. The most frequent side effects reported after intradetrusor BonT/A injection are bladder pain and urinary infections [214, 427, 471]. Hematuria may also occur, most of the times mild in nature. The most dangerous one, paralysis of the striated musculature due to circulatory leakage of the toxin, has never been reported. Transient muscle weakness was, nevertheless, reported with abobotA application in several studies [12, 214, 822]. Among 199 NDO patients followed during 8 years, 5 developed hypostenia when injected with after abotbotA 1,000 U [214]. In another study with 44 patients, three adults also treated with 1,000 U developed muscular weakness which subsided after 5–7 weeks [12]. No such cases were reported with onabotA [427]. The reason for the lack of transient muscle weakness among BoNT/A-treated patients is unclear, but might be related with the larger size of its molecule which limits diffusion into the blood stream. Caution should be used in selecting high-risk patients for botulism including children, patients with low pulmonary reserve, or patients with myasthenia gravis. Aminoglycosides should be avoided during BoNT-A treatment since they might blockade motor plates and therefore enhance BoNT/A effect.

The most feared complication of BoNT/A application in patients with voluntary voiding is urinary retention and a transient necessity to perform clean intermittent catheterization (CIC). It is, therefore, strongly recommended that in patients with spontaneous voiding BoNT/A administration is preceded by a complete information of this risk. Caregivers should ideally teach CIC to each patient before toxin injection.

In the study by Nitti et al. [585], the majority of adverse effects occurred in the first 12 weeks (15.5 % with onabotA vs. 5.9 % with placebo). The most frequently reported adverse effect was uncomplicated urinary tract infection with no upper urinary tract involvement. Other adverse effects were dysuria (12.2 %), bacteriuria (5.0 %), and urinary retention (5.4 %). Post void residual (PVR) urine volume significantly increased with onabotA vs. placebo, with the highest volume at week 2 post-treatment, and 8.7 % of patients had an increase from baseline of ≥ 200 mL in PVR urine volume at any time following the initial toxin treatment (none with placebo). The proportion of patients who initiated CIC at any time during treatment cycle 1 was 6.1 % vs. none in the placebo group; for over half the patients who initiated CIC (10/17), the duration of CIC was ≤ 6 weeks. This value is lower than those reported in previous studies on idiopathic DO. In the study of Nitti et al. [585] discontinuation rates due to adverse effects were low in both the onabotulinumtoxinA (1.8 %) and in the placebo (1.4 %) groups.

Capsaicin and Resiniferatoxin
Rationale for Intravesical Vanilloids
The rationale for intravesical vanilloid application in patients with detrusor overactivity (DO) was offered by the demonstration that capsaicin, following bladder C-fiber desensitization, suppresses involuntary detrusor contractions dependent upon a sacral micturition reflex [202]. The C-fiber micturition reflex is usually inactive but it was shown that it is enhanced in patients with chronic spinal-cord lesions above sacral segments [202] in those with chronic bladder outlet obstruction [134] and in those with IDO [696]. In the bladders of NDO patients, the enhancement of the micturition reflex is accompanied by an increase in the number of sub-urothelial C-fibers expressing TRPV1 [101]. Curiously, NDO patients who responded better to intravesical resiniferatoxin (RTX) exhibited a significant decrease in the density of TRPV1 immunoreactive fibers, whereas non-responders experience a non-significant variation [101]. A decrease in TRPV1 expression in urothelial cells

of NDO patients was also demonstrated after intravesical application of RTX [57, 58, 60].

Changes in sub-urothelial C-fiber innervation expressing neuropeptides [705] or TRPV1 [493] were also reported in patients with sensory urgency. In IDO patients, responders to intravesical RTX are closely associated with the overexpression of the receptor in the bladder mucosa [493]. In women with sensory urgency, TRPV1 mRNA expressed in trigonal mucosa was not only increased but also inversely correlated with the bladder volume at first sensation of filling during cystometry, further indicating that TRPV1 play a role in premature bladder sensation [494].

Intravesical Capsaicin
Intravesical capsacin for NDO was studied in six non-controlled [195, 199, 209, 276, 278, 297] and one controlled clinical trial [211]. Capsaicin was dissolved in 30 % alcohol and 100–125 mL (or half of the bladder capacity if lower than that volume) of 1–2 mM solutions were instilled into the bladder and left in contact with the mucosa for 30 min. Best clinical results were found among patients with incomplete spinal cord lesions, in whom clinical improvement could be observed in up to 70–90 % of the patients [195, 209, 276]. In patients with complete spinal cord lesions the success rate was much lower [297].

Only one small randomized controlled study compared capsaicin against 30 % ethanol, the vehicle solution. Ten patients received capsaicin and found a significant regression of the incontinence and urge sensation. In contrast, only 1 among the 10 patients who received ethanol had clinical improvement [211].

The pungency of alcoholic capsaicin solutions has prevented the widespread use of this compound. In particular, the possibility of triggering autonomic dysreflexia with capsaicin, especially in patients with higher spinal cord lesions, has progressively restrained its use. The relevance of capsaicin might, however, be back with a recent observation by de Sèze et al. [210] with a new capsaicin formulation. They conducted a double-blind placebo-controlled study with a glucidic solution of capsaicin in 33 NDO

patients. The glucidic-capsaicin-treated group showed improvement both in symptoms and urodynamic parameters above the comparator arm. The global tolerance of this new capsaicin formulation was excellent [210].

RTX in NDO
Resiniferatoxin (RTX) has the advantage over capsaicin in being much less pungent [195]. Intravesical RTX application in NDO patients was evaluated in five small open-label studies [195, 467, 475, 476, 697]. Different RTX concentrations, 10, 50, 100 nM, and 10 μM, were tested. RTX brought a rapid improvement or disappearance of urinary incontinence in up to 80 % of the selected patients and a 30 % decrease in their daily urinary frequency. Furthermore, RTX also increased the volume to first detrusor contraction and maximal cystometric capacity. In general, in patients receiving 50–100 nM RTX the effect was long-lasting, with a duration of more than 6 months being reported. In patients treated with 10 μM doses, transient urinary retention may occur [476].

In a placebo-controlled study, the urodynamic effects of RTX in NDO patients were specifically evaluated. Only in the RTX arm a significant increase in first detrusor contraction and maximal cystometric capacity was found [699]. RTX also caused a significant improvement in urinary frequency and incontinence [699].

RTX, 600 nM was compared against BONT/A (Botox, 300 U) in a study involving 25 patients with NDO due to chronic SCI. Both neurotoxins were capable of significantly reducing the number of daily incontinence episodes and improving maximum bladder capacity, although BONT/A turned out to be more effective.

RTX in IDO
The first study with intravesical RTX in IDO patients was designed as a proof-of-concept study and involved 13 patients. Intravesical RTX 50 nmol/L was associated with an improvement in volume to FDC from 170 ± 109 to 440 ± 153 mL at 30 days, and to 391 ± 165 mL at 90 days. An increase in mean MCC from 291 ± 160 to 472 ± 139 mL at 30 days and to 413 ± 153 mL at

90 days was also observed. These improvements were accompanied by a decrease in episodes of urgency incontinence and of daily frequency [696]. Subsequent small open label studies confirmed these observations using either a single high (50–100 nM) or multiple low (10 nM) dose approaches [221, 467, 469].

The effect of RTX on refractory IDO was evaluated in two randomized clinical trials [472, 635]. Kuo et al. [472] randomized 54 patients to receive 4 weekly instillations of a low concentration RTX solutions (10 nmol/L) or the vehicle solution, 10 % ethanol in saline. Three months after completing the four intravesical treatments, the RTX treated group had 42.3 % and 19.2 % of patients feeling much better or improved, respectively. This was significantly more than in the placebo group, 14.2 % and 7.1 %, respectively. At 6 months treatment remained effective in 50 % patients in the RTX group, but only in 11 % in the placebo group [472]. Such clinical and urodynamic findings could not be reproduced in another study in which patients were randomly assigned to receive a single intravesical dose of 100 mL of either RTX 50 nM or placebo. Patients were followed up only for 4 weeks. During this period a single 50 nM intravesical dose of RTX was not better than placebo for the treatment of women with IDO and urgency incontinence [635].

RTX and Urgency

The involvement of bladder C-fibers in IDO has led some investigators to explore the role of these sensory afferents to the genesis of urgency. In a non-controlled study involving 12 male patients with LUTS associated with BPH, mean IPSS halved following intravesical administration of RTX (50 nmol/L). The decrease in IPSS was largely due to improvements in scores related to urgency, in addition to improvement in nocturia and frequency [222]. In another open-label study 15 patients with intractable urgency and frequency, with or without urgency incontinence or bladder pain/discomfort, and without urodynamic evidence of DO received one single 50 nM RTX solution. A trend towards an improvement of urgency was noticed [58].

In a quasi-randomized study, 23 OABs patients with refractory urgency entered a 30-day run-in period in which medications influencing the bladder function were interrupted. At the end of this period patients filled a 7-day bladder diary. Then, patients were instilled with 100 mL of 10 % ethanol in saline (vehicle solution) and 30 days later a second 7-day diary was collected. Finally, patients were instilled with 100 mL of 50 nM RTX in 10 % ethanol in saline and additional bladder diaries were collected at 1 and 3 months. After vehicle instillation, the mean number of episodes of urgency per week was 56 ± 11. At 1 and 3 months after RTX instillation the number of episodes of urgency decreased to 39 ± 9 ($p = 0.002$) and 37 ± 6 ($p = 0.02$), respectively [698].

Other Drugs

Baclofen

Gamma-amino-butyric acid (GABA) is a ubiquitous inhibitory neurotransmitter in the CNS that can inhibit the micturition reflex in several points along its central pathway [202, 614]. Experimental data suggest the GABAergic system as an interesting target for bladder dysfunction therapy. Baclofen intrathecally attenuated oxyhemoglobin-induced detrusor overactivity, suggesting that the inhibitory actions of GABA (B) receptor agonists in the spinal cord may be useful for controlling micturition disorders caused by C-fiber activation in the urothelium and/or suburothelium [614]. In spinal intact rats, intrathecal application of bicuculline induced detrusor-sphincter dyssynergia (DSD)-like changes, whereas intrathecal application of baclofen induced urethral relaxation during isovolumetric bladder contractions [557]. After SCI, Miyazato et al. [557] found signs of hypofunction of the GABAergic system (glutamate decarboxylase 67 mRNA levels in the spinal cord and dorsal root ganglia were decreased) and showed that activation of GABA(A) and GABA(B) receptors in the spinal cord inhibited DO as evidenced by a reduction in non-voiding contractions. GABA(B) receptor activation preferentially reduced DO prior to inhibiting voiding contractions, while GABA(A) receptor activation inhibited DO and voiding contraction at the same concentration.

As a GABA agonist on GABA(B) receptors, *baclofen* was used orally in IDO patients. However, its efficacy was poor, eventually dictated by the fact that baclofen does not cross the blood–brain barrier [755]. Baclofen is one of the most effective drugs for the treatment of spasticity following SCI, traumatic or hypoxic brain injury, and cerebral palsy [596], and *intrathecal* baclofen was shown to be useful in some patients with spasticity and bladder dysfunction [110]. Baldo et al. [75] found a rapid (24 h) and persistent increment in the volume to first detrusor contraction and of the maximal cystometric, whereas maximal detrusor pressure decreased. At 10 days the volume to first detrusor contraction had increased from 143 to 486 mL. In selected patients with spasticity and bladder dysfunction, intrathecal baclofen seems to be an effective therapy.

Combinations

α₁-AR Antagonists with Antimuscarinics

Traditionally, male LUTS were thought to result from BPO secondary to benign prostatic enlargement (BPE). However, male LUTS may arise from prostatic pathology, bladder dysfunction, or both. Thus, diagnosis and appropriate treatment of men with OAB symptoms are complex and difficult. α₁-AR antagonists remain the most widely used pharmacologic agents for relief of bladder outflow resistance, as they relax prostatic and urethral smooth muscle tone, the dynamic component of BPO [43, 486]. In contrast, antimuscarinics, which function by competitively blocking the muscarinic receptors, are the first-line pharmacologic treatment for OABs [39]. Given the prevalence of combined voiding and OAB symptoms as well as the finding that the QoL of these patients is affected primarily by the symptoms of OABs, it might be logical for this category of patients to be given antimuscarinic drugs [657].

A variety of such combinations have been evaluated. Several randomized, controlled trials demonstrated that the combination treatment of antimuscarinic drugs and α₁-AR antagonist was more effective at reducing male LUTS than α₁-AR antagonists alone in men with OABs and coexisting BPO [68, 423, 424, 426, 479, 481, 665]. Therapeutic benefit of combining an antimuscarinic agent (propiverine) with α₁-AR antagonists (tamsulosin), as compared to α₁-AR antagonists alone, was reported by Saito and colleagues [665]. The rates of improvement in daytime frequency, incontinence, and urgency were greater in the combination group than the α₁-AR antagonist-alone group. The post-void residual (PVR) was unchanged in both groups, and there was only one case (1.5 %) of acute urinary retention (AUR) with the combined treatment.

Subsequently, Lee et al. [479] compared the efficacy and safety of combination therapy with propiverine and doxazosin in 211 men with urodynamically confirmed bladder outlet obstruction (BOO) and OAB symptoms for 8 weeks. Compared with the doxazosin arm, the patients in the combination therapy group showed greater improvement in urinary frequency, average micturition volume, and storage and urgency scores of IPSS. Patient satisfaction was significantly higher in the combination group. There was also a significant increase in PVR (+20.7 mL) in the combination group, but no case of urinary retention was reported.

A large-scale, multicenter, randomized, double-blind, placebo-controlled trial (the TIMES study) demonstrated the efficacy and safety of tolterodine extended release (ER) alone, tamsulosin alone, and the combination of both in 879 men with OABs and BPO [424]. In the primary efficacy analysis, 172 men (80 %) receiving tolterodine ER plus tamsulosin reported treatment benefits by week 12 ($p < 0.001$ vs. placebo; $p = 0.001$ vs. tolterodine ER; $p = 0.03$ vs. tamsulosin). In the secondary efficacy analysis, patients receiving tolterodine ER plus tamsulosin compared with placebo experienced small but significant reductions in urgency incontinence, urgency episodes, daytime frequency, and nocturia. However, there were no significant differences between tamsulosin monotherapy and placebo for any diary variables at week 12. Patients receiving tolterodine ER plus tamsulosin demonstrated significant improvements in total IPSS (−8.02 vs. placebo, −6.19, $p=0.003$) and QoL (−1.61 vs. −1.17, $p=0.003$). Although there were significant improvements in the total IPSS among patients who received tamsulosin alone, the differences in total IPSS among patients who received tolterodine ER vs. placebo were not significant. The combination of antimuscarinics and α_1-AR antagonists may be the most effective therapy in men with OAB symptoms in the presence of BPO.

A subanalysis [651, 652] of data from the TIMES study focused on the urgency perception scale and concluded that the group of 217 men who received tolterodine plus tamsulosin showed significantly improved urgency variables and patient-reported outcomes. Moreover, this group of patients reported increased satisfaction with the treatment as well as willingness to continue the treatment. Another subanalysis [423, 426] of data from the TIMES study examined the effects of the drugs on urinary symptoms as assessed by the IPSS. Based on this subanalysis, the authors concluded that tolterodine ER plus tamsulosin was significantly more effective than placebo in treating storage LUTS, including OAB symptoms. However, these results should be considered with caution, as they were derived from post hoc analysis of the TIMES data.

Maruyama et al. [528] reported different results in their prospective, randomized, controlled study in which naftopidil (25–75 mg/day), an α_{1D}-AR antagonist, alone or in combination with propiverine hydrochloride (10–20 mg/day) or oxybutynin hydrochloride (2–6 mg/day), was administered for 12 weeks to 101 BPH patients. In the study, the IPSS and QoL index improved significantly in both groups, with no marked differences between groups. Maximum flow rate (Q_{max}) and PVR tended to improve in both groups, again with no differences between groups. However, median post-therapeutic PVR was significantly large in the combination group (45.0 mL) than in the monotherapy group (13.5 mL, $p=0.021$). There were significantly more patients with increased

residual urine volume relative to unchanged residuals in the combination therapy (22.9 %) group vs. the monotherapy group (5.0 %, $p=0.038$). The authors of this study concluded that combination therapy with a low-dose antimuscarinic agent was not more effective than monotherapy. Moreover, although they did not encounter any cases of urinary retention, the percentage of patients with increased residual urine volume was significantly greater in the combination therapy group than the monotherapy group.

The results of another study using low-dose antimuscarinic therapy was published by Kang et al. [419]. They evaluated the efficacy and safety of combined treatment with tamsulosin 0.2 mg and propiverine hydrochloride 10 mg compared with tamsulosin monotherapy. After 3 months, both groups showed significant improvements in IPSS, QoL, voided volume, Q_{max}, and PVR, but only the QoL index was significantly different between groups in favor of the combination group. No cases of AUR were recorded in this low-dose study.

Medical therapy to reduce detrusor overactivity in a neurogenic bladder has focused on antimuscarinic therapy, which increases bladder capacity, decreases bladder filling pressure, and improves compliance [315, 727]. Although antimuscarinics combined with CIC is the most commonly recommended medical therapy for neurogenic bladder, the results are sometimes unsatisfactory, and many patients continue to have poor bladder compliance and remain incontinent [631]. McGuire and Savastano [539] reported that α-AR antagonists decreased bladder pressure with filling and increased capacity, and that the addition of an antimuscarinic enhanced these effects, indicating that α-AR antagonists and the antimuscarinic had a synergistic effect on detrusor tone in the decentralized bladder. This finding led to the widespread use of α_1-AR antagonists in the treatment of neurogenic bladder [1, 137, 738]. Swierzewski treated 12 patients with SCI who had poor bladder compliance, despite therapy with CIC and an antimuscarinic, with 5 mg terazosin for bladder management [738]. After 4 weeks, compliance increased by 73 %, bladder pressure decreased by 36 cm H_2O, and capacity increased by 157 mL. These results support the assumption that α_1-AR antagonists and antimuscarinics may have a synergistic effect on the bladder in the neurogenic population.

In a retrospective chart review, combination therapy with an antimuscarinic agent, an α1-AR antagonist, and imipramine produced superior results to those obtained using a single agent in patients with neurogenic bladder dysfunction [113]. These patients showed significant improvement in clinical parameters and compliance and decreased bladder pressures at capacity. It has been shown that in the decentralized human detrusor, there may be an increase in α-AR receptor sites and a switch to α-AR-mediated contractile function from the typical β-AR-mediated relaxation function during bladder filling [735]. The tricyclic antidepressant imipramine is a muscarinic receptor agonist and a direct smooth muscle inhibitor that decreases bladder overactivity by blocking the reuptake of serotonin. Other effects include the peripheral blockade of noradrenaline, stimulating the β-ARs at the dome of the bladder, and decreasing bladder contractility [366]. These results suggest that targeting multiple receptors may maximize the effectiveness of pharmacological treatment of neurogenic bladder and should be considered in patients in whom treatment with antimuscarinics alone fails.

β_3-AR Antagonists with Antimuscarinics

β_3-AR agonists exert their therapeutic effects through stimulation of adenylyl cyclase and activation of potassium K+ channels. The former leads to an increase in cyclic adenosine monophosphate and the latter to hyperpolarization, both of which result in relaxation. The beneficial effects of modulation of these pathways are: inhibition of spontaneous activity, increased bladder compliance (decreased bladder tone during filling), greater distension needed to activate the micturition reflex (increased bladder capacity), and decreased afferent activity, with no effect on voiding contraction (no risk for urinary retention).

These mechanisms are distinct from those of antimuscarinic therapies used to treat OABs. As such, the combination of these two types of medications is being investigated to determine whether concomitant use can result in increased efficacy with an acceptable profile of safety and tolerability. Based on results with an animal model, it was concluded that the "combination of antimuscarinics and β_3-adrenoceptor agonists can result in increased efficacy and potency and supports the hypothesis that combining these compound classes in the clinic could have beneficial effects in treating urinary bladder dysfunction" [632]. Indeed, the results of a phase II clinical study (the Symphony study) evaluating the combination of solifenacin and mirabegron in 1,307 patients with OABs [7]. The subjects were randomized to receive one of six combinations: mirabegron 25 or 50 mg in combination with solifenacin 2.5, 5, or 10 mg; monotherapy with mirabegron or solifenacin (at each of the same doses studied in the combinations); or placebo. The study duration was 12 weeks. The primary efficacy variable was change in mean volume voided (MVV) per micturition; secondary variables included change in micturition frequency (MF) and incontinence episode frequency (IEF) per 24 h. The investigators reported that mirabegron combination therapy with solifenacin (the latter at a dose of >5 mg) demonstrated greater efficacy than solifenacin 5 mg alone on MVV and MF [7]. The enhanced efficacy with the combination was of a magnitude that is probably similar to the enhanced efficacy one might expect from uptitrating the dose of the antimuscarinic. However, the combination was not associated with the adverse effects one would expect to encounter with higher doses of antimuscarinics. In this study, all six combinations appeared to be well tolerated and there appeared to be no safety concern or significant increase in adverse effects with the combination treatment compared with either monotherapy [7].

Combined Antimuscarinics

Although antimuscarinic agents are the first choice of treatment for patients with OAB symptoms, these drugs do not always lead to the desired effect of detrusor stability and continence, especially for patients with SCI or neurologic diseases such as multiple sclerosis or meningomyelocele. In these patients, the goal of urological therapy is to maintain continence and to reduce intravesical pressure. When antimuscarinic treatment fails, however, invasive procedures such as the injection of BoNT/A, intravesical application of drugs, or surgery are necessary.

A combined antimuscarinic regimen was evaluated as a non-invasive alternative by Amend et al. [21] for patients who had neurogenic bladder dysfunction with incontinence, reduced bladder capacity, and increased intravesical pressure. They added secondary antimuscarinics to the existing double-dosed antimuscarinics for patients who previously demonstrated unsatisfactory outcomes with double-dosed antimuscarinic monotherapy. The study drugs were tolterodine, oxybutynin, and trospium. After a 4-week combined regimen, incontinence episodes decreased and reflex volume, maximal bladder capacity, and detrusor compliance increased. Side effects were comparable to those seen with normal-dosed antimuscarinics. Those positive findings were speculated to be due to: (1) synergistic activation of different muscarinic receptors or interactions of receptors on different parts of the bladder wall, (2) undiscovered faster metabolism of antimuscarinics requiring an increased dosage of different antimuscarinic drugs, and/or (3) down-regulation of subdivisions of antimuscarinic receptors under monotherapy that may lead to better susceptibility of other subdivisions when treated by the second drug. The combined regimen needs further investigation to verify its efficacy as a non-invasive alternative for patients in whom antimuscarinic monotherapy fails.

Antimuscarinics and 5a-Reductase Inhibitors

The standard first-line medical therapy for men with moderate-to-severe LUTS is an α_1-AR antagonist, a 5α-reductase inhibitor, or combination therapy with both. Both α_1-AR antagonist and 5α-reductase inhibitors alleviate LUTS in men by reducing bladder outlet resistance. α_1-AR antagonists decrease smooth muscle tone in the prostate and bladder neck, while 5α-reductase inhibitors reduce prostate volume. As mentioned, several trials have demonstrated the efficacy and safety of the combination therapy of antimuscarinics and α_1-AR antagonist for patients with

OABs and coexisting BPO. However, post-hoc analyses of the TIMES study [424] suggested that men with smaller prostates benefit more from antimuscarinic therapy than those with larger prostates [643–645]. Chung et al. [172] conducted an open-label, fixed-dose study to assess the efficacy and safety of tolterodine ER in combination with dutasteride in men with a large prostate (≥30 g) and persistent OAB symptoms after α_1-AR antagonist therapy who had been unsuccessfully treated with dutasteride alone. At the start of the study, all patients had been on dutasteride 0.5 mg daily for at least 6 months and α_1-AR antagonist therapy had failed. All patients were given 4 mg tolterodine ER daily for 12 weeks and had discontinued α_1-AR antagonist before the start of the study. At 12 weeks, the frequency (−3.2/24 h, $p < 0.02$), urgency (19.2 %, $p < 0.03$), number of severe OABs episodes (71.4 %, $p < 0.05$), and incidence of nighttime voiding (−0.9, $p < 0.003$) were found to have decreased significantly from baseline. The IPSS decreased with dutasteride treatment (from 19.3 to 14.3) and further decreased with the addition of tolterodine to 7.1 ($p < 0.001$). Storage symptoms decreased from 9.8 to 4.5 ($p < 0.001$). Dry mouth occurred in four (7.5 %) subjects, constipation in one (2 %), and decreased sexual function in two (3.9 %). Post-void residual increased by 4.2 mL, Q_{max} decreased by 0.2 mL/s, and no patients went into retention. The authors concluded that the combination of tolterodine and dutasteride was effective, safe, and well-tolerated in men with large prostates with persistent OAB symptoms and LUTS secondary to BPO.

The results of this study indicate that antimuscarinics are safe and effective in selected patients with OABs and BPO when used in combination with 5α-reductase inhibitors. Further studies are required to verify the efficacy of antimuscarinics combined with 5α-reductase inhibitors in these patients.

$5\alpha_1$-AR Antagonists with 5a-Reductase Inhibitors

It has been well established that the combinations of α_1-AR antagonists with 5-α reductase inhibitors (doxazosin finasteride: MTOPS; dutasteride + tamsulosin: CombAT) can improve clinical outcomes and reduce the incidence of BPH and LUTS progression measured as symptom worsening, retention, or progression to surgery [537, 646].

Future Possibilities

Peripherally Acting Drugs
Vitamin D₃ Receptor Analogues

It is well known that vitamin D affects skeletal muscle strength and functional efficiency, and vitamin D insufficiency has been associated with notable muscle weakness. The levator ani and coccygeus skeletal muscles are critical components of the pelvic floor and may be affected by vitamin D nutritional status. Weakened pelvic floor musculature is thought to be associated with the development of urinary incontinence and fecal incontinence symptoms. Aging women are at increased risk for both pelvic floor dysfunction and vitamin D insufficiency; to date, only small case reports and observational studies have shown an association between insufficient vitamin D and pelvic floor dysfunction symptom severity [612]. Rat and human bladders were shown to express receptors for vitamin D [193], which makes it conceivable that the bladder may also be a target for vitamin D. Analogues of vitamin D₃ have also been shown to inhibit BPH cell proliferation and to counteract the mitogenic activity of potent growth factors for BPH cells [191, 192, 194]. Experiments in rats with bladder outflow obstruction [677] showed that one of the analogues, BXL-628, at non-hypercalcemic doses, did not prevent bladder hypertrophy, but reduced the decrease in contractility of the bladder smooth muscle which occurred with increasing bladder weight [677]. The mechanism of action for the effects has not been clarified. However, elocalcitol was shown to have an inhibitory effect on the RhoA/Rho kinase pathway [562]. Upregulation of his pathway has been associated with bladder changes associated with diabetes, outflow obstruction, and DO [168, 618]. In rats with outflow obstruction, previous elocalcitol-treatment improved the effects of tolterodine on bladder compliance [728]. It was suggested that in rats

elocalcitol exerted additional beneficial actions on outflow obstruction-induced functional changes during the filling phase of micturition. If valid in humans, combined therapy with the drug would be of value.

The effect of elocalcitol on prostate volume was evaluated in patients with BPH, and it was found that elocalcitol was able to arrest prostate growth within 12 weeks in men aged ≥50 years with prostatic volume ≥40 mL [182]. In an RCT enrolling 120 female patients with OABs, where the primary endpoint was an increase in the MVV, a significant increase vs. placebo (22 % vs. 11 %) was demonstrated [181]. Whether or not vitamin D receptor agonism (monotherapy or in combination) will be a useful alternative for the treatment of LUTS/OABs requires further RCTs. However, currently, the development of the drug seems to be stopped [763].

TRP Channel Antagonists

The transient receptor potential (TRP) channel superfamily has been shown to be involved in nociception and mechanosensory transduction in various organ systems, and studies of the LUT have indicated that several TRP channels, including TRPV1, TRPV2, TRPV4, TRPM8, and TRPA1, are expressed in the bladder and may act as sensors of stretch and/or chemical irritation [44, 63, 64, 262]. TRPV1 and TRPV4 channels have been found to be expressed in the urinary bladder [92, 299, 767]. TRPV1 is present and active both in the urothelium and in the nerve fibers of several species including humans [166, 401]. TRPV4 was initially described in the urothelium of rodents and humans [399]. Co-expression of the two receptors was observed in 20 % of rat urothelial cells [466]. Recent observations indicate, however, that TRPV4 may also be expressed in bladder afferents. In fact, about 30 % of L6 dorsal root ganglia neurons that project to the urinary bladder co-express TRPV1 and TRPV4 [116]. The physiological meaning of this observation is unclear.

TRPV1 KO mice have a normal or quasi-normal phenotype. In awake animals, the only change detected in TRPV1 KO mice was a smaller volume per void when compared with wild-type (WT) controls [92]. In cystometries performed under anesthesia, the TRPV1 KO mice phenotype seems also very benign. Some studies reported that these animals have totally normal cystometric traces [164]. However, other studies showed that TRPV1 KO mice develop a few non-voiding contractions preceding the voiding contraction [92, 287]. Accordingly, TRPV1 antagonists (GRC 6211) did not show any relevant effect on bladder activity of intact rodents [165]. In contrast with TRPV1 KO mice, the micturition phenotype of TRPV4 KO animals is clearly abnormal. TRPV4 KO mice are incontinent, most probably due to incomplete bladder emptying [299]. Cystometric studies carried out under physiological conditions revealed that TRPV4 KO mice have a marked increase in the inter-contraction interval when compared to wild-type (WT) littermates [93, 299]. Likewise, TRPV4 antagonists (HC-067047) decreased the frequency of bladder contractions and increased the inter-contraction interval [263]. These observations indicated that TRPV4 has a role in the control of normal micturition reflex.

Indisputably, TRPV1 or TRPV4 have a role in the increase of micturition frequency associated with cystitis [164, 263]. While inflamed WT mice exhibit bladder hyperactivity and intense spinal Fos expression after different forms of bladder inflammation, including acetic acid or bacterial extracts, TRPV1 KO mice have normal cystometries and normal spinal c-fos expression [164]. The same holds true for TRPV4. In fact, TRPV4 KO mice exhibit significantly lower voiding frequencies and larger voided volumes than WT after inflammation with cyclophosphamide [263].

The blockade of TRPV1 and TRPV4 with specific antagonist confirm the observations carried out in knock-out animals. As a matter of fact, the TRPV1 antagonist GRC 6211 or the TRPV4 antagonist HC-067047 both abolish the increase of micturition frequency associated with chemical cystitis [165, 263]. Systemic co-administration of TRPV1 and TRPV4 antagonist was more effective in treating the cystitis-induced increase of micturition frequency than the individual application of each antagonist [70]. In particular,

the effect could be observed at very low doses of the TRPV1 and TRPV4 antagonists, which had no effect when given isolated. This observed effect might be the answer to overcome the eventual adverse events related with the application of some of these antagonists [622]. Just to mention a few, TRPV1 antagonists are associated with hyperthermia and increased risk of cardiac ischemia [70], while TRPV4 antagonists may eventually precipitate urinary retention and overflow incontinence [299].

It is known for long that TRPV1 is involved in the emergence of neurogenic detrusor overactivity following spinal cord transaction [71]. A TRPV1 antagonist, GRC 6211, has been shown to decrease reflex detrusor overactivity in rats after chronic spinal cord transaction. With increasing doses it was possible to obtain a total suppression of bladder activity [673].

There seem to be several links between activation of different members of the TRP superfamily and LUTS/DO/OABs, and further exploration of the involvement of these channels in LUT function, normally and in dysfunction, may be rewarding. However, proof of concept studies in humans is still lacking.

Prostanoid Receptor Agonists/Antagonists

Developments in the field of prostanoid receptors may open new possibilities to use selective prostanoid receptor antagonists for OABs/DO treatment [56, 403]. There is evidence suggesting that PGE2 contributes to the pathophysiology of OABs/DO: PGE2 infused into the bladder induces DO in humans and animals, increases PGE2 production in DO models, and there are high concentrations of PGE2 in the urine of patients with OABs [536]. PGE2 is an agonist at EP receptors 1–4, all G-protein coupled, which mediate its physiological effects. Based on studies using knockout (KO) mice and EP1 receptor antagonists, it was suggested that the effects of PGE2 on bladder function were mediated through EP1 receptors [678]. EP receptors can be found on urothelium/urothelium, in detrusor smooth muscle, and in intramural ganglia [627, 628, 804]. Functionally, it has been proposed that modulation of bladder activity exerted via EP1 receptors occurs via an afferent mechanism. Schroder et al. [678] found no difference in urodynamic parameters between unobstructed EP1 receptor KO and WT mice. However, EP1 receptor KO mice did not respond to intravesical PGE2 instillation, while WT mice developed DO. The lack of EP1 receptor did not prevent bladder hypertrophy due to partial bladder outflow obstruction but after obstruction WT mice had pronounced DO, while this was negligible in EP1 receptor KO mice.

Lee et al. [478] found that in normal rats a selective EP receptor antagonist significantly increased bladder capacity, micturition volume, and micturition intervals. The antagonist significantly decreased the stimulatory effects of PGE2 and decreased the frequency and amplitude of non-voiding contractions in animals with BOO. It has been shown that also EP3 receptor KO mice have a diminished response to bladder infusion of PGE2 and demonstrate an enhanced bladder capacity under basal conditions [403]. This findings suggest an important contribution for EP3 receptors in the modulation of bladder function under physiological conditions as well as under conditions of enhanced PGE2 production evoking DO. Thus, EP1 and EP3 receptors may have a role in PGE2-mediated DO.

Interestingly, activation of EP3 receptors evoked diuresis and EP3 receptor antagonism was found to induce an antidiuretic effect [406]. Thus, to modulate bladder activity, it appears that the EP3 receptor has a role in regulating urine production. Both effects may be useful for treatment of OABs/DO. It cannot be denied that EP1/EP3 receptors constitute interesting and promising targets for drugs aimed at OABs/DO treatment. However, a randomized, double-blind, placebo-controlled phase II study to investigate the efficacy and safety of the EP-1 receptor antagonist, ONO-8539, in patients with the OAB suggests that the role of EP1 receptor antagonism in the management of the OAB syndrome is minimal [144].

Intraprostatically Injected Drugs

(a) *NX-1207*. NX-1207 is a new drug under investigation for the treatment of LUTS associated with BPH. It is a new therapeutic protein of proprietary composition with selective pro-apoptotic properties [694]. The drug is injected directly into the transitional zone of the prostate as a single administration to induce focal cell loss in prostate tissue through apoptosis, leading to non-regressive prostate shrinkage and both short- and long-term symptomatic improvement. Information about the drugs is scarce and mostly published in abstract form and not yet in the peer-reviewed literature. Two US Phase II trials have been performed [694]. One of them was a multicenter, randomized, non-inferiority study involving 32 clinical sites with 85 subjects and two dose ranges (2.5 and 0.125 mg) and an active open-label comparator (finasteride). Subjects and investigators on NX-1207 were double-blind as to dosage. The primary endpoint was change in AUASI at 90 and 180 days for a single injection of NX-1207 as compared to finasteride on a non-inferiority basis. Inclusion criteria included an AUA Symptom Score ‡ 15, diminished peak urine flow (<15 mL/s), and a prostate size of >30 and <70 mg. The mean AUA Symptom Score improvement after 90 days in the intent-to-treat group was 9.71 points for 2.5 mg NX-1207 (n=48) vs. 4.13 points for finasteride (n=24) (p=0.001) and 4.29 for 0.125 mg NX-1207 (n=7) (p=0.034). The 180-day results also were positive (NX-1207 2.5 mg non-inferior to open-label finasteride).

No significant changes were found in serum testosterone or serum prostate-specific antigen (PSA) levels in the NX-1207 cohorts. There were no reported adverse effects on sexual function. Two US multicenter, double-blind, placebo-controlled Phase III studies are currently under way. The results of such studies are needed to assess whether or not this therapeutic principle is a useful addition to the current treatment alternatives.

(b) *PRX302*. PRX302 is a modified form of pro-aerolysin, a highly toxic bacterial pore-forming protoxin that requires proteolytic processing by PSA [702]. The safety and efficacy of PRX302 was evaluated in men with moderate-to-severe BPH [217]. The patients were refractory, intolerant, or unwilling to undergo medical therapies for BPH and had an IPSS >12, a quality of life (QoL) score >3, and prostate volumes between 30 and 80 g. Fifteen patients were enrolled in phase 1 studies, and 18 patients entered phase 2 studies. Subjects received intraprostatic injection of PRX302 into the right and left transition zone via a transperineal approach in an office-based setting. Phase 1 subjects received increasing concentrations of PRX302 at a fixed volume; phase 2 subjects received increasing volumes per deposit at a fixed concentration. Out to day 360, sixty percent of men in the phase 1 study and 64 % of men in the phase 2 study treated with PRX302 had >30 % improvement in IPSS compared to baseline. Patients also experienced improvement in QoL and reduction in prostate volume out to day 360. Patients receiving >1 mL of PRX302 per deposit had the best response overall. There was no deleterious effect on erectile function. Adverse events were mild to moderate and transient in nature. The major study limitation was the small sample size.

Elhilali et al. [254] conducted a phase IIb double-blind safety and efficacy evaluation of intraprostatic injection of PRX302 in 92 patients with I-PSS 15 or greater, peak urine flow 12 mL or less per second, and prostate volume 30–100 mL. The patients were randomized 2:1 to a single ultrasound-guided intraprostatic injection of PRX302 vs. vehicle (placebo). It was concluded that PRX302 produced clinically meaningful and statistically significant improvement in patient subjective (I-PSS) and quantitative objective (peak urine flow) measures sustained for 12 months.

Cannabinoids

There is increasing evidence that cannabinoids can influence micturition in animals as well as in humans, both normally and in bladder dysfunction [656]. The effects of the cannabinoids are exerted via two types of well-defined receptors, CB1 and CB2, distributed widely in the body. However, additional receptor subtypes cannot be excluded [617, 656]. Both in the CNS and in peripheral tissues, CB1 and CB2 receptors

have been identified; centrally CB1 and peripherally CB2 receptors seem to be predominant [617, 656]. CBI as well as CB2 receptors have been identified in all layers of the human bladder [321, 547, 773, 798]; their expression in the urothelium was found to be significantly higher than in the detrusor, and the expression of CB1 was higher than that of CB2 [773]. Gratzke et al. [321] found higher expression of CB2 receptors, but not CB1 receptors, in the mucosa than in the detrusor. Compared to the detrusor, larger amounts of CB2 receptor containing nerves that also expressed TRPV1 or CGRP were observed in the suburothelium. Nerve fibers containing CB2 receptors and VAChT (cholinergic neurons) were located in the detrusor. In general, activation of CB1 peripherally has been associated with vasodilation and motility changes via suppression of release of neurotransmitters, whereas activation of CB2 appears to induce anti-inflammatory, antinociceptive, and immunosuppressive actions [617, 656]. Several animal studies have suggested a modulatory role of CB2 receptors in both afferent signaling and cholinergic nerve activity [321–323]. Thus, in vivo the selective CB2 receptor agonist, cannabinor, increased micturition intervals and volumes and increased threshold and flow pressures, suggesting that peripheral CB2 receptors may be involved in sensory functions. In rats with partial urethral obstruction treated daily for 14 days with cannabinor, bladder weight was lower, the ability to empty the bladder was preserved, and non-voiding contraction frequency was low compared to those in controls.

The key enzyme for the degradation of anandamide and other endogenous cannabinoids is fatty acid amide hydrolase (FAAH) (Fig. 13.9). FAAH was found to be expressed in rat and human urothelium and was coexpressed with CB2 receptors. In rats, a FAAH inhibitor altered urodynamic parameters that reflect sensory functions, suggesting a role for the endocannabinoid system in bladder mechanoafferent functions [731].

It has not been established whether the effects of the cannabinoids are exerted in the CNS (brain, spinal cord) or peripherally. A preliminary report

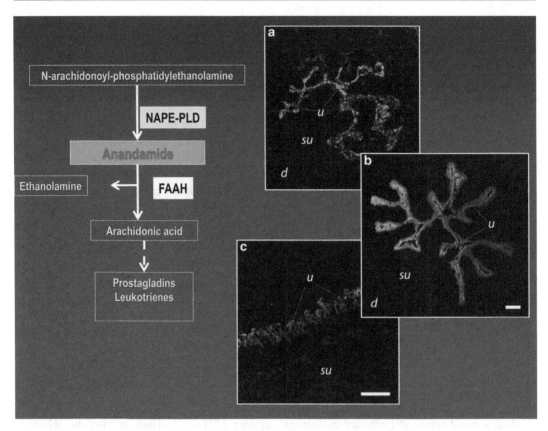

Fig. 13.9 Metabolism of and distribution of fatty acid amide hydrolase (FAAH; cannabinoid degrading enzyme) immunoreactivity in the rat urothelium

[96] demonstrated an effect of combined CB1/ CB2 receptor activation on detrusor overactivity in rats with spinal cord transection, which seemed to exclude the brain as a main site of action.

The clinical experiences of the cannabinoid treatment of micturition disturbances including LUTS are limited [656], but both open-label and placebo-controlled studies have demonstrated that orally administered cannabinoid modulators may alleviate neurogenic OAB symptoms refractory to first-line treatment [102, 283, 430]. Brady et al. [102] evaluated the efficacy of two whole plant extracts (δ9-tetrahydrocannabinol and cannabidiol) of Cannabis sativa in patients with advanced MS and refractory LUTS. Urinary urgency, the number and volume of incontinence episodes, frequency, and nocturia decreased significantly following treatment. Freeman et al. [283] tested in a subanalysis of a multicenter trial (the

CAMS study) whether cannabinoids could decrease urge incontinence episodes without affecting voiding in patients with MS. The CAMS study randomized 630 patients to receive oral administration of the cannabis extract δ9-tetrahydrocannabinol or matched placebo. Based on incontinence diaries a significant decrease in incontinence episodes was demonstrated.

Kavia et al. [430] assessed the efficacy, tolerability, and safety of Sativex(®) (nabiximols) as an add-on therapy in alleviating bladder symptoms in patients with MS. They performed a 10-week, double-blind, randomized, placebo-controlled, parallel-group trial on 135 randomized subjects with MS and OABs. The primary endpoint, reduction in daily number of urinary incontinence episodes from baseline to end of treatment (8 weeks), showed little difference between Sativex and placebo. However, four out

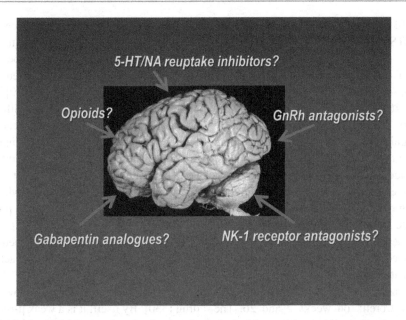

Fig. 13.10 OABs drugs with a central mode of action. Several principles seem to work, but currently used drugs have low efficacy and/or unacceptable side effects. However, there is great potential for further developments

of seven secondary endpoints were significantly in favor of Sativex, including number of episodes of nocturia, number of voids/day, and number of daytime voids. The improvement in I-QOL was in favor of Sativex, but did not reach statistical significance.

Systemic cannabinoids have effects on the LUT that may have a therapeutic potential; local delivery (intravesical, spinal) may be possible, but more information is needed. The mechanisms of cannabinoid receptors in control of the human LUT is incompletely known, and further research is necessary for the development of novel cannabinoid drugs for treatment of LUT disorders.

Centrally Acting Drugs

Many parts of the brain seem to be activated during storage and voiding (see, [277, 325–327]), and there is increasing interest in drugs modulating the micturition reflex by a central action [48] (Fig. 13.10). Several drugs used for pain treatment also affect micturition; morphine and some antiepileptic drugs being a few examples. However, central nervous mechanisms have so far not been preferred targets for drugs aimed to treat OABs, since selective actions may be difficult to obtain. Holstege [369], reviewing some of the cen-

tral mechanisms involved in micturition, including the periaqueductal gray (PAG) and the pontine micturition center (PMC), suggested that "the problem in OAB or urgency-incontinence is at the level of the PAG or PMC and their connections, and possible treatments for this condition should target the micturition pathways at that level."

Gonadotropin-releasing hormone antagonists. The beneficial effects of the 5α-reductase inhibitors, finasteride and dutasteride, in the treatment of male LUTS are well documented. The efficacy of other hormonal treatments, for example, anti-androgens or gonadotropin-releasing hormone (GnRH; also known as luteinizing hormone-releasing hormone: LHRH) agonists, is either poor or at the expense of unacceptable side effects such as medical castration associated with hot flushes, decrease of potency and libido, and negative effects on bone density following long-term androgen ablation [99, 261, 619, 679]. With GnRH antagonists submaximal, non-castrating blockade of the androgen testosterone and consequently of dihydrotestosterone (DHT) can be achieved, thus avoiding medical castration. Several GnRH antagonists—such as cetrorelix, ozarelix, and teverelix—have been tested in

Phase IIA/IIB clinical trials for their ability to improve LUTS in patients with BPH [183].

Debruyne et al. [213] demonstrated in a phase 2 RCT that the LHRH antagonist cetrorelix, given subcutaneously weekly for 20 weeks to 140 men with LUTS (IPSS ≥ 13, peak urinary flow rates 5–13 mL/s), rapidly caused a significant improvement in the mean IPSS: the peak decrease was −5.4 to −5.9 vs. −2.8 for placebo. All dosage regimens tested were well tolerated, and the authors concluded that the drug offered a safe and effective treatment of male LUTS.

Due to these results, two phase III studies were conducted in the United States and Europe (AEterna Zentaris); in the US study, 637 men were randomized to receive either two doses of placebo or cetrorelix on weeks 2 and 26. The drug showed no statistically significant benefit in improving IPSS. In addition, cetrorelix did not have a significant effect on peak flow rate or prostate volume vs. placebo. It is difficult to reconcile this lack of efficacy given favorable prior results. A subsequent multicenter European trial also failed to show any treatment-related efficacy of cetrorelix. The experience with cetrorelix highlights the importance of randomized, placebo-controlled trials that are appropriately powered to show clinical benefit and safety.

Gabapentin. Gabapentin is one of the new first-generation antiepileptic drugs that expanded its use into a broad range of neurologic and psychiatric disorders [730]. It was originally designed as an anticonvulsant GABA mimetic capable of crossing the blood–brain barrier [517]. The effects of gabapentin, however, do not appear to be mediated through interaction with GABA receptors, and its mechanism of action remains controversial [517]. It has been suggested that it acts by binding to a subunit of the $\alpha_2\delta$ unit of voltage-dependent calcium channels [296, 730]. Gabapentin is also widely used not only for seizures and neuropathic pain, but for many other indications, such as anxiety and sleep disorders, because of its apparent lack of toxicity.

Carbone et al. [118] reported on the effect of gabapentin on neurogenic DO. They found a positive effect on symptoms and significant improvement in urodynamic parameters and suggested that the effects of the drug should be explored in further controlled studies in both neurogenic and non-neurogenic DO. Kim et al. [450] studied the effects of gabapentin in patients with OABs and nocturia not responding to antimuscarinics. They found that 14 out of 31 patients improved with oral gabapentin. The drug was generally well tolerated, and the authors suggested that it can be considered in selective patients when conventional modalities have failed. It is possible that gabapentin and other $\alpha_2\delta$ ligands (e.g., pregabalin and analogs) will offer new therapeutic alternatives, but convincing RTC are still lacking.

Tramadol. Tramadol is a well-known analgesic drug [330]. By itself, it is a weak µ-receptor agonist, but it is metabolized to several different compounds, some of them almost as effective as morphine at the µ-receptor. However, the drug (metabolites) also inhibits serotonin (5-HT) and noradrenaline reuptake [330]. This profile is of particular interest, since both µ-receptor agonism and amine reuptake inhibition may be useful principles for treatment of LUTS/OABs/DO, as shown in a placebo-controlled study with duloxetine [722].

In rats, tramadol abolished experimentally induced DO caused by cerebral infarction [633]. Tramadol also inhibited DO induced by apomorphine in rats [615]—a crude model of bladder dysfunction in Parkinson's disease. Singh et al. [701] gave tramadol epidurally and found the drug to increase bladder capacity and compliance, and to delay filling sensations without adverse effects on voiding. Safarinejad and Hosseini [659] evaluated in a double-blind, placebo-controlled, randomized study the efficacy and safety of tramadol in patients with idiopathic DO. A total of 76 patients 18 years or older were given 100 mg tramadol sustained release every 12 h for 12 weeks. Clinical evaluation was performed at baseline and every 2 weeks during treatment. Tramadol significantly ($p<001$) reduced the number of incontinence periods per 24 h from 3.2±3.3 to 1.6±2.8 and induced improvements in urodynamic parameters. The main adverse event was nausea. It was concluded that in patients with non-neurogenic DO, tramadol provided beneficial clinical and urodynamic effects. Even if tramadol may not be the best suitable drug for treatment of LUTS/OABs, the study suggests efficacy for modulation of micturition via the μ-receptor.

NK1-receptor antagonists. The main endogenous tachykinins, substance P (SP), neurokinin A (NKA), and neurokinin B (NKB), and their preferred receptors, NK1, NK2, and NK3, respectively, have been demonstrated in various CNS regions, including those involved in micturition control [189, 477, 660, 685]. NK1 receptor expressing neurons in the dorsal horn of the spinal cord may play an important role in DO, and tachykinin involvement via NK1 receptors in the micturition reflex induced by bladder filling has been demonstrated [395] in normal, and more clearly, rats with bladder hypertrophy secondary to BOO. Capsaicin-induced detrusor overactivity was reduced by blocking NK1 receptor-expressing neurons in the spinal cord, using intrathecally administered substance P-saponin conjugate [395]. Furthermore, blockade of spinal NK1 receptor could suppress detrusor activity induced by dopamine receptor (L-DOPA) stimulation [397].

In conscious rats undergoing continuous cystometry, antagonists of both NK1 and NK2 receptors inhibited micturition, decreasing micturition pressure and increasing bladder capacity at low doses, and inducing dribbling incontinence at high doses. This was most conspicuous in animals with outflow obstruction [332]. Intracerebroventricular administration of NK1 and NK2 receptor antagonists to awake rats suppressed detrusor activity induced by dopamine receptor (L-DOPA) stimulation [396]. Taken together, available information suggests that spinal and supraspinal NK1 and NK2 receptors may be involved in micturition control.

Aprepitant, an NK-1 receptor antagonist used for treatment of chemotherapy-induced nausea and vomiting [529], significantly improved symptoms of OAB in postmenopausal women with a history of urgency incontinence or mixed incontinence (with predominantly urgency urinary incontinence), as shown in a well-designed pilot RCT [324]. The primary end-point was percent change from baseline in average daily micturitions assessed by a voiding diary. Secondary endpoints included average daily total urinary incontinence and urgency incontinence episodes, and urgency episodes. Aprepitant significantly ($p < 0.003$) decreased the average daily number of micturitions (-1.3 ± 1.9) compared with placebo (-0.4 ± 1.7) at 8 weeks. The average daily number of urgency episodes was also significantly ($p < 0.047$) reduced (-23.2 ± 32 %) compared to placebo (-9.3 ± 40 %), and so were the average daily number of urgency incontinence and total urinary incontinence episodes, although the difference was not statistically significant. Aprepitant was generally well tolerated and the incidence of side effects, including dry mouth, was low. Since this initial proof of concept study suggested that NK-1 receptor antagonism hold promise as a potential treatment approach for OAB symptoms, a randomized, double-blind, multicenter trial enrolled 557 adults with overactive bladder (8 or more average daily micturitions and 1 or more daily urge incontinence episodes) [285]. After a 1-week placebo run-in the patients were randomized to treatment with 8 weeks of daily 0.25, 1, or 4 mg serlopitant, 4 mg tolterodine extended release, or placebo. Patients kept 7-day voiding diaries. The primary endpoint was change from baseline in micturitions per day. Secondary endpoints included urgency, total incontinence, urge incontinence episodes, and incidence of dry mouth. Of the 557 patients randomized, 476 completed the trial and had valid efficacy data for analysis. Mean change from baseline in daily micturitions was significantly greater for 0.25 (-1.1) and 4 mg (-1.1) serlopitant, and for tolterodine (-1.5) than for placebo (-0.5), but not for 1 mg serlopitant (-0.8). No serlopitant dose response was demonstrated. Tolterodine was numerically superior to all doses of serlopitant in mean micturitions per day and secondary endpoints. The incidence of dry mouth on serlopitant (3.3 %) was comparable to placebo (4.6 %) and lower than tolterodine (8.8 %). Serlopitant was generally well tolerated.

NK-1 receptor antagonists may have a role in the treatment of overactive bladder but at least the compounds tested so far does not offer advantages in efficacy compared to tolterodine.

A different approach, modulation of neuropeptide release rather than NK receptor blockade, was tested in a pilot study with cizolirtine, which is a substance-P and CGRP release modulator at the spinal cord level. The modulation of substance-P and CGRP is probably related to the increase of extracellular levels of noradrenaline and serotonin. Cizolirtine 200 and 400 mg were compared to placebo in 79 OABs patients. Although the decrease in key OAB symptoms was significantly higher in the active arms, adverse events were reported in 68 and 81 % of the patients on cizorlitine 200 and 400 mg. More commonly reported side effects were gastrointestinal in nature, including dry mouth and vomiting [527].

Drugs Used for Treatment of Stress Incontinence in Women

Many factors seem to be involved in the pathogenesis of stress urinary incontinence (SUI) in women: urethral support and function, bladder neck support and function of the nerves and musculature of the bladder, urethra, and pelvic floor [155, 215, 459, 567]. Pure structural factors cannot be treated pharmacologically. However, SUI in women is generally thought to be characterized by decreases in urethral transmission pressure and, in most cases, resting urethral closure pressure [351, 363, 459]. It, therefore, seems logical that increasing urethral pressure should improve the condition.

Factors which may contribute to urethral closure include the tone of the urethral smooth and striated muscle (the rhabdosphincter) and the passive properties of the urethral lamina propria, in particular its vasculature. The relative contribution to intraurethral pressure of these factors is still subject to debate. However, there is ample pharmacological evidence that a substantial part of urethral tone is mediated through stimulation of α-ARs in the urethral smooth muscle by released noradrenaline [24, 52, 53]. A contributing factor to SUI, mainly in elderly women with lack of estrogen, may be lack of mucosal function. The pharmacological treatment of SUI (Table 13.2) aims at increasing intraurethral closure forces by increasing the tone in the urethral smooth and striated musculature, either directly or through increased motorneuron activity. Several drugs may contribute to such an increase [53], but relative lack of efficacy or/and side effects have limited their clinical use.

α-Adrenoceptor Agonists

Several drugs with agonistic effects on peripheral α-ARs have been used in the treatment of SUI. Relatively recently, a central role of noradrenaline (NA) in increasing the excitability of urethral rhabdosphincter motorneurons in the rat analogue of Onuf's nucleus has been observed, an effect

Table 13.2 Drugs used in the treatment of stress incontinence

Drug	Level of evidence	Grade of recommendation
Clenbuterol	3	C
Duloxetine	1	B
Ephedrine	3	D
Estrogen	2	D
Imipramine	3	D
Methoxamine	2	D
Midodrine	2	C
Norephedrine (phenylpropanolamine)	3	D

Assessments according to the Oxford system (modified)

due at least in part to α_1-AR receptor-dependent depolarization. This could contribute to the mechanism by which NA reuptake inhibitors improve SUI [828]. Ephedrine and norephedrine (phenylpropanolamine; PPA) seem to have been the most widely used [53]. The original United States Agency for Healthcare Policy and Research Guidelines [9] reported eight randomized controlled trials with PPA, 50 mg twice daily for SUI in women. Percent cures (all figures refer to percent effect on drug minus percent effect on placebo) were listed as 0–14 %, percent reduction in continence as 19–60 %, and percent side effects and percent dropouts as 5–33 % and 0–4.3 %, respectively. The most recent Cochrane review on the subject [14], reprinted virtually unchanged in 2008) assessed randomized or quasi-randomized controlled trials in adults with stress urinary incontinence which included an adrenergic agonist drug in at least one arm of the trial. There were no controlled studies reported on the use of such drugs in men. Twenty-two eligible trials were identified, 11 of which were crossover trials, which included 1,099 women, 673 of whom received an adrenergic drug (PPA in 11, midrodrine in 2, norepinephrine in 3, clenbuterol in 3, terbutaline in 1, eskornade in 1, and RO 115-1240 in 1). The authors concluded, "there was weak evidence to suggest that use of an adrenergic agonist was better than placebo in reducing the number of pad changes and incontinence episodes, as well as, improving subjective symptoms." There was not enough evidence to evaluate the merits of an adrenergic agonist compared with estrogen, whether used alone or in combination. Regarding adverse events, the review reported similar numbers with adrenergic, placebo, or alternative drug treatment. Over 25 % of subjects reported such effects, but when these consisted of effects due to adrenergic stimulation, they caused discontinuation in only 4 % of the total.

Ephedrine and PPA lack selectivity for urethral α-ARs and can increase blood pressure and cause sleep disturbances, headache, tremor, and palpitations [53]. Kernan et al. [442] reported the risk of hemorrhagic stroke to be 16 times higher in women less than 50 years of age who had been taking PPA as an appetite suppressant (statistically significant) and three times higher in women who had been taking the drug for less than 24 h as a cold remedy (not statistically significant). There was no increased risk in men. PPA has been removed from the market in the United States. It is still allowed as a treatment for SUI in a few countries. Numerous case reports of adverse reactions due to ephedra alkaloids exist, and some [85] had suggested that sale of these compounds as a dietary supplement be restricted or banned. In December 2003, the Food and Drug Administration (FDA) of the US decreed such a ban, a move which has survived legal appeal.

Midodrine and methoxamine stimulate α_1-ARs with some degree of selectivity. According to the RCTs available, the effectiveness of these drugs is moderate at best, and the clinical usefulness seems to be limited by adverse effects [15, 626, 809].

Attempts continue to develop agonists with relative selectivity for the human urethra. Musselman et al. [572] reported on a phase 2 randomized crossover study with RO 115-1240, a peripheral active selective $\alpha_{1A/1L}$-AR partial agonist [95] in 37 women with mild-to-moderate SUI. A moderate, positive effect was demonstrated, but side effects have apparently curtailed further development of the drug. PF-3774076, a CNS penetrating partial α_{1A}-AR agonist, increased peak urethral pressure in dogs and was selective with respect to α_{1B} and α_{1D} receptors, but heart rate and blood pressure changes caused significant concern [184]. Furuta et al. [291] reported that the α_2-AR can inhibit the release of glutamate presynaptically in the spinal cord and proposed that α_2-AR antagonists would be useful as a treatment for SUI. This hypothesis awaits testing.

β-Adrenoceptor Agonists

Clenbuterol. β-AR stimulation is generally conceded to decrease urethral pressure [24], but β_2-AR agonists have been reported to increase the contractility of some fast contracting striated muscle fibers and suppress that of slow contracting fibers of others [268]. Some β-AR agonists also stimulate skeletal muscle hypertrophy—in fast twitch more so than slow twitch fibers [451]. Clenbuterol has been reported to potentiate the field stimulation-induced contraction in rabbit isolated periurethral muscle preparations, an action which is suppressed by propanolol and greater than that produced by isoprotererol [454]. These authors were the first to report an increase in urethral pressure with clinical use of clenbuterol and to speculate on its potential for the treatment of SUI. Yaminishi et al. [826] reported an inotropic effect of clenbuterol and terbutaline on the fatigued striated urethral sphincter of dogs, abolished by β-AR blockade.

Yasuda et al. [829] described the results of a double-blind placebo-controlled trial with this agent in 165 women with SUI. Positive statistical significance was achieved for subjective evaluation of incontinence frequency, pad usage per day, and overall global assessment. Pad weight decreased from 11.7 ± 17.9 to 6.0 ± 12.3 g for drug and from 18.3 ± 29.0 to 12.6 ± 24.7 g for placebo, raising questions about the comparability of the two groups. The "significant" increase in maximal urethral closure pressure (MUCP) was from 46.0 ± 18.2 to 49.3 ± 19.1 cm H_2O, vs. a change of -1.5 cm H_2O in the placebo group. 56/77 patients in the Clenbuterol group reported some degree of improvement vs. 48/88 in the placebo group. The positive effects were suggested to be a result of an action on urethral striated muscle and/or the pelvic floor muscles. Ishiko et al. [394] investigated the effects of clenbuterol on 61 female patients with stress incontinence in a 12-week randomized study, comparing drug therapy to pelvic floor exercises (PFEs). The frequency and volume of stress incontinence and the patient's own impression were used as the basis for the assessment of efficacy. The improvement of incontinence was 76.9 %, 52.6 %, and 89.5 % in the respective groups. In an open study, Noguchi et al. [590] reported positive results with clenbuterol (20 mg BID for 1 month) in 9 of 14 patients with mild-to-moderate stress incontinence after radical prostatectomy. Further well-designed RTCs investigating effects of clenbuterol are needed to adequately assess its potential as a treatment for stress incontinence.

β-Adrenoceptor Antagonists

The theoretical basis for the use of β-AR antagonists in the treatment of stress incontinence is that blockade of urethral β-As may enhance the effects of noradenaline on urethral α-ARs. Propranolol has been reported to have beneficial effects in the treatment of stress incontinence [312, 414], but there are no RCTs supporting such an action. In the Gleason et al. [312] study, the beneficial effects become manifest only after 4–10 weeks of treatment, a difficult to explain phenomenon. Donker and Van der Sluis [238] reported that β-blockade did not change UPP in normal women. Although suggested as an alternative to α-AR agonists in patients with SUI and hypertension, these agents may have major potential cardiac and pulmonary side effects of their own, related to their therapeutic β-AR blockade.

Serotonin-Noradrenaline Uptake Inhibitors

Imipramine

Imipramine, among several other pharmacological effects, has classically been reported to inhibit the re-uptake of noradrenaline and serotonin in adrenergic nerve endings. In the urethra this could be expected to enhance the contractile effects of noradrenaline on urethral smooth muscle. Gilja et al. [305] reported in an open study on 30 women with stress incontinence that imipramine, 75 mg daily, produced subjective continence in 21 patients and increased mean MUCP from 34 to 48 mmHg. A 35 % cure rate was reported by pad test and, in an additional 25 %, a 50 % or more improvement. Lin et al. [490] assessed the efficacy of imipramine (25 mg imipramine three times a day for 3 months) as a treatment of genuine stress incontinence in 40 women with genuine stress incontinence. A 20-min pad test, uroflowmetry, filling and voiding cystometry, and stress urethral pressure profile were performed before and after treatment. The efficacy of "successful treatment" was 60 % (95 % CI 11.8–75.2). There are

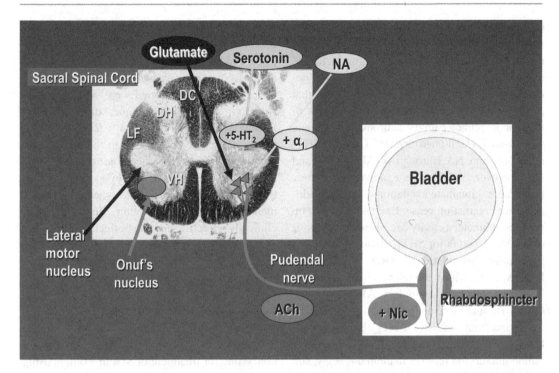

Fig. 13.11 The striated urethral sphincter is innervated by the pudendal nerve, which contains the axons of motor neurons whose cell bodies are located in Onuf's nucleus. Glutamate exerts a tonic excitatory effects on these motor neurons, and this effect is enhanced by noradrenaline (NA) and serotonin (5-HT), acting on α1-adrenoceptors and 5-HT2-receptors, respectively. By inhibition of the reuptake of noradrenaline and serotonin, duloxetine increases the contractile activity in the striated sphincter (nicotinic receptors: + Nic). *DC* dorsal commissure, *DH* dorsal horn, *VH* ventral horn, *LF* lateral funiculus, *ACh* acetylcholine

no RCTs on the effects of imipramine on SUI. No subsequent published reports have appeared.

Interestingly, Gillman [308] reported that clomipramine had far greater 5HT reuptake inhibition than imipramine and roughly similar NA reuptake inhibition. Desipramine and reboxetine had greater NA reuptake inhibition (desipramine superior), with less effects than imipramine on 5HT uptake (desipramine superior).

Duloxetine

Duloxetine hydrochloride is a combined norepinephrine and serotonin reuptake inhibitor, which has been shown to significantly increase sphincteric muscle activity during the filling/storage phase of micturition (Fig. 13.11) in the cat acetic acid model of irritated bladder function [429, 757]. Bladder capacity was also increased in this model, both effects mediated centrally through both motor efferent and sensory afferent modulation [279]. The sphincteric effects were reversed by α₁ adrenergic (praxosin) and 5HT2 serotonergic (LY 53857) antagonism, while the bladder effects were mediated by temporal prolongation of the actions of serotonin and norephinephrine in the synaptic cleft [279]. Duloxetine is lipophilic, well absorbed, and extensively metabolized (CYP2D6). Its plasma half-life is approximately 12 h [690].

Thor et al. [758] described the mechanisms of action and the physiologic effects of duloxetine. 5HT (serotonin) and NA terminals are dense in spinal areas associated with LUT functioning especially around the pudendal nerve neurons in Onuf's nucleus. These are projections from separate areas in the brain stem.

Glutamate is the primary excitatory neurotransmitter in the spinal cord, activating the pudendal neurons in Onuf's nucleus causing contraction of the urethral rhabdosphincter. The rhabdosphincter innervation is proposed as distinct from that of the levator ani [756]. The responsiveness of the rhabdosphincter motor neurons to glutamate is modulated (facilitated) by 5HT (through $5HT_2$ receptors) and NA (through α_1-ARs). 5HT and NA, however, only modulate, and when micturition occurs, glutamate excitation and the rhabdosphincter contraction cease. Excitatory effects on urethral sphincter activity are shared to a lesser extent by receptors for $5HT_{1A}$ (indirect through a supraspinal stimulation), TRH, Vasopressin, NMDA, and AMPA; inhibitory effects are similarly mediated by κ_2 opioid, α_1 ARs, GABA-A, GABA-B, and glycine receptors [756]. Some CNS penetrant selective $5HT_{2C}$ agonists have been found to increase urethral muscle tone and inhibit micturition reflexes in animal models, and these are additional candidates for clinical development for the treatment of SUI [756].

Several RTCs have documented the effect of duloxetine SUI [229, 554, 593, 780]. A Cochrane review of the effects of duloxetine for stress urinary incontinence in women is available; the last substantive amendment listed as 25 May, 2005 [521]. Fifteen reports were deemed eligible for analysis, nine primary studies and six additional reports related to one or two of the primary references. An additional analysis "performed under the auspices of the Cochrane Incontinence Group" was performed on just the nine primary trials comparing duloxetine and placebo and published separately [521]. The results can be summarized as follows. Subjective "cure" in the duloxetine 80 mg daily (40 mg BID) was higher than in the placebo group (10.8 % vs. 7.7 %, overall RR = 1.42; 95 % CI, 1.02–1.98; $p = 0.04$). The estimated absolute size of effect was about 3 more patients cured of every 100 treated. Objective cure data, available from only one trial, showed no clear drug/placebo difference. Duloxetine showed greater improvement in I-QOL (WMD for 80 mg: 4.5; 95 % CI 2.83–6.18, $p < 0.00001$). Adverse effects in six trials were analyzed. These were reported by 71 % of

drug subjects and 59 % of those allocated to placebo. Nausea was the most common adverse event and the incidence ranged from 23 to 25 % and was the main reason for discontinuation. Other side effects reported were vomiting, constipation, dry mouth, fatigue, dizziness, and insomnia, overall RR 1.30 (95 % CI, 1.23–1.37). Across these six trials 17 % in the drug group withdrew, 4 % in the placebo arm. In the 2007 article, the authors conclude by saying that further research is needed as to whether management policies incorporating duloxetine are clinically effective and cost-effective compared to other current minimally invasive and more invasive approaches in patients with varying severity of SUI, and that "longer term experience is now a priority to determine whether there is sustained efficacy during and after duloxetine use and to rule out complications."

Hurley et al. [380] characterized the safety of duloxetine for treatment of SUI in women, using an integrated database generated from four published placebo-controlled clinical trials. The database included 1,913 women randomized to duloxetine ($N = 958$) or placebo ($N = 955$), examining adverse events (AEs), serious adverse events (SAEs), vital signs, electrocardiograms (ECGs), and laboratory analytes. AEs occurring initially or worsening during the double-blind treatment period were considered treatment-emergent (TEAE). Differences between duloxetine-treated and placebo-treated groups were compared statistically. Common TEAEs included: nausea (23.2 %), dry mouth (13.4 %), fatigue (12.7 %), insomnia (12.6 %), constipation (11.0 %), headache (9.7 %), dizziness (9.5 %), somnolence (6.8 %), and diarrhea (5.1 %). Most TEAEs that emerged early were mild to moderate, rarely worsened, and resolved quickly. Overall AE discontinuation rates were 20.5 % for duloxetine and 3.9 % for placebo ($P < 0.001$). Most discontinuations (83 %) occurred within the first month of treatment. SAEs were uncommon and did not differ between treatments. Statistically significant, but clinically unimportant mean increases in heart rate (2.4 bpm) and systolic and diastolic blood pressure (≤ 2 mmHg) occurred. No arrhythmogenic potential was observed and any rare, transient, asymptomatic increases in hepatocellular enzymes normalized. The authors concluded that duloxetine was safe and tolerable, although transient AEs were not uncommon. Hashim and Abrams [345] suggested, to reduce the risk of nausea, to begin with a dose of 20 mg twice daily for 2 weeks, then to increase to the recommended 40 mg BID dosage.

Ghoneim et al. [300] randomized women with SUI to one of four treatment combinations: duloxetine alone (40 mg BID), pelvic floor muscle training, combination, and placebo. Overall, drug with or without PFMT was superior to PFMT alone or placebo, while pad results and QOL data favored combination therapy to single treatment. Cardozo et al. [123] reported that 20 % of women awaiting continence surgery changed their minds while taking duloxetine. Duckett et al. [246] offered a 4-week course to women awaiting a TVT operation. Thirty-seven percent (of 73) declined. Excluding women for whom concomitant prolapse surgery was planned, 8/33 (24 %) scheduled for incontinence surgery alone came off the list. Sixteen (48 %) discontinued duloxetine because of AEs, 9 (27 %) found the drug ineffective.

Bent et al. [84] reported on the effects of 12 weeks of duloxetine (40 mg BID) vs. placebo in a large group of women with MUI. For SUI episodes, the mean IEF per week decreased 58.9 % with drug (7.69 to 3.93) vs. 43.3 % for placebo (8.93 to 6.05). Interestingly, corresponding decreased for UUI episodes were 57.7 % vs. 39.6 %. Both sets of values are statistically significant, but the baselines are different and the absolute change for SUI amounted to −3.76 episodes per week for drug, −2.87 for placebo. Nausea was reported by 18 % of patients on drug, 4.5 % on placebo. Corresponding percents for other AEs include dry mouth (12 vs. 2.8), dizziness (9.7 vs. 2.4), constipation (8.3 vs. 4.2), and fatigue (6.7 vs. 2.8). Nausea and dizziness were less common in a subgroup taking concurrent antidepressants. Women 65 years and older with SUI or stress predominant MUI (S-MUI) were given duloxetine (40 mg BID after a 2-week start on 20 mg BID) or placebo for 12 weeks by Schagen van Leeuwen et al. [674]. They

conclude, "this study supports the use of duloxetine in elderly women with SUI or S-MUI." The data show an absolute change in SUI + S-MUI episodes of −11.7 and −6.9 IEF/ week (drug and placebo) and median percent changes of −52.5 % vs. −36.7 % from 24 h diaries, both significant at $p < 0.001$. However, the changes for SUI alone were −53 % vs. −42 % (NS), while for S-MUI alone they were −51.6 % vs. −32.7 % ($p < 0.001$). Nausea was less than in other trials (7.5 % vs. 3.1 %), perhaps due to the lower starting dose. Other AEs included fatigue (14.2 % vs. 5.4 %), constipation (10.4 vs. 0.8), dizziness (9.0 vs. 4.6), and excess sweating (5.2 vs. 0).

Persistence on duloxetine was studied by Vella et al. [787] who found that only 31 % of an original cohort of 228 were still taking drug beyond 4 weeks, 12 % at 4 months, 10 % at 6 months, and 9 % at 1 year. Fifty-six percent of the discontinuations were attributed to side effects, 33 % to lack of efficacy; Bump et al. [109], however, reported that the positive effects of duloxetine were maintained in patients who continued treatment up to 30 months, but admitted that this subgroup was likely to include predominantly patients who had favorable responses. The number decreased from 1,424 in this cohort at 3 months to 368 at 30 months.

Shaban et al. [689] concluded that duloxetine is "optional second line for women not willing or unfit for surgery after warning against side effects as recommended by NICE guidelines in the UK." Similar sentiments are expressed by Robinson and Cardozo [638].

Duloxetine is licensed at 40 mg twice daily for the treatment of SUI in the European Union (European Medicines Agency, Scientific Discussion, 2005) in women with moderate-to-severe incontinence (defined as 15 or more episodes per week). It was withdrawn from the FDA consideration process in the United States for the treatment of SUI, but is approved for the treatment of major depressive disorder (20–30 mg BID initially, 60 mg once daily maintenance), diabetic peripheral neuropathic pain (60 mg once daily), generalized anxiety disorder (60 mg once daily), fibromyalgia (c0 mg once daily initially, 60b mg once daily maintenance), and chronic musculoskeletal pain (30 mg once daily initially,

60 mg once daily as maintenance). The product information contains a "black box" warning of "increased risk of suicidal thinking and behavior in children, adolescents and young adults taking antidepressants for major depressive disorder and other psychiatric disorders," noting also that "depression and certain other psychiatric disorders are themselves associated with increases in the risk of suicide" (Prescribing Information, revised September 2011, Eli Lilly and Company, Indianapolis, Indiana 46285). Other warnings and precautions in the U.S. in the United States Product Information for psychiatric indications, not SUI, include hepatotoxicity (not to be used in patients with substantial alcohol use or chronic liver disease), orthostatic hypotension, serotonin syndrome (general statement regarding SSRIs and SNRIs), abrupt discontinuation (may result in dizziness, paresthesias, irritability, and headache), inhibitors of CYP1A2 (such as ciprofloxacin), thioridaxine (do not administer concomitantly), potent inhibitors of CYP2D6 (may increase concentration), and others. Adverse events for 6,801 drug and 4,487 placebo-treated patients reported in the US Product Information (treatment for the indications mentioned) are nausea (24 % vs. 8 %), dry mouth (13 vs. 5), fatigue (10 vs. 5), somnolence (10 vs. 3), insomnia (10 vs. 6), constipation (10 vs. 4), and dizziness (10 vs. 5).

Stress Urinary Incontinence in Men

Although a problem of significant magnitude, especially after radical prostatectomy (RP) for cancer, the pharmacologic treatment of male SUI is an area that has received relatively little attention.

Intrinsic sphincter function is the most important outlet factor maintaining continence in men. Urethral support is less important, and there is no entity similar to the hypermobility phenomenon in women. The proximal urethral sphincter extends from the bladder neck through the prostatic urethra. Its function is removed by radical prostatectomy. The distal urethral sphincter includes the rhabdosphincter, urethral smooth muscle, and extrinsic paraurethral skeletal muscle, extending from the prostatic urethra

below the verumontanum through the membranous urethra [459]. Tsakiris et al. [770] searched for articles on drug treatment of male SUI published between 1966 and June 2007 and did a generalized database search in addition. Nine trials were identified using alpha adrenergic agonists, beta-2 antagonists, or SNRSs. Only one of these included a comparison arm [270], 40 mg BID duloxetine plus PFE vs. PFE with placebo. The results suggested a positive effect of drug, but were a bit confusing. Of those patients completing the 4-month trial (92/112), 78 % of the drug-treated patients vs. 52 % of those in the placebo group were "dry." However, 1 month after the end of the study, the corresponding figures were 46 % vs. 73 %, a shift still observed 2 months later. The authors of the review article suggested further larger and well-designed studies on duloxetine for this potential usage.

Cornu et al. [188] reported a series of post-RP men with SUI or MUI (stress predominant) randomized to duloxetine (I5) and placebo (16) after a 2-week placebo run in. Dosage was 20 mg BID for 7 days, 40 mg BID for 67 days, 20 mg for 14 days. Subjects were at least 1 year post-surgery. Outcome measures included percent decrease in IEF, 1 h pad test and various QOL measures. Statistical significance for IEF percent decrease occurred only at week 8 and 12 [$(-)52.2 \pm 38.6$ % vs. $(+)19 \pm 43.5$ %], but there was clearly a trend at 4 weeks. There was no statistical difference in 1 h pad test weights, but there was in various QOL scores. A 50–100 % decrease in IEF was seen at 12 weeks in over half of the patients. Adverse events for drug and placebo included fatigue (50 % vs. 13 %), insomnia (25 vs. 7), libido loss (19 vs. 7), constipation (13 vs. 7), nausea (13 vs. 7), diarrhea (13 vs. 7), dry mouth (6 vs. 0), anorexia (6 vs. 0), and sweating (25 vs. 20). Drawbacks and concerns are the small number (the original proposed sample size was 90) and the lack of any placebo effect on IEF and QOL. There were four men with MUI in the drug group, five in the placebo group. Results for SUI and UUI were not separated. One would logically not expect improvement to continue after drug withdrawal unless a permanent change occurred in behavior, anatomy, or neuromuscular function. In an uncontrolled usage study on men with post-RP SUI, Collado Serra et al. [179] reported that the benefit remained in 85 % after the drug was stopped. In that series, 25 % of patients withdrew because of AEs and 33 % because of lack of effect.

Usage of duloxetine for SUI in the male is universally off-label. A drug for this indication would be welcome. Larger controlled and better designed studies are necessary to provide conclusive positive or negative data on this subject.

Drugs to Treat Overflow Incontinence/Acute Urinary Retention

Urinary incontinence most often results from involuntary bladder contractions and/or too little resistance generated by the bladder outflow tract during the storage phase of the micturition cycle (urgency incontinence and stress incontinence, respectively). More rarely, incontinence can also occur because of too little pressure generation and/or too much outflow resistance, which can lead to a markedly distended bladder and urinary retention and, secondarily, overflow incontinence [4].

Based upon theoretical reasoning, animal studies [331, 416], and reports of drugs that can cause overflow incontinence [22], a variety of medical approaches to the treatment of overflow incontinence have been proposed [173, 223, 342]. Treatment may aim to increase bladder contractility, decrease bladder outlet resistance, or both. Theoretically, all drugs that improve decreased sensation (and increase afferent activity) or drugs that increase detrusor contractile force could be useful. Alternatively, agents that decrease outflow resistance, thereby restoring an appropriate balance between detrusor strength and urethral resistance, could be used.

These drugs include direct or indirect muscarinic receptor agonists, α_1-adrenoceptor antagonists, choline esterase inhibitors, prostaglandins (PG), and skeletal muscle relaxants [223]. The use of muscarinic receptor agonists, such as bethanechol, to stimulate detrusor muscarinic receptors, or choline esterase inhibitors, such as distigmine, to reduce the degradation of acetylcholine, is based upon the idea that stimulation of muscarinic receptors may overcome a hypocontractile detrusor [77]. However, a recent systematic review of controlled clinical studies that used direct and indirect parasympathetic agonists in patients with an underactive detrusor reported that these drugs do not provide consistent benefits and may even be harmful. The available information indicates that muscarinic receptor agonists and choline esterase inhibitors have little, if any, beneficial effects on preventing and treating detrusor underactivity. While there is a theoretical basis for the use of β-agonists to relax the sphincter, no definite improvements in symptoms have yet been demonstrated [10, 77, 200, 634]. As bethanechol exerts its effect on intact smooth muscle cells only, it is of limited use for the treatment of bladder atony. Idiopathic detrusor atony is poorly responsive to medical treatment [589].

The use of α_1-AR antagonists has repeatedly been shown to be beneficial in patients with AUR due to BPE [272, 540, 541]. These drugs are believed to facilitate bladder emptying by relaxing tone at the bladder neck. Administration of alfuzosin 10 mg daily almost doubles the likelihood of a successful trial without a catheter, even in patients who are elderly with a PVR > 100 mL. Continued use of alfuzosin significantly reduced the risk of BPH surgery in the first 3 months; however, this effect was not significant after 6 months [258, 273, 415]. Thus, α_1-AR antagonists provide rapid symptom relief from outlet obstruction caused by BPE and delay the time to AUR; however, they do not decrease the overall risk of AUR or surgery [252, 257, 272].

AUR may occur after surgery. Buckley and Lapitan [108] reviewed drugs used for treatment of post-operative urinary retention either alone or in combination, assessing cholinergic agents, α_1-AR blockers, sedatives, and prostaglandins. A statistically significant association between intravesically administered prostaglandins and successful voiding was detected, but no such association was found for the other drugs investigated. When cholinergic agents were combined with sedative there was an improved likelihood of spontaneous voiding compared with placebo.

There are some potential new agents for the treatment of an underactive bladder. Misoprostol, a cholinesterase inhibitor, and cholinergic agents are potential candidates for the treatment of the underactive bladder, but their safety and lack of benefit is of concern. The prokinetics used in gastroenterology and the smooth muscle ionotropics used in cardiology warrant consideration. The use of trophic factors such as insulin-like growth factor and NGF may improve muscle and nerve function in the LUT. Furthermore, the use of stem cells, regenerative medicine, and gene therapy might facilitate improved contractility in a weak detrusor [139].

However, these agents have never been tested systematically in patients with overflow incontinence; there have been no randomized controlled trials to demonstrate the effectiveness and safety of these agents. Therefore, there is no empirical basis to select medical treatments for overflow incontinence and all previously recommended treatments must be rated as "expert opinion" at best. Better systemic studies are required to determine the best medical treatment for overflow incontinence. Any medical treatment for overflow incontinence should be compared to catheterization or surgery.

Hormonal Treatment of Urinary Incontinence

Estrogens

Estrogens and the Continence Mechanism

The estrogen-sensitive tissues of the bladder, urethra and pelvic floor all play an important role in the continence mechanism. For women to remain continent the urethral pressure must exceed the intra-vesical pressure at all times except during micturition. The urethra has four estrogen-sensitive functional layers all of which have a role in the maintenance of a positive urethral pressure (1) epithelium, (2) vasculature, (3) connective tissue, (4) muscle.

Two types of estrogen receptor (α and β) have been identified in the trigone of the bladder, urethra, and vagina as well as in the levator ani muscles and fascia and ligaments within the pelvic floor [186, 295, 709]. After the menopause estrogen receptor α has been shown to vary depending upon exogenous estrogen therapy [289]. In addition exogenous estrogens affect the remodeling of collagen in the urogenital tissues resulting in a reduction of the total collagen concentration with a decrease in the cross-linking of collagen in both continent and incontinent women [265, 435]. Studies in both animals and humans have shown that estrogens also increase vascularity in the peri-urethral plexus which can be measured as vascular pulsations on urethral pressure profilometry [259, 641, 790].

Estrogens for Stress Urinary Incontinence

The role of estrogen in the treatment of stress urinary incontinence has been controversial despite a number of reported clinical trials [358]. Some have given promising results but this may have been because they were small observational and not randomized, blinded or controlled. The situation is further complicated by the fact that a number of different types of estrogen have been used with varying doses, routes of administration, and duration of treatment.

Fantl et al. [266] treated 83 hypo-estrogenic women with urodynamic stress incontinence and/or detrusor overactivity with conjugated equine estrogens (CEEs) 0.625 mg and medroxyprogesterone 10 mg cyclically for 3 months. Controls received placebo tablets. At the end of the study period the clinical and quality of life variables had not changed significantly in either group. Jackson et al. [398] treated 57 post-menopausal women with urodynamic stress or mixed incontinence with estradiol 2 mg or placebo daily for 6 months. There was no significant change in objective outcome measures, although both the active and placebo groups reported subjective benefit.

Two meta-analyses of early data have been performed. In the first, a report by the Hormones and Urogenital Therapy (HUT) committee, the use of estrogens to treat all causes of incontinence in post-menopausal women was examined [267]. Of 166 articles identified, which were published in English between 1969 and 1992, only six were controlled trials and 17 uncontrolled series. The results showed that there was a significant subjective improvement for all patients and those with urodynamic stress incontinence. However, assessment of the objective parameters revealed that there was no change in the volume of urine lost. Maximum urethral closure pressure increased significantly but this result was influenced by only one study showing a large effect.

In the second meta-analysis Sultana and Walters [734] reviewed eight controlled and 14 uncontrolled prospective trials and included all types of estrogen treatment. They also found that estrogen therapy was not an efficacious treatment for stress urinary incontinence, but may be useful for the often associated symptoms of urgency and frequency. Estrogen when given alone therefore does not appear to be an effective treatment for stress urinary incontinence.

Several studies have shown that estrogen may have a role in combination with other therapies, e.g., α-adrenoceptor agonists. However, phenylpropamalamine (the most widely used α-adrenoceptor agonist in clinical practice) has now been restricted or banned by the FDA.

In a randomized trial Ishiko et al. [393] compared the effects of the combination of PFE and estriol (1 mg/day) in 66 patients with post-menopausal stress urinary incontinence. Efficacy was evaluated every 3 months based on stress scores obtained from a questionnaire. They found a significant decrease in stress score in mild and moderate stress incontinent patients in both groups 3 months after the start of therapy and concluded that combination therapy with estriol plus PFE was effective and could be used as first line treatment for mild stress urinary incontinence. Unfortunately this has not been reproduced in other clinical trials.

Thus even prior to the more recently reported secondary analyses of the heart and estrogens/progestogen replacement study (HERS) [320] and Women's Health Initiative (WHI) [349] it was already recognized that estrogen therapy had little effect in the management of urodynamic stress incontinence [13, 637].

Estrogens for Urgency Urinary Incontinence and Overactive Bladder Symptoms

Estrogen has been used to treat post-menopausal urgency and urge incontinence for many years but there have been few controlled trials to confirm that it is of benefit [358]. A double-blind multicenter study of 64 post-menopausal women with "urge syndrome" failed to show efficacy [119]. All women underwent pre-treatment urodynamic investigation to ensure that they had either sensory urgency or detrusor overactivity. They were randomized to treatment with oral estriol 3 mg daily or placebo for 3 months. Compliance with therapy was confirmed by a significant improvement in the maturation index of vaginal epithelial cells in the active but not the placebo group. Estriol produced subjective and objective improvements in urinary symptoms but was not significantly better than placebo.

Another randomized controlled trial from the same group using 25 mg estradiol implants confirmed the previous findings [655], and furthermore found a high complication rate in the estradiol treated patients (vaginal bleeding).

Symptoms of an overactive bladder increase in prevalence with increasing age and LUTS and recurrent urinary tract infections are commonly associated with urogenital atrophy. Whilst the evidence supporting the use of estrogens in LUT dysfunction remains controversial there are considerable data to support their use in urogenital atrophy and the vaginal route of administration correlates with better symptom relief by improving vaginal dryness, pruritis and dyspareunia, greater improvement in cytological findings and higher serum estradiol levels [119]. Overall vaginal estradiol has been found to be the most effective in reducing patient symptoms although conjugated estrogens produced the most cytological change and the greatest increase in serum estradiol and estrone. The most recent meta-analysis of intravaginal estrogen treatment in the management of urogenital atrophy was reported by the Cochrane group in 2003 [732]. Overall 16 trials including 2,129 women were included and intravaginal estrogen was found to be superior to placebo in terms of efficacy although there were no differences between types of formulation. Fourteen trials compared safety between the different vaginal preparations and found a higher risk of endometrial stimulation with CEEs as compared to estradiol.

Thus, theoretically there could be a role for combination treatment with an anti muscarinic agent and vaginal estrogen in post-menopausal women. However, the two clinical trials which have been reported to date differ in their outcome. Tseng et al. [771] showed superior efficacy in terms of symptom improvement for the overactive bladder when tolterodine was used with vaginal estrogen cream as opposed to tolterodine alone. However, Serati et al. [686] found no difference between tolterodine with or without topical estrogen in women with symptomatic detrusor overactivity.

Evidence Regarding Estrogens and Incontinence from Large Clinical Trials

The HERS study included 763 post-menopausal women under the age of 80 years with coronary heart disease (CHD) and intact uteri [320]. It was designed to evaluate the use of estrogen in secondary prevention of cardiac events. In a secondary analysis 1,525 participants who reported at least one episode of incontinence per week at baseline were included. Participants were randomly assigned to 0.625 mg of conjugated estrogens plus 2.5 mg of medroxyprogesterone acetate (MPA) in one tablet ($N = 768$) or placebo ($N = 757$) and were followed for a mean of 4.1 years. Severity of incontinence was classified as improved, unchanged or worsened. The results showed that incontinence improved in 26 % of the women assigned to placebo compared to 21 % assigned to hormones whilst 27 % of the placebo group worsened compared with 39 % of the hormone group ($P = 0.001$). This difference was evident by 4 months of treatment, for both urgency and stress urinary incontinence. The number of incontinence episodes per week increased an average of 0.7 in the hormone group and decreased by 0.1 in the placebo group ($p < 0.001$). The authors concluded that daily oral estrogen plus progestogen therapy was associated with worsening urinary incontinence in older

post-menopausal women with weekly incontinence and did not recommend this therapy for treatment of incontinence. However, it is possible that the progestogen component may have had an influence on the results of this study.

The WHI was a multicenter double-blind placebo controlled randomized clinical trial of menopausal hormone therapy in 27,347 post-menopausal women age 50–79 years enrolled between 1992 and 1998 for whom urinary incontinence symptoms were known in 23,296 participants at baseline and 1 year [349]. The women were randomized based on hysterectomy status to active treatment or placebo. Those with a uterus were given 0.625 mg/day of CEE plus 2.5 mg/day of medroxyprogesterone acetate (CEE + MPA), whereas those who had undergone hysterectomy received estrogen alone (CEE). At 1-year hormone therapy was shown to increase the incidence of all types of urinary incontinence among women who were continent at baseline. The risk was highest for stress urinary incontinence CEE + MPA: RR, (1.7 95 % continence interval) CI (1.61–2.18); CEE alone RR 2.15 mg, 95 % CI, 1.77–2.62, followed by mixed urinary incontinence CEE + MPA: RR 1.49 95 % CI 1.10–2.01. On CEE alone RR was 1.79 95 % CI, 1.26–2.53. The combination of CEE and MPA had no significant effect on developing urge urinary incontinence RR, 1.15; 95 % CI, 0.99–1.34 but CEE alone increased the risk RR 1.32; 95 % CI, 1.10–1.58. For those women experiencing urinary incontinence at baseline frequency worsened in both active groups CEE + MPA; RR, 1.38 95 % CI 1.28–1.49; CEE alone: RR, 1.47 95 % CI, 1.35–1.61. Quantity of urinary incontinence worsened at 1 year in both active groups, CEE + MPA: RR, 1.20 95 % CI, 1.06–1.76; CEE alone: RR, 1.59 95 % CI, 1.39–1.82. Those women receiving hormone therapy were more likely to report that urinary incontinence limited their daily activities CEE + MPA: RR 1.18 95 % CI, 1.06–1.32. CEE alone: RR 1.29 95 % CI, 1.15–1.45 at 1 year. Thus based on this secondary analysis of data from a huge study CEE alone or in combination with MPA was shown to increase the risk of urinary incontinence amongst continent women and worsen urinary incontinence amongst asymptomatic women after 1 year of therapy.

The Nurses Health Study [329] was a biennial postal questionnaire starting in 1976. In 1996, 39,436 post-menopausal women aged 50–75 years was reported no urinary leakage at the start of the study were followed up for 4 years to identify incident cases of urinary incontinence. Five thousand and sixty cases of occasional and 2,495 cases of frequent incontinence were identified. The risk of developing urinary incontinence was increased among post-menopausal women taking hormones compared to women who had never taken hormones (oral estrogen: RR1.54 95 % CI 1.44, 1.65; transdermal estrogen: RR1.68, 95 % CI 1.41, 2.00; oral estrogen with progestin: RR1.34, 95 % CI 1.24, 1.44; transdermal estrogen with progestin: RR1.46, 95 % CI 1.16, 1.84). After cessation of hormone therapy there was a decreased risk of incontinence such that 10 years after stopping hormones the risk was identical in women who had and who never had taken hormone therapy.

The most recent meta analysis of the effect of estrogen therapy on the LUT has been performed by the Cochrane Group [175] and is notable as the conclusions are starkly different from those drawn from the previous review [558]. Overall 33 trials were identified including 19,313 incontinent women (1,262 involved in trials of local administration) of which 9,417 received estrogen therapy.

Systemic administration (of unopposed oral estrogens—synthetic and CEEs) resulted in worse incontinence than placebo (RR1.32; 95 % CI: 1.17–1.48). Although this is heavily influenced by the size of the WHI study [349]. When considering combination therapy there was a similar worsening effect on incontinence when compared to placebo (RR1.11; 95 % CO: 1.04–1.08). There was some evidence suggesting that the use of local estrogen therapy may improve incontinence (RR0.74; 95 % CI: 0.64–0.86) and overall there were 1–2 fewer voids in 24 h and less frequency and urgency.

The authors conclude that local estrogen therapy for incontinence may be beneficial although there was little evidence of long-term effect. The evidence would suggest that systemic hormone replacement using CEEs may make incontinence worse. In addition they report that

there are too few data to comment reliably on the dose type of estrogen and route of administration.

Other Hormones

Progesterone and progestogens are thought to increase the risk of urinary incontinence. LUTS especially stress urinary incontinence have been reported to increase in the progestogenic phase of the menstrual cycle [359]. In similar studies progesterone has been shown to increase beta adrenergic activity leading to a decrease in the urethral closure pressure in female dogs [630]. However, in the WHI there appeared to be no difference whether or not progestin was given in addition to estrogen [349].

Selective estrogen receptor modulators (SERMS) have been reported to have varying effects. Each of the SERMS has receptor ligand conformations that are unique and have both estrogenic and anti estrogenic effects. In the clinical trials of levormeloxifene there was a fourfold increase in the incidence of incontinence leading to cessation of the clinical trial [350]. However raloxifene has not been shown to have any effect at all on urinary incontinence [794]. There are no reported clinical trials evaluating the effect of androgens, and in particular Testosterone, on urinary incontinence in women.

Conclusions. Estrogen has an important physiological effect on the female LUT and its deficiency is an etiological factor in the pathogenesis of a number of conditions. However the use of estrogen either alone or in combination with progestogen has yielded poor results. The current level 1 evidence against the use of estrogen for the treatment of urinary incontinence comes from studies powered to assess their benefit in the prevention of cardiovascular events and therefore the secondary analyses have only been based on self reported symptoms of urinary leakage without any objective data (Table 13.3). Despite this all of these large randomized controlled trials show a worsening of pre-existing urinary incontinence both stress and urgency and an increased new incidence of urinary incontinence with both estrogen and estrogen plus progestogen.

Table 13.3 ICI assessments 2008: Oxford guidelines (modified)

Levels of evidence

Level 1: Systematic reviews, meta-analyses, good quality randomized
controlled clinical trials (RCTs)

Level 2: RCTs, good quality prospective cohort studies

Level 3: Case–control studies, case series

Level 4: Expert opinion

Grades of recommendation

Grade A: Based on level 1 evidence (highly recommended)

Grade B: Consistent level 2 or 3 evidence (recommended)

Grade C: Level 4 studies or "majority evidence" (optional)

Grade D: Evidence inconsistent/inconclusive (no recommendation possible) or the evidence indicates that the drug should not be recommended

However, the majority of subjects in all of these studies were taking combined equine estrogen and this may not be representative of all estrogens taken by all routes of administration.

In a systematic review of the effects of estrogens for symptoms suggestive of an overactive bladder the conclusion was that estrogen therapy may be effective in alleviating OAB symptoms, and that local administration may be the most beneficial route of administration [124, 125]. It is quite possible that the reason for this is that the symptoms of urinary urgency, frequency and urge incontinence may be a manifestation of urogenital atrophy in older post-menopausal women rather than a direct effect on the LUT [637]. Whilst there is good evidence that the symptoms and cytological changes of urogenital atrophy may be reversed by low dose (local) vaginal estrogen therapy there is currently no evidence that estrogens with or without progestogens should be used in the treatment of urinary incontinence.

Desmopressin

The endogenous hormone vasopressin (also known as anti-diuretic hormone) has two main functions: it causes contraction of vascular smooth muscle and stimulates water reabsorption in the renal medulla. These functions are mediated by two specific vasopressin receptors of which there are two major subtypes, namely the V_1 and V_2 receptors. The V_2 subtype is particularly important for the anti-diuretic effects of vasopressin. A genetic or acquired defect in making and secreting vasopressin leads to central diabetes insipidus, and genetic defects in the gene encoding the V_2 receptor can cause nephrogenic diabetes insipidus [390]. Accordingly, decreased vasopressin levels are believed to be important in the pathophysiology of polyuria, specifically nocturnal polyuria, which can lead to symptoms such as nocturia [532, 813]. Nocturia is currently defined by the ICS as the complaint that an individual has to wake at night one or more times to void. It is, however, "an underreported, understudied, and infrequently recognized problem in adults" [812]. Nocturia leads to decreased quality of life [473], and has been associated with both increased morbidity and mortality [474, 574]. While it remains largely unknown in which fraction of patients nocturia can indeed be explained by too little vasopressin, the presence of nocturnal polyuria in the absence of behavioral factors explaining it (such as excessive fluid intake) is usually considered as an indication that a (relative) lack of vasopressin may exist. While it remains largely unknown in what fraction of patients nocturia is explained by too little vasopressin, the presence of nocturnal polyuria in the absence of behavioral factors that can explain it (e.g., excessive fluid intake) is usually considered to indicate decreased vasopressin levels [100, 812]. Based upon these considerations, vasopressin receptor agonists have been used to treat nocturia, both in children and in adults. Desmopressin is the most common vasopressin analogue used to treat nocturia. Desmopressin shows selectivity for anti-diuretic over vasopressor effects. It has a more powerful and longer-lasting antidiuretic action than vasopressin. It is available in formulations for oral, parenteral, and nasal administration. It has a fast onset of action, with urine production decreasing within 30 min of oral administration [636]. Because of symptomatic hyponatremia with water intoxication which is the only SAE reported in children, occurred after intranasal or intravenous administration of desmopressin [642, 759, 778], the FDA and the European Medicines Agency (EMA) removed the indication for the treatment of primary nocturnal enuresis from all intranasal preparations of desmopressin. An oral lyophilisate (MELT) formulation requiring no concomitant fluid intake is currently available. In a recent open-label, randomized, cross-over study, desmopressin MELT was shown to have similar levels of efficacy and safety at lower doses than the tablet formulation of desmopressin in children. A recent study confirmed the superior pharmacodynamic characteristics of desmopressin MELT to desmopressin tablets [204].

The use of desmopressin in children with nocturnal enuresis was comprehensively reviewed by the Cochrane Collaboration in 2002 [310]. These authors evaluated 47 randomized controlled trials involving 3,448 children, of whom 2,210 received desmopressin. According to their analysis, desmopressin was effective relative to placebo in reducing bed-wetting e.g., a dose of 20 μg resulted in a reduction of 1.34 wets/night (95 % CI 1.11; 1.57), and children were more likely to become dry with desmopressin (98 %) than with placebo (81 %). However, there was no difference between desmopressin and placebo after discontinuation of treatment, indicating that desmopressin suppresses symptom enuresis but does not cure the underlying cause. Additionally, not all children responded sufficiently to desmopressin monotherapy. The combination of desmopressin and an enuresis alarm resulted in a greatly improved short-term success rate and decreased relapse rates [18]. The combination of desmopressin and antimuscarinics resulted in better short- and long-term success rates as well as a lower relapse rate than desmopressin alone [17, 69]. For non-responders to desmopressin, replacement of desmopressin with other medications such as tricyclic antidepressants or loop diuretics could be of benefit, whereas muscarinic receptor antagonists may be ineffective in such children [205, 576].

Other studies have explored a possible treatment role for desmopressin in the treatment of nocturia in adults. A search for these studies in Medline using the terms "desmopressin" and "nocturia" was performed and limited to clinical studies of de novo nocturia, i.e., those that excluded subjects in whom childhood enuresis persisted into adulthood. Several previous studies investigated the use of desmopressin for the treatment of nocturia in the context of multiple sclerosis [250, 251]. One study with single dose administration reported a reduction in nocturnal polyuria, but by design did not assess nocturia [250]. Three placebo-controlled double-blind studies with a small patient number (16–33 patients total per study) reported a significant reduction in nocturia [251, 363, 777]. Other controlled studies of similar size, most with a cross-over design, used micturition frequency within the first 6 h after desmopressin administration rather than nocturia as their primary endpoint. These studies consistently reported that desmopressin treatment for up to 2 weeks was efficacious [282, 372, 453]. While desmopressin treatment was generally well tolerated, 4 of 17 patients in one study discontinued treatment due to asymptomatic or minimally symptomatic hyponatremia [777]. Accordingly, desmopressin is now registered for the treatment of nocturia in multiple sclerosis patients [197]. In a small open-label study, desmopressin was also reported to reduce nocturnal polyuria in SCI patients [841].

Further studies have explored the use of desmopressin in adults with nocturia in the apparent absence of neurological damage. The recruited patient populations were based upon different criteria, including having at least two nocturia episodes per night or having nocturnal polyuria. Earlier studies mostly used a desmopressin dose of 20 μg given either orally [66] or intranasally [115, 364] and tended to be very small (≤25 patients). Later studies, as part of the NOCTUPUS program, were considerably larger, involving a total of 1,003 screened patients, and higher oral doses (0.1–0.4 mg) were administered for a period of 3 weeks of double-blind treatment in adults [497, 498, 533, 782]. A total of 632 patients entered the dose-titration phase and 422 patients the double-blind phase of the three NOCTUPUS trials. To counter the argument that the study was performed in desmopressin responders after the dose titration phase, all patients in the NOCTUPUS trials were washed out following the dose-titration phase, and in order to be randomized, it was a requirement that the patients returned to baseline nocturnal diuresis before inclusion in the double-blind phase. The trials showed that oral desmopressin (0.1, 0.2 or 0.4 mg) is effective in both men and women aged ≥ 18 years with nocturia. The number of nocturnal voids decreased from 3 to 1.7 in the desmopressin group compared to 3.2 to 2.7 in the placebo group. In women, the number of nocturnal voids in the desmopressin group decreased from 2.92 to 1.61, whereas that in the placebo group decreased from 2.91 to 2.36. When clinical response was defined as ≥ 50 % reduction in nocturnal voids from baseline, 34 % of men experienced clinical response with desmopressin, compared with 3 % of men who received placebo. In women, 46 % of desmopressin-treated patients experienced a clinical response, compared with 7 % of patients on placebo.

The efficacy of desmopressin for the treatment of nocturia was confirmed in a long-term (10–12 months) open-label study involving 249 patients, which was an extension of the randomized studies in known desmopressin responders. However, a rebound effect was seen when treatment was withdrawn, confirming the association between continued treatment and response [498]. An open-label pilot study in a nursing home setting also reported that desmopressin had beneficial effects [402].

Around 75 % of community-dwelling men and women with nocturia (≥ 2 voids/night) have nocturnal polyuria (NP) [633, 739]. The key urological factors most relevant to nocturia are NP and OABs in women [391], and NP and BPH in men. About 74 % of women with OABs have nocturia and 62 % of patients with OABs and nocturia have NP. Among men with nocturia, 83 % have NP, 20 % have NP alone, and 63 % have NP in combination with another factor such as a small nocturnal bladder capacity or bladder outlet obstruction [143]. Therefore, desmopressin combination therapy with α_1-AR antagonists and/or antimuscarinics should be considered for patients with treatment-resistant nocturia. Seventy-three percent of α_1-AR antagonist-resistant BPH patients experienced a ≥ 50 % reduction in nocturnal voids with oral desmopressin [633, 833]. A randomized, double-blind, placebo-controlled study evaluating the long-term (1, 3, 6, and 12 months) efficacy and safety of low-dose (0.1 mg) oral desmopressin in elderly (≥ 65 years) patients reported that low-dose oral desmopressin led to a significant reduction in the number of nocturnal voids and nocturnal urine volume in patients with BPH [803].

Because nocturia can be caused by different factors, several studies have investigated whether desmopressin may be beneficial in patients with other symptoms in addition to nocturia. In a small, non-randomized pilot study of men believed to have BPH, desmopressin was reported to improve not only nocturia, but also to reduce the overall IPSS [136]. An exploratory, placebo-controlled double-blind study in women with daytime urinary incontinence reported that intranasal administration of 40 µg desmopressin increased the number of leakage-free episodes 4 h after drug administration [639]. One double-blind, placebo-controlled pilot study in patients with OABs treated with 0.2 mg oral desmopressin reported a reduction in voids along with an improvement in quality of life (QoL) [346]. While these data indicate that desmopressin may be effective in treating voiding dysfunction not limited to nocturia, they are too sparse to allow treatment recommendations.

Desmopressin was well tolerated in all the studies and resulted in significant improvements compared to placebo in reducing nocturnal voids and increasing the hours of undisturbed sleep. There was also an improvement in QoL. However, one of the main clinically important side effects of demopressin usage is hyponatremia. Hyponatremia can lead to a variety of adverse events ranging from mild headache, anorexia, nausea, and vomiting to loss of consciousness, seizures, and death. Hyponatremia usually occurs soon after treatment is initiated. The risk of hyponatremia appears to increase with age, cardiac disease, and increasing 24-h urine volume [633]. Based on a meta-analysis, the incidence is around

7.6 % [805]. Increased age and female gender are well-known risk factors for the development of desmopressin-induced hyponatremia. Bae et al. [72] assessed the effects of long-term oral desmopressin on serum sodium and baseline antidiuretic hormone secretion in 15 elderly male patients with severe nocturia (greater than 3 voids nightly), who did not show hyponatremia within 7 days of administration of 0.2 mg desmopressin. Desmopressin (0.2 mg) was administered orally nightly for 1 year. Before and 1 month after the 1-year medication 24-h circadian studies were performed to monitor changes in antidiuretic hormone. Every 3 months during the 1-year medication, serum changes and timed urine chemistry were monitored. The results showed that long-term desmopressin administration gradually decreased serum sodium and induced statistically, but not clinically significant, hyponatremia after 6 months of treatment. Administration of desmopressin for 1 year did not affect baseline antidiuretic hormone secretion. The authors recommended that for long-term desmopressin administration serum sodium should be assessed regularly, at least every 6 months.

Little focus has been on exploring gender differences in the antidiuretic response to desmopressin. Juul et al. [410] found an increasing incidence of hyponatremia with increasing dose, and at the highest dose level of 100 µg, decreases in serum sodium were approximately twofold greater in women over 50 year of age than in men. A new dose recommendation stratified by gender was suggested in the treatment of nocturia: for men, 50- to 100 µg melt was suggested to be an efficacious and safe dose, while for women a dose of 25 µg melt was recommended as efficacious with no observed incidences of hyponatremia. Initiation of desmopressin is currently not indicated for patients aged ≥65 years. The mechanisms behind desmopressin-induced hyponatraemia are well understood, and serum sodium monitoring at baseline and early during treatment of older patients for whom treatment with desmopressin is indicated can greatly reduce their risk of developing the condition. Other advice regarding treatment administration, such as restriction of evening fluid intake and adherence

to recommended dosing, should be followed to minimize the risk of hyponatremia [784].

Desmopressin is useful for patients with nocturia as well as for children with nocturnal enuresis. The drug has been proven to be well-tolerated and effective by several randomized, placebo-controlled trials and is recommended as a first-line treatment (either as monotherapy or in combination with other agents) for patients who have been appropriately evaluated and whose nocturia is related to NP, whether or not this is accompanied by BPH or OABs. For assessment, see Table 13.1.

Appendix

Antimuscarinics with "Specific" Action

Below data on the different antimuscarinics are presented. These drugs are assumed to block only muscarinic receptors (motivating the term "specific"). The amount of information for the individual drugs varies, and so does the degree of details from the different studies presented. However, the information has been chosen to give a reasonable efficacy and adverse effect profile of each individual drug.

Atropine Sulfate

Atropine (DL-hyoscyamine) is rarely used for treatment of OABs/DO because of its systemic side effects, which preclude its use as an oral treatment. However, in patients with neurogenic DO, intravesical atropine may be effective for increasing bladder capacity without causing any systemic adverse effects, as shown in open pilot trials [212, 253, 260, 264, 314]. It appears that intravesical atropine may be as effective as intravesical oxybutynin in patients with neurogenic DO [264].

The pharmacologically active antimuscarinic component of atropine is L-hyoscyamine. Although still used, few clinical studies are available to evaluate the antimuscarinic activity of L-hyoscyamine sulfate [571]. For assessment, see Table 13.1.

Darifenacin Hydrobromide

Darifenacin is a tertiary amine with moderate lipophilicity, well absorbed from the gastrointestinal tract after oral administration, and extensively metabolized in the liver by the cytochrome P450 isoforms CYP3A4 and CYP2D6, the latter saturating within the therapeutic range [704]. UK-148,993, UK-73,689, and UK-88862 are the three main circulating darifenacin metabolites of which only UK-148,993 is said to have significant antimuscarinic activity. However, available information suggests that various metabolites of darifenacin contribute little to its clinical effects [549]. The metabolism of darifenacin by CYP3A4 suggests that co-administration of a potent inhibitor of this enzyme (e.g., ketoconazole) may lead to an increase in the circulating concentration of darifenacin [441].

Darifenacin is a relatively selective muscarinic M_3 receptor antagonist. In vitro, it is selective for human cloned muscarinic M_3 receptors relative to M_1, M_2, M_4, or M_5 receptors. Theoretically, drugs with selectivity for the M_3 receptor can be expected to have clinical efficacy in OABs/DO with reduction of the adverse events related to the blockade of other muscarinic receptor subtypes [27]. However, the clinical efficacy and adverse effects of a drug are dependent not only on its profile of receptor affinity, but also on its pharmacokinetics, and on the importance of muscarinic receptors for a given organ function.

Darifenacin has been developed as a controlled-release formulation, which allows once-daily dosing. Recommended dosages are 7.5 and 15 mg/day. The clinical effectiveness of the drug has been documented in several RCTs [6, 122, 138, 140, 148, 150, 152, 154, 161, 163, 248, 274, 338, 339, 361, 721, 848; for reviews, see 153, 162, 334, 594, 844]. Haab et al. [339] reported a multicenter, double-blind, placebo-controlled, parallel-group study which enrolled 561 patients (19–88 years; 85 % female) with OAB symptoms for more than 6 months and included some patients with prior exposure to antimuscarinic agents. After washout and a 2-week placebo run-in, patients were randomized (1:4:2:3) to once-daily oral darifenacin controlled-release tablets: 3.75 mg (n=53), 7.5 mg (n=229), or 15 mg

(n=115) or matching placebo (n=164) for 12 weeks. Patients recorded daily incontinence episodes, micturition frequency, bladder capacity (MVV), frequency of urgency, severity of urgency, incontinence episodes resulting in change of clothing or pads and nocturnal awakenings due to OABs using an electronic diary during weeks 2, 6, and 12 (directly preceding clinic visits). Tolerability data were evaluated from adverse event reports. Darifenacin 7.5 and 15 mg had a rapid onset of effect, with significant improvement compared with placebo being seen for most parameters at the first clinic visit (week 2). Darifenacin 7.5 mg and 15 mg, respectively, were significantly superior to placebo for (median) improvements in micturition frequency (7.5 mg: −1.6; 15 mg: −1.7; placebo −0.8), frequency of urgency per day (−2.0; −2.0; −0.9) and number of incontinence episodes leading to a change in clothing or pads (−4.0; −4.7; −2.0). There was no significant reduction in nocturnal awakenings due to OABs. The most common adverse events were mild-to-moderate dry mouth and constipation with a CNS and cardiac safety profile comparable to placebo. No patients withdrew from the study as a result of dry mouth and discontinuation related to constipation was rare (0.6 % placebo vs. 0.9 % darifenacin).

In a dose titration study on 395 OABs patients, darifenacin, allowing individualized dosing (7.5 or 15 mg), was found to be effective and well-tolerated [721]. A 2-year open label extension study of these investigations (i.e., [339, 721]) confirmed a favorable efficacy, tolerability, and safety profile [338].

A review of the pooled darifenacin data from the three phase III, multicenter, double-blind clinical trials in patients with OABs was reported by Chapple et al. [152, 154, 161]. After a 4-week washout/run-in period, 1,059 adults (85 % female) with symptoms of OAB (urgency incontinence, urgency, and frequency) for at least 6 months were randomized to once-daily oral treatment with darifenacin: 7.5 mg (n=337) or 15 mg (n=334) or matching placebo (n=388) for 12 weeks. Efficacy was evaluated using electronic patient diaries that recorded incontinence episodes (including those resulting in a change of clothing or pads), frequency and severity of urgency, micturition frequency, and bladder capacity (volume voided). Safety was evaluated by analysis of treatment-related adverse events, withdrawal rates, and laboratory tests. Relative to baseline, 12 weeks of treatment with darifenacin resulted in a dose-related significant reduction in median number of incontinence episodes per week (7.5 mg, -8.8 [-68.4 %; placebo -54 %, $P < 004$]; 15 mg, -10.6 [-76.8 %; placebo 58 %, $p < 0.001$]). Significant decreases in the frequency and severity of urgency, micturition frequency, and number of incontinence episodes resulting in a change of clothing or pads were also apparent, along with an increase in bladder capacity. Darifenacin was well tolerated. The most common treatment-related adverse events were dry mouth and constipation, although together these resulted in few discontinuations (darifenacin 7.5 mg 0.6 % of patients; darifenacin 15 mg 2.1 %; placebo 0.3 %). The incidences of CNS and cardiovascular adverse events were comparable to placebo. The results were confirmed in other RCTs, including also a pooled analysis of three phase III studies in older patients (≥ 65 years), showing that darifenacin (7.5 and 15 mg) had an excellent efficacy, tolerability, and safety profile [274, 361, 849].

The time-to-effect with darifenacin was analyzed in a pooled analysis of efficacy and safety data from 1,059 patients participating in three double-blind 12-week studies [447]. Darifenacin significantly improved all OAB symptoms as early as 6–8 days.

One of the most noticeable clinical effects of antimuscarinics is their ability to reduce urgency and allow patients to postpone micturition. A study was conducted to assess the effect of darifenacin, on the "warning time" associated with urinary urgency. Warning time was defined as the time from the first sensation of urgency to the time of voluntary micturition or incontinence. This was a multicenter, randomized, double-blind, placebo-controlled study consisting of 2 weeks' washout, 2 weeks' medication-free run-in, and a 2-week treatment phase [122]. Warning time was defined as the time from the first

sensation of urgency to voluntary micturition or incontinence and was recorded via an electronic event recorder at baseline (visit 3) and study end (visit 4) during a 6-h clinic-based monitoring period, with the subject instructed to delay micturition for as long as possible. During each monitoring period, up to three urgency-void cycles were recorded. Of the 72 subjects who entered the study, 67 had warning time data recorded at both baseline and study end and were included in the primary efficacy analysis (32 on darifenacin, 35 on placebo). Darifenacin treatment resulted in a significant ($p < 0.004$) increase in mean warning time with a median increase of 4.3 min compared with placebo (darifenacin group from 4.4 to 1.8 min; placebo from 7.0 to -1.0 min). Overall, 47 % of darifenacin-treated subjects compared with 20 % receiving placebo achieved a 30 % increase in mean warning time. There were methodological problems associated with this study; it utilized a dose of 30 mg (higher than the dose recommended for clinical use), the treatment period was short, it was conducted in a clinical-centered environment, the methodology carried with it a significant potential training effect, and the placebo group had higher baseline values than the treatment group. In another warning time study [848] on 445 OABs patients, darifenacin treatment (15 mg) resulted in numerical increases in warning time; however, these were not significant compared to placebo.

Further studies have demonstrated that darifenacin treatment is associated with clinically relevant improvements on health-related quality of life (HRQoL) in patients with OABs [6], and such improvements were sustained as shown in a 2-year extension study [248]. It was shown that neither the positive effects on micturition variables, nor on HRQoL produced by darifenacin (7.5 and 15 mg) were further enhanced by a behavioral modification program including timed voiding, dietary modifications, and Kegel exercises [138, 140].

Since darifenacin is a substrate for the P-glycoprotein drug efflux transporter [142, 555], which is present both in the blood–brain and blood-ocular barriers, several clinical studies have been devoted to investigate possible effect of darifenacin on cognition. Neither in healthy volunteers (19–44 years) and healthy subjects (≥60 years), nor in volunteers 65 years or older could any effect of darifenacin (3.75–15 mg daily) be demonstrated, compared to placebo [142, 432–434, 491].

To study whether darifenacin had any effect on QT/QTc intervals, Serra et al. [688] performed a 7-day, randomized, parallel-group study ($n = 188$) in healthy volunteers receiving once-daily darifenacin at steady-state therapeutic (15 mg) and supratherapeutic (75 mg) doses, alongside controls receiving placebo or moxifloxacin (positive control, 400 mg) once daily. No significant increase in QTcF interval could be demonstrated compared with placebo. Mean changes from baseline at pharmacokinetic T_{max} vs. placebo were −0.4 and −2.2 ms in the darifenacin 15 mg and 75 mg groups, respectively, compared with +11.6 ms in the moxifloxacin group ($P < 0.01$). The conclusion was that darifenacin does not prolong the QT/QTc interval.

Darifenacin 15 mg/day given to healthy volunteers did not change heart rate significantly compared to placebo [604].

Assessment. Darifenacin has a well-documented beneficial effect in OABs/DO (Table 13.1), and tolerability and safety seem acceptable.

Fesoterodine Fumarate

Fesoterodine functions as an orally active pro-drug that is converted to the active metabolite 5-hydroxymethyltolterodine (5-HMT) by non-specific esterases [511, 548]. This compound, which is chemically identical to the 5-hydroxy metabolite of tolterodine, is a non-subtype selective muscarinic receptor antagonist [577]. All of the effects of fesoterodine in man are thought to be mediated via 5-HMT, since the parent compound remains undetectable upon oral dosing. 5-HMT is metabolized in the liver, but a significant part of 5-HMT is excreted renally without additional metabolism. Since the renal clearance of 5-HMT is about 250 mL/min, with >15 % of the administered fesoterodine dose excreted as unchanged 5-HM, this raises the possibility that 5-HMT also could work from the luminal side of

the bladder [548]. The bioavailability of fesoterodine, averaging 52 %, was independent of food intake and the drug may be taken with or without a meal [514]. Peak plasma concentration of 5-HMT is reached at 5 h following oral administration and has a half-life of 7–9 h [513]. The suggested starting dose, 4 mg/day, can be used in patients with moderately impaired renal or hepatic function due to the combination of renal excretion and hepatic metabolism of 5-HMT [207, 510].

The clinical efficacy and tolerability of fesoterodine have been documented in several RCTs [148, 150, 163, 226, 232, 233, 357, 421, 425, 586, 588; see 216]. In a multicenter, double-blind, double-dummy RCT with tolterodine ER, 1,132 patients were enrolled and received treatment [148, 150, 163]. The trial showed that both the 4 and 8 mg doses of fesoterodine were effective in improving symptoms of OAB, with the 8 mg dose having a greater effect at the expense of a higher rate of dry mouth. There appeared to be little difference between fesoterodine 4 mg and tolterodine ER. Only one subject from the fesoterodine 8 mg group and one subject from the tolterodine ER group withdrew from the study due to dry mouth. The dose–response relationship was confirmed in another study that pooled data from two phase III RCTs [448]. Fesoterodine 8 mg performed better than the 4 mg dose in improving urgency and urge UI as recorded by 3-day bladder diary, offering the possibility of dose titration.

A head-to-head placebo controlled trial has been completed comparing fesoterodine 8 mg to tolterodine-extended release 4 mg and placebo [357]. The study randomized 1,590 patients to assess the primary outcome of reduced urgency incontinence episodes at 12 weeks. Fesoterodine produced statistically significant improvements in urgency incontinence episodes, complete dry rates (64.0 % vs. 57.2 %, $p = 0.015$), mean voided volume per void (+32.9 mL vs. +23.5 mL, $p = 0.005$), and in patients' assessments of bladder-related problems as measured by OABs questionnaire (except sleep domain), Patient Perception of Bladder Condition (40 % vs. 33 % with >2 point improvement, $p < 0.001$), and

Urgency Perception Scale (46 % vs. 40 % with improvement, $p=0.014$) compared with tolterodine. The clinical significance of these statistically significant findings is questionable as there was no difference between agents with respect to number of micturitions, urgency episodes, and frequency-urgency sum per 24 h. The improved efficacy of fesoterodine came at the cost of greater dry mouth (27.8 % vs. 16.4 %), headache (5.6 % vs. 3.4 %), constipation (5.4 % vs. 4.1 %), and withdrawal rates (6 % vs. 4 %). Nonetheless, this first head-to-head trial comparing two drugs in class supports the use of fesoterodine 8 mg for additional benefit over tolterodine ER 4 mg.

Wyndaele et al. [821] reported the first flexible-dose open-label fesoterodine trial, which was conducted at 80 different centers worldwide and comprised 516 participants (men and women) >18 years who self-reported OAB symptoms for at least 3 months before screening and had been treated with either tolterodine or tolterodine ER within 2 years without symptom improvement. Approximately 50 % opted for dose escalation to 8 mg at week 4. Significant improvements from baseline to week 12 were observed in micturitions, urgency urinary incontinence episodes, micturition-related urgency episodes, and severe micturition-related urgency episodes per 24 h. Significant improvements from baseline were observed in QoL parameters. Dry mouth (23 %) and constipation (5 %) were the most common adverse events; no safety issues were identified.

The largest double-blind, double-dummy, flexible-dose fesoterodine RCT, which was conducted at 210 different centers with a total of 2,417 patients enrolled, was performed by Kaplan et al. [421]. All patients were healthy, >18 years of age, and self-reported OAB symptoms for at least 3 months. The 960 patients who received fesoterodine 8 mg showed significantly greater mean improvements at week 12 in most efficacy parameters (diary variables) than those receiving either tolterodine ER or placebo; UUI and urgency episodes, micturition frequency, and MVV. No statistically significant changes were shown in reduction of nocturnal micturitions compared with the tolterodine group, whereas when comparing the mean changes in nighttime

micturition with the placebo group a significant difference was found. This phase III study confirmed the superiority of fesoterodine 8 mg over tolterodine ER 4 mg for improving UUI and urgency episodes and 24-h micturitions but not for MVV and nocturia. In another RCT of flexible-dose fesoterodine, Dmchowski et al. reported statistically significant improvements at week 12 in the mean number of micturition per 24 h and in both UUI and urgency episodes. Between groups, difference in nocturnal micturition was not statistically significant.

Nitti et al. [588] determined whether the presence of DO in patients with OABs and urgency urinary incontinence was a predictor of the response to treatment with fesoterodine in a phase 2 randomized, multicenter, placebo-controlled trial. They concluded that regardless of the presence of DO, the response to fesoterodine treatment was dose-proportional and associated with significant improvements in OAB symptoms, indicating that *the response to OABs pharmacotherapy in patients with UUI was independent of the urodynamic diagnosis of DO.*

Kelleher et al. [439] evaluated the effect of fesoterodine on HRQoL in patients with OAB syndrome. Pooled data from two randomized placebo-controlled phase III studies [148, 150, 163, 586] were analyzed. Eligible patients were randomized to placebo or fesoterodine 4 or 8 mg for 12 weeks; one trial also included tolterodine-extended release (tolterodine-ER) 4 mg. By the end of treatment, all active-treatment groups had significantly improved HRQoL compared with those on placebo. In a post hoc analysis of data pooled from these studies, significant improvements in all KHQ domains, ICIQ-SF scores, and bladder-related problems were observed at months 12 and 24 compared to open label baseline [438]. The authors concluded that treatment satisfaction was high throughout the open-label treatment regardless of gender and age.

Malhotra et al. [515] performed a thorough QT study to investigate the effects of fesoterodine on cardiac repolarization in a parallel-group study. Subjects were randomly assigned to receive double-blind fesoterodine 4 mg, fesoterodine 28 mg, or placebo or open-label moxifloxacin 400 mg (positive control) for 3 days. ECGs were obtained on Days −1 (baseline), 1, and 3. The primary analysis was the time-averaged changes from baseline for Fridericia's-corrected QT interval (QTcF) on Day 3. Among 261 subjects randomized to fesoterodine 4 mg ($n=64$), fesoterodine 28 mg ($n=68$), placebo ($n=65$), or moxifloxacin 400 mg ($n=64$), 256 completed the trial. The results indicated that fesoterodine is not associated with QTc prolongation or other ECG abnormalities at either therapeutic or supratherapeutic doses.

Assessment. Fesoterodine has a well-documented beneficial effect in OABs (Table 13.1), and the adverse event profile seems acceptable.

Imidafenacin

Imidafenacin (KRP-197/ONO-8025, 4-(2-methyl-1H-imidazol-1-yl)-2,2-diphenylbutanamide) is an antagonist for the muscarinic ACh receptor with higher affinities for M_3 and M_1 receptors than for the M_2 receptor. Metabolites of imidafenacin (M-2, M-4, and M-9) had low affinities for muscarinic ACh receptor subtypes [458]. The drug blocks pre- as well as postjunctional muscarinic receptors and was shown to block both detrusor contractions and acetylcholine release [570]. The receptor-binding affinity of imidafenacin in vitro was found to be significantly lower in the bladder than submaxillary gland or colon [823], and in rats orally administered imidafenacin distributes predominantly to the bladder and exerts more selective and longer-lasting effect here than on other tissues. Whether this can be translated to the human situation has to be established before claims of clinical bladder selectivity can be made.

Imidafenacin is well absorbed from the gastrointestinal tract and its absolute bioavailability in human is 57.8 % [601, 602]. It is rapidly absorbed with maximum plasma concentration occurring 1–3 h after oral administration [602]. Metabolites in the plasma are produced mainly by first-pass effects. The major enzymes responsible for the metabolism of the drug are CYP3A4 and UGT1A4. The oxidative metabolism is reduced by concomitant administration of CYP3A4 inhibitors. In contrast, imidafenacin

and its metabolites have no inhibitory effect on the CYP-mediated metabolism of concomitant drugs [418].

Kitagawa et al. [455] reported that the subjective efficacy of imidafenacin was observed from 3 days after the commencement of administration and that mean total overactive bladder symptom score (OABSS) decreased gradually during 2 weeks after administration.

A randomized, double-blind, placebo-controlled phase II dose-finding study in Japanese OABs patients was performed to evaluate the efficacy, safety/tolerability, and dose–response relationship of imidafenacin [371]. Overall, 401 patients were enrolled and randomized for treatment with 0.1 mg of imidafenacin/day (99 patients), 0.2 mg of imidafenacin/day (100), 0.5 mg of imidafenacin/day (101), or a placebo (101). After 12 weeks of treatment, the number of incontinence episodes was reduced in a dose-dependent manner, and a significant difference between the imidafenacin treatment and the placebo was observed ($P<0.0001$). Compared with the placebo, imidafenacin caused significant reductions in urgency incontinence, voiding frequency, and urinary urgency, and a significant increase in the urine volume voided per micturition. Imidafenacin was also well tolerated. The incidence of dry mouth in the imidafenacin groups increased dose-dependently. Even though the percentage of patients receiving 0.5 mg/day who discontinued treatment due to dry mouth was high (8.9 %), the percentages in the 0.1 and 0.2 mg/day groups (1.0 % and 0.0 %, respectively) were comparable with that in the placebo group (0.0 %).

A randomized, double-blind, placebo- and propiverine-controlled trial of 781 Japanese patients with OAB symptoms was conducted by Homma et al. [370]. They were randomized to imidafenacin (324), propiverine (310), or a placebo (147). After 12 weeks of treatment, a significantly larger reduction in the mean number of incontinence episodes was observed in the imidafenacin group than in the placebo group ($P<0.0001$). The non-inferiority of imidafenacin compared with propiverine was confirmed for the reduction in using incontinence episodes ($P=0.0014$, non-inferiority margin: 14.5 %).

Imidafenacin was well tolerated. The incidence of adverse events with imidafenacin was significantly lower than with propiverine ($P=0.0101$). Dry mouth, the most common adverse event, was significantly more common in the propiverine group than in the imidafenacin group. There were no significant increases in either the imidafenacin or placebo group in the mean QTc interval, whereas there was a significant increase in the mean QTc interval in the propiverine group ($P<0.0001$). However, there were no clinical arrhythmia and clinical arrhythmic events in any of the treatment groups.

The long-term safety, tolerability, and efficacy of imidafenacin were studied in Japanese OABs patients [370], of whom 478 received treatment and 376 completed a 52-week program. Imidafenacin was well tolerated, the most common adverse event being a dry mouth (40.2 % of the patients). Long-term treatment did not produce an increase in the frequency of adverse events compared with short-term treatment. A significant efficacy of the drug was observed from week 4 through week 52. After 52 weeks, imidafenacin produced mean changes from baseline in the number of incontinence episodes (−83.51 %), urgency incontinence episodes (−84.21 %), voiding frequency (−2.35 micturitions/day), urgency episodes (−70.53 %), and volume voided per micturition (28.99 mL). There were also significant reductions from baseline in all domains of the King's Health Questionnaire. Imidafenacin had no significant effects on the corrected QT interval, vital signs, results from laboratory tests, or post-void residual volume.

A 52-week prospective, open randomized comparative study to evaluate the efficacy and tolerability of imidafenacin (0.2 mg/day) and solifenacin (5 mg/day) was conducted in a total of 41 Japanese patients with untreated OABs [842]. They were randomly assigned to imidafenacin and solifenacin groups. There was no difference in OABSS and KHQ scores between the two groups, but the severity and incidence of adverse events caused by the drugs showed increased differences between the groups with time. The severity of dry mouth and the incidence of constipation were significantly lower in the

imidafenacin group ($P=0.0092$ and $P=0.0013$, respectively). An important limitation of this study is the low number of patients. Only 25 patients (17 males, 8 females) were available for long-term analysis.

Assessment. Imidafenacin seems to be effective and to have an acceptable tolerability. However, the documentation is relatively scarce and the drug is not yet available in the Western countries.

Propantheline Bromide

Propantheline is a quaternary ammonium compound, non-selective for muscarinic receptor subtypes, which has a low (5–10 %) and individually varying biological availability. It is metabolized (metabolites inactive) and has a short half-life (less than 2 h) [82]. It is usually given in a dose of 15–30 mg four times daily, but to obtain an optimal effect, individual titration of the dose is necessary, and often higher dosages are required. Using this approach in 26 patients with detrusor overactivity contractions [94] in an open study obtained a complete clinical response in all patients but one, who did not tolerate more than propantheline 15 mg four times daily. The range of dosages varied from 7.5 to 60 mg four times daily. In contrast, Thüroff et al. [760] comparing the effects of oxybutynin 5 mg three times daily, propantheline 15 mg three times daily, and placebo in a randomized, double-blind, multicenter trial on the treatment of frequency, urgency, and incontinence related to DO (154 patients) found no differences between the placebo and propantheline groups. In another randomized comparative trial with crossover design (23 women with idiopathic DO), and with dose titration, Holmes et al. [368] found no differences in efficacy between oxybutynin and propantheline. Controlled randomized trials ($n=6$) reviewed by Thüroff et al. [761] confirmed a positive, but varying, response to the drug.

Assessment. Although the effect of propantheline on OABs/DO has not been well documented in controlled trials satisfying standards of today, it can be considered effective, and may, in individually titrated doses, be clinically useful (Table 13.1). No new studies on the use of this drug for treatment of OABs/DO seem to have been performed during the last decade.

Solifenacin Succinate

Solifenacin succinate (YM905) is a tertiary amine and well absorbed from the gastrointestinal tract (absolute bioavailability 90 %). The mean terminal half-life is 45–68 h [465, 710, 711]. It undergoes significant hepatic metabolism involving the cytochrome P450 enzyme system (CYP3A4). In subjects who received a single oral dose of 10 mg solifenacin on day 7 of a 20-day regimen of ketoconazole administration (200 mg), C_{max} and AUC_{0-inf} were increased by only approximately 40 % and 56 %, respectively [737]. Solifenacin has a modest selectivity for M3 over M2 (and M1) receptors [2]. Supporting an effect on sensory function by solifenacin, 15 women with DO receiving 10 mg/day of the drug showed an increase in the area under the bladder-volume sensation curve [501]. Solifenacin also increased maximum bladder capacity, a finding in agreement with other studies [374, 751].

Two large-scale phase 2 trials with parallel designs, comprising men and women, were performed [146, 708]. The first dose-ranging study evaluated solifenacin 2.5, 5, 10, and 20 mg and tolterodine (2 mg twice daily) in a multinational placebo-controlled study of 225 patients with urodynamically confirmed DO [146]. Patients received treatment for 4 weeks followed by 2 weeks of follow-up. Inclusion criteria for this and subsequent phase 3 studies of patients with OABs included at least 8 micturitions/24 h and either one episode of incontinence or one episode of urgency daily as recorded in 3-day micturition diaries. Micturition frequency, the primary efficacy variable, was statistically significantly reduced in patients taking solifenacin 5 mg (−2.21), 10 mg (−2.47), and 20 mg (−2.75), but not in patients receiving placebo (−1.03) or tolterodine (−1.79). This effect was rapid with most of the effect observed at the earliest assessment visit, 2 weeks after treatment initiation. In addition, there were numerically greater reductions in episodes of urgency and incontinence when compared with placebo. Study discontinuations due to adverse events were similar across treatment groups, albeit highest in the 20-mg solifenacin group. As the 5 and 10 mg doses caused lower rates of dry mouth than tolterodine, and superior efficacy outcomes relative to placebo, these dosing strengths were selected for further evaluation in large-scale phase 3 studies.

The second dose-ranging study of solifenacin 2.5–20 mg was carried out in the United States (USA) [708]. This trial included 261 evaluable men and women receiving solifenacin or placebo for 4 weeks followed by a 2-week follow-up period. Micturition frequency was statistically significantly reduced relative to placebo in patients receiving 10 and 20 mg solifenacin. The number of micturitions per 24 h showed reductions by day 7 and continued to decrease through day 28; day 7 was the earliest time point tested in solifenacin trials and these findings demonstrate efficacy as early as 1 week. The 5, 10, and 20 mg dosing groups experienced statistically significant increases in volume voided; the 10 mg solifenacin dose was associated with statistically significant reductions in episodes of incontinence.

In one of the early RCTs, a total of 1,077 patients were randomized to 5 mg solifenacin, 10 mg solifenacin, tolterodine (2 mg twice daily), or placebo [160]. It should be noted that this study was powered only to compare active treatments to placebo. Compared with placebo (−8 %), mean micturitions/24 h were significantly reduced with solifenacin 10 mg (−20 %), solifenacin 5 mg (−17 %), and tolterodine (−15 %). Solifenacin was well tolerated, with few patients discontinuing treatment. Incidences of dry mouth were 4.9 % with placebo, 14.0 % with solifenacin 5 mg, 21.3 % with solifenacin 10 mg, and 18.6 % with tolterodine 2 mg twice daily.

Cardozo et al. [124, 125] randomized 911 patients to 12-week once daily treatment with solifenacin 5 mg, solifenacin 10 mg or placebo. The primary efficacy variable was change from baseline to study endpoint in mean number of micturitions per 24 h. Secondary efficacy variables included changes from baseline in mean number of urgency, nocturia, and incontinence episodes per 24 h, and MVV per micturition. Compared with changes obtained with placebo (−1.6), the number of micturitions per 24 h was statistically significantly decreased with solifenacin 5 mg (−2.37) and 10 mg (−2.81). A statistically significant decrease was observed in the number of all incontinence episodes with both solifenacin doses (5 mg: −1.63, 61 %; 10 mg: −1.57, 52 %), but not with placebo (−1.25, 28 %). Of patients reporting incontinence at baseline, 50 % achieved continence after treatment with solifenacin (based on a 3-day micturition diary, placebo responses not given). Episodes of nocturia were statistically significantly decreased in patients treated with solifenacin 10 mg vs. placebo. Episodes of urgency and MVV per micturition were statistically significantly reduced with solifenacin 5 and 10 mg. Treatment with solifenacin was well tolerated. Dry mouth, mostly mild in severity, was reported in 7.7 % of patients receiving solifenacin 5 mg and 23 % receiving solifenacin 10 mg (vs. 2.3 % with placebo). A 40-week follow-up of these studies (i.e., [124, 125, 160]) demonstrated that the favorable profile, both in terms of efficacy and tolerability, was maintained over the study period [337].

The STAR trial [148, 150, 152, 154, 161, 163] was a prospective, double-blind, double-dummy, two-arm, parallel-group, 12-week study which was conducted to compare the efficacy and safety of solifenacin 5 or 10 mg and TOLT-ER 4 mg once daily in OABs patients. The primary effect variable was micturition frequency. After 4 weeks of treatment patients had the option to request a dose increase, but were dummied throughout as approved product labeling only allowed an increase for those on solifenacin. The results showed that solifenacin, with a flexible dosing regimen, was "non-inferior" to tolterodine concerning the primary effect variable, micturition frequency. However, solifenacin showed significant greater efficacy to tolterodine in decreasing urgency episodes (−2.85 vs. −2.42), incontinence (−1.60 vs. −0.83), urgency incontinence (−1.42 vs. −0.83), and pad usage (−1.72 vs. −1.19). More solifenacin-treated patients became continent by study endpoint (59 vs. 49 %) and reported improvements in perception of bladder condition (−1.51 vs. −1.33) assessments. However, this was accompanied by an adverse event incidence which was greater with solifenacin than

with tolterodine. Dry mouth and constipation (mild + moderate + severe) were the most common (solifenacin 30 and 6.4 %, tolterodine 23 and 2.5 %). The majority of side effects were mild to moderate in nature, and discontinuations were comparable and low (5.9 and 7.3 %) in both groups.

Luo et al. (2012) performed a systematic review and meta-analysis of solifenacin RCTs and provided a comprehensive assessment regarding the efficacy and safety of the drug. Their results which largely confirmed what could be deduced from previously published information indicated that solifenacin could significantly decrease the number of urgency episodes per 24 h, micturitions per 24 h, incontinence episodes per 24 h, nighttime micturitions per 24 h, and UUI episodes per 24 h and improve volume voided per micturitions compared with the placebo or tolterodine treatment.

A number of studies and reviews have further documented the effects of solifenacin [120, 147, 148, 150, 159, 163, 519, see also 153, 162, 503, 594, 687, 765, 785], including men with OABs without bladder outlet obstruction [421]. In a pooled analysis of four RCTs, Abrams and Swift [8] demonstrated positive effects on urgency, frequency, and nocturia symptoms in OABs dry patients. In an analysis of four phase III clinical trials, Brubaker and FitzGerald [105] confirmed a significant effect of solifenacin 5 and 10 mg on nocturia in patients with OABs (reductions of nocturia episodes with 5 mg: −0.6, $p < 0.025$; with 10 mg: −0.6, $p < 0.001$ vs. placebo: −0,4) but without nocturnal polyuria. A positive impact on nocturia and sleep quality in patients with OABs treated with solifenacin has also been reported in other studies [742, 831]. Kelleher et al. [437] and Staskin and Te [720] presented data showing efficacy in patients with mixed incontinence.

A pooled analysis of four studies confirmed the efficacy and tolerability of solifenacin 5 and 10 mg in elderly (≥65 years) patients and also showed a high level of persistence in a 40-week extension trial [797]. Post hoc analysis of two 12-week, open label, flexible-dosing studies on 2,645 patients over 65 years of age with OABs revealed that solifenacin was associated with improvements in measures assessing patients' perception of their bladder problems, symptom bother, and aspects of health-related quality of life [117]. Solifenacin was equally well tolerated in younger (<65 years) and older (>65 years) patients [356]. An exploratory pilot study with single doses of solifenacin 10 mg to 12 elderly volunteers suggested no clear propensity to impair cognitive functions [815].

Improvement of QoL by solifenacin treatment has been documented in several studies [294, 436]. In 30 patients with multiple sclerosis, van Rey and Heesakkers [783] improved OAB symptoms as well as neurogenic disease-specific QoL measures.

Information on solifenacin treatment in children is scarce. In a prospective open label study in 72 children (27 with neurogenic bladders) Bolduc et al. [98] improved urodynamic capacity and improved continence. Chart review of 138 children with therapy-resistant OABs treated with solifenacin increased mean voided volume and improved continence [365].

In female volunteers, aged 19–79 years, the effect of 10 and 30 mg solifenacin on the QT interval was evaluated at the time of peak solifenacin plasma concentration in a multi-dose, randomized, double-blind, placebo, and positive-controlled (moxifloxacin 400 mg) trial. The QT interval prolonging effect appeared greater for the 30 mg (8 ms, 4, 13: 90%CI) compared to the 10 mg (2 ms, −3, 6) dose of solifenacin. Although the effect of the highest solifenacin dose (three times the maximum therapeutic dose) studied did not appear as large as that of the positive control moxifloxacin at its therapeutic dose, the confidence intervals overlapped. This study was not designed to draw direct statistical conclusions between the drugs or the dose levels.

Michel et al. [551] studied cardiovascular safety and overall tolerability of solifenacin in routine clinical use in a 12-week, open-label, postmarketing surveillance study. They concluded that "in real-life conditions, i.e., with inclusion of large numbers of patients with cardiovascular co-morbidities and taking comedications, therapeutically

effective doses of solifenacin did not increase heart rate or blood pressure."

Assessment. Solifenacin has a well-documented beneficial effect in OABs/DO (Table 13.1), and the adverse event profile seems acceptable.

Tolterodine Tartrate

Tolterodine is a tertiary amine, rapidly absorbed, and extensively metabolized by the cytochrome P450 system (CYP 2D6). The major active 5-hydroxymethyl metabolite (5-HMT) has a similar pharmacological profile as the mother compound [579] and significantly contributes to the therapeutic effect of tolterodine [106, 107]. Both tolterodine and 5-HMT have plasma half-lifes of 2–3 h, but the effects on the bladder seem to be more long-lasting than could be expected from the pharmacokinetic data. Urinary excretion of tolterodine accounted for <1–2.4 % of the dose; 5–14 % of 5-HMT is eliminated in the urine [107]. Whether or not the total antimuscarinic activity of unchanged tolterodine and 5-HMT excreted in urine is sufficient to exert any effect on the mucosal signaling mechanisms has not been established. However, the preliminary studies by Kim et al. [450] and Chuang et al. [171] do not support such an effect.

The relatively low lipophilicity of tolterodine and even lesser one of 5-HMT implies limited propensity to penetrate into the CNS, which may explain a low incidence of cognitive side effects [174, 362, 668]. However, tolterodine may disturb sleep in subjects unable to form the even less lipophilic 5-HMT due to a low activity of CYP 2D6 [219].

Tolterodine has no selectivity for muscarinic receptor subtypes, but is claimed to have functional selectivity for the bladder over the salivary glands [578, 713]. In healthy volunteers, orally given tolterodine in a high dose (6.4 mg) had a powerful inhibitory effect on micturition and also reduced stimulated salivation 1 h after administration of the drug [713]. However, 5 h after administration, the effects on the urinary bladder were maintained, whereas no significant effects on salivation could be demonstrated.

Animal experiments have suggested that antimuscarinics may affect signaling from the bladder [33]. Cirfirming data in humans were found by Vijaya et al. [791]. In a randomized, placebo-controlled study, they evaluated the effect of tolterodine on urethral and bladder afferent nerves in women with DO in comparison to placebo, by studying the changes in the current perception threshold (CPT). They found a significantly increased CPT value at 5 (described as urgency) and 250 Hz upon both urethral and bladder stimulation after 1 week of treatment. When compared with placebo, women taking tolterodine had significantly increased bladder CPT values at 5 Hz (P-value <0.05).

Tolterodine is available as immediate-release (TOLT-IR; 1 or 2 mg; twice daily dosing) and extended-release (TOLT-ER) forms (2 or 4 mg; once daily dosing). The ER form seems to have advantages over the IR form in terms of both efficacy and tolerability [781].

Several randomized, double-blind, placebo-controlled studies on patients with OABs/DO (both idiopathic and neurogenic DO) have documented a significant reduction in micturition frequency and number of incontinence episodes [174, 362, 668]. Comparative RCTs such as the OBJECT (Overactive Bladder: Judging Effective Control and Treatment) and the OPERA (Overactive Bladder; Performance of Extended Release Agents) studies have further supported its effectiveness.

The OBJECT trial compared oxybutynin ER (OXY-ER) 10 mg once daily with TOLT-IR 2 mg twice daily [62] in a 12-week randomized, double-blind, parallel-group study including 378 patients with OABs. Participants had between 7 and 50 episodes of urgency incontinence per week and 10 or more voids in 24 h. The outcome measures were the number of episodes of urgency incontinence, total incontinence, and micturition frequency at 12 weeks adjusted for baseline. At the end of the study, OXY-ER was found to be significantly more effective than TOLT-IR in each of the main outcome measures adjusted for baseline (see also below: oxybutynin chloride). Dry mouth, the most common adverse event, was reported by 33 % and 28 % of participants taking

OXY-ER and TOLT-IR, respectively. Rates of CNS and other adverse events were low and similar in both groups. The authors concluded that OXY-ER was more effective than TOLT-IR and that the rates of dry mouth and other adverse events were similar in both treatment groups.

In the OPERA study [224], OXY-ER at 10 mg/day or TOLT-ER at 4 mg/day were given for 12 weeks to women with 21–60 urgency incontinence episodes per week and an average of 10 or more voids per 24 h. Episodes of incontinence episodes (primary endpoint), total (urgency and non-urgency) incontinence, and micturition were recorded in seven 24-h urinary diaries at baseline and at weeks 2, 4, 8, and 12 and compared. Adverse events were also evaluated. Improvements in weekly urgency incontinence episodes were similar for the 790 women who received OXY-ER ($n = 391$) or TOLT-ER ($n = 399$). OXY-ER was significantly more effective than TOLT-ER in reducing micturition frequency, and 23.0 % of women taking OXY-ER reported no episodes of urinary incontinence compared with 16.8 % of women taking TOLT-ER. Dry mouth, usually mild, was more common with OXY-ER. Adverse events were generally mild and occurred at low rates, with both groups having similar discontinuation of treatment due to adverse events. The conclusions were that reductions in weekly urgency incontinence and total incontinence episodes were similar with the two drugs. Dry mouth was more common with OXY-ER, but tolerability was otherwise comparable, including adverse events involving the CNS.

In the ACET (Antimuscarinic Clinical Effectiveness Trial) [736] study, which consisted of two trials, patients with OABs were randomized to 8 weeks of open-label treatment with either 2 or 4 mg of once-daily TOLT-ER (study one) and to 5 or 10 mg of OXY-ER (study two). A total of 1,289 patients were included. Fewer patients prematurely withdrew from the trial in the TOLT-ER 4 mg group (12 %) than either the OXY-ER 5 mg (19 %) or OXY-ER 10 mg groups (21 %). More patients in the OXY-ER 10 mg group than the TOLT-ER 4 mg group withdrew because of poor tolerability (13 % vs. 6 %). After 8 weeks, 70 % of patients in the TOLT-ER 4 mg group perceived an improved bladder condition, compared with 60 % in the TOLT-ER 2 mg group, 59 % in the OXY-ER 5 mg group, and 60 % in the OXY-ER 10 mg group. Dry mouth was dose-dependent with both agents, although differences between doses reached statistical significance only in the oxybutynin trial (OXY-ER 5 mg vs. OXY-ER 10 mg; $p = 0.05$). Patients treated with TOLT-ER 4 mg reported a significantly lower severity of dry mouth compared with OXY-ER 10 mg. The conclusion that the findings suggest improved clinical efficacy of TOLT-ER (4 mg) than of OXY-ER (10 mg) is weakened by the open label design of the study.

Zinner et al. [847] evaluated the efficacy, safety, and tolerability of TOLT-ER in older (≥ 65) and younger (<65) OABs patients, in a 12-week RCT including 1,015 patients with urgency incontinence and urinary frequency. Patients were randomized to treatment with TOLT-ER 4 mg once daily ($n = 507$) or placebo ($n = 508$) for 12 weeks. Efficacy, measured with micturition charts (incontinence episodes, micturitions, volume voided per micturition) and subjective patient assessments, safety, and tolerability endpoints, was evaluated, relative to placebo. Compared with placebo, significant improvements in micturition chart variables with TOLT-ER showed no age-related differences. Dry mouth (of any severity) was the most common adverse event in both the TOLT-ER and placebo treatment arms, irrespective of age (<65: ER 22.7 %, placebo 8.1 %; ≥ 65: ER 24.3 %, placebo 7.2 %). A few patients (<2 %) experienced severe dry mouth. No CNS (cognitive functions were not specifically studied), visual, cardiac (per ECG), or laboratory safety concerns were noted in this study. Withdrawal rates due to adverse events on TOLT-ER 4 mg QD were comparable in the two age cohorts (<65: 5.5 %; ≥ 65: 5.1 %).

The central symptom in the OAB syndrome is urgency. Freeman et al. [284] presented a secondary analysis of a double-blind, placebo-controlled study evaluating the effect of once-daily TOLT-ER on urinary urgency in patients with OABs. Patients with urinary frequency (8 or more micturitions per 24 h) and urgency incontinence (5 or more episodes per week) were

randomized to oral treatment with TOLT-ER 4 mg once daily ($n = 398$) or placebo ($n = 374$) for 12 weeks. Efficacy was assessed by use of patient perception evaluations. Of patients treated with TOLT-ER, 44 % reported improved urgency symptoms (compared with 32 % for placebo), and 62 % reported improved bladder symptoms (placebo, 48 %). The proportion of patients unable to hold urine upon experiencing urgency was decreased by 58 % with TOLT-ER, compared with 32 % with placebo ($P < 0.001$).

In the Improvement in Patients: Assessing symptomatic Control with Tolterodine ER (IMPACT) study [255], the efficacy of TOLT-ER for patients' most bothersome OAB symptom was investigated in an open label, primary care setting. Patients with OAB symptoms for ≥ 3 months received TOLT-ER (4 mg once daily) for 12 weeks. By week 12, there were significant reductions in patients' most bothersome symptom: incontinence, urgency episodes, nocturnal and daytime frequency. The most common adverse events were dry mouth (10 %) and constipation (4 %), and it was concluded that in primary care practice, bothersome OAB symptoms can be effectively and safely treated with TOLT-ER, even in patients with comorbid conditions.

Various aspects of the efficacy and tolerability of tolterodine have been further documented in a number of RCTs [87, 167, 190, 225, 228, 647, 651; see further: 153, 162, 594]. Importantly, the QTc effects of tolterodine were determined in a crossover-designed QT study of recommended (2 mg twice daily) and supratherapeutic (4 mg twice daily) doses of tolterodine, moxifloxacin (400 mg once daily), and placebo. No subject receiving tolterodine exceeded the clinically relevant thresholds of 500 ms absolute QTc or 60 ms change from baseline, and it was concluded that tolterodine does not have a clinically significant effect on QT interval [512].

Olshansky et al. [604] compared the effects on heart rate of TOLT-ER 4 mg/day with those of darifenacin 15 mg/day in healthy volunteers. They found that tolterodine, but not darifenacin, significantly increased mean heart rate per 24 h. The proportion of subjects with an increase >5 beats/min was significantly greater in those receiving TOLT-ER (25 % than with darifenacin (8.9 %)).

Hsiao et al. [374] compared the urodynamic effects, therapeutic efficacy, and safety of solifenacin (5 mg) vs. tolterodine ER (4 mg) treatment in women with the OAB syndrome. Both solifenacin and tolterodine had similar urodynamic effects, therapeutic efficacy and adverse events; however, tolterodine had a greater effect in increasing heart rate than solifenacin.

In a prospective, open study, Song et al. [712] compared the effects of bladder training and/or tolterodine as first-line treatment in female patients with OABs. One hundred and thirty-nine female patients with OABs were randomized to treatment with bladder training (BT), tolterodine (2 mg twice daily) or both for 12 weeks. All treatments were efficacious; however, combination therapy was the most effective. Mattiasson et al. [534] compared the efficacy of tolterodine 2 mg twice daily plus simplified bladder training (BT) with tolterodine alone in patients with OABs in a multicenter single-blind study. At the end of the study the median percentage reduction in voiding frequency was greater with tolterodine + BT than with tolterodine alone (33 % vs. 25 %; $p < 0.001$), while the median percentage increase in volume voided per void was 31 % with tolterodine + BT and 20 % with tolterodine alone ($p < 0.001$). There was a median of 81 % fewer incontinence episodes than at baseline with tolterodine alone, which was not significantly different from that with tolterodine + BT (−87 %). It was concluded that the effectiveness of tolterodine 2 mg twice daily can be augmented by a simplified BT regimen. However, Millard et al. [553] investigated whether the combination of tolterodine plus a simple pelvic floor muscle exercise program would provide improved treatment benefits compared with tolterodine alone in 480 patients with OABs. Tolterodine therapy for 24 weeks resulted in significant improvement in urgency, frequency, and incontinence; however, no additional benefit was demonstrated for a simple pelvic floor muscle exercise program. In a 16-week, multicenter, open label study tolterodine-extended release plus behavioral intervention resulted in high treatment satisfaction and improved bladder diary variables in patients who had previously been treated and were dissatisfied with tolterodine or other antimuscarinics [457].

Abrams et al. [5] studied the safety and tolerability of tolterodine for the treatment of OAB symptoms in men with BOO. They found that tolterodine did not adversely affect urinary function in these men. Urinary flow rate was unaltered, and there was no evidence of clinically meaningful changes in voiding pressure and PVR or urinary retention. It was suggested that antimuscarinics can be safely administered in men with BOO. Lee et al. [483] reviewed the safety and efficacy of antimuscarinic agents in treating men with BOO and OABs and emphasized their safety and efficacy. They also concluded that combination therapy of antimuscarinic and α_1-AR antagonists improves the symptoms effectively without increasing the incidence of AUR.

The beneficial effect of TOLT-ER in men with BPE and LUTS, including OABs, has been well documented. Both as monotherapy, but in particularly in combination with α_1-adenoceptor (AR) antagonist, TOLT-ER was found effective [367, 423, 424, 426, 644, 645, 651, 652]. This effect was obtained irrespective of prostate size and was not associated with increased incidence of AUR [644, 645]. A large, 26-week, multicenter, randomized, double-blind, placebo-controlled, three-period crossover study enrolled women aged ≥18 years who were diagnosed with OABs and reported ≥8 micturitions/24 h and ≥4 urgency episodes/week on 5-day bladder diary at baseline [520]. Subjects were randomized to 1 of 10 treatment sequences and received three of five treatments, each for 4 weeks with 4-week washout periods: standard-dose pregabalin/tolterodine ER (150 mg twice daily [BID]/4 mg once daily [QD], $n = 102$), pregabalin alone (150 mg BID, $n = 105$), tolterodine ER alone (4 mg QD, $n = 104$), low-dose pregabalin/tolterodine ER (75 mg BID/2 mg QD, $n = 105$), and placebo ($n = 103$). Subjects completed 5-day diaries at the end of treatment and washout periods. The primary endpoint was change from baseline to week 4 in mean voided volume (MVV) per micturition. Baseline-adjusted changes in MVV were significantly greater after treatment with standard-dose pregabalin/tolterodine ER (39.5 mL) vs. tolterodine ER alone (15.5 mL; $P < 0.0001$), and with pregabalin alone (27.4 mL) vs. tolterodine ER alone ($P=0.005$) and placebo (11.9 mL; $P=0.0006$). Treatments were generally well tolerated; discontinuation rates due to adverse events were 4 %, 2 %, 5 %, 0 %, and 1 % with standard- and low-dose pregabalin/tolterodine ER, pregabalin, tolterodine ER, and placebo, respectively. (See further section on "Combinations"]).

Assessment. Both the IR and ER forms of tolterodine have a well-documented effect in OABs/DO (Table 13.1) and are well tolerated.

Trospium Chloride

Trospium is a quaternary ammonium compound with a biological availability less than 10 % [240, 292]. The drug has a plasma half-life of approximately 20 h and is mainly (60 % of the dose absorbed) eliminated unchanged in the urine. The concentration obtained in urine seems to be enough to affect the mucosal signaling system in a rat model [452]. Whether or not it contributes to the clinical efficacy of the drug remains to be established.

Trospium is not metabolized by the cytochrome P450 enzyme system [81, 240]. It is expected to cross the blood–brain to a limited extent since it is a substrate for the drug-efflux transporter P-glycoprotein, which restricts its entry into the brain [716]. This was demonstrated by Staskin et al. [716], showing that trospium chloride levels in CSF samples were undetectable on Day 10 at steady-state peak plasma concentration concurrent with measureable peak plasma values. Clinically, trospium seems to have no negative cognitive effects [142, 292, 716, 764, 816].

Trospium has no selectivity for muscarinic receptor subtypes. In isolated detrusor muscle, it was more potent than oxybutynin and tolterodine to antagonize carbachol-induced contractions [776].

Several RCTs have documented positive effects of trospium both in neurogenic [507, 545, 725] and non-neurogenic DO [16, 121, 235, 341, 407, 653, 719, 846]. In a placebo-controlled, double-blind study on patients with neurogenic DO [725], the drug was given twice daily in a dose of 20 mg over a 3-week period. It increased maximum cystometric capacity, decreased maximal detrusor pressure, and increased compliance in the treatment group, whereas no effects were noted in the placebo group. Side effects were few and comparable in both groups. In another RCT including patients with spinal cord injuries and neurogenic DO, trospium and oxybutynin were equieffective; however, trospium seemed to have fewer side effects [507].

The effect of trospium in urgency incontinence has been documented in several RCTs. Allousi et al. [16] compared the effects of the drug with those of placebo in 309 patients in a urodynamic study of 3-week duration. Trospium 20 mg was given twice daily. Significant increases were noted in volume at first involuntary contraction and in maximum bladder capacity. Cardozo et al. [121] investigated 208 patients with DO, who were treated with trospium 20 mg twice daily for 2 weeks. Also in this study, significant increases were found in mean volume at first unstable contraction (from 233 to 299 mL; placebo 254–255 mL) and in maximum bladder capacity (from 329 to 356 mL; placebo 345–335 mL) in the trospium-treated group. Trospium was well tolerated with similar frequency of adverse effects as in the placebo group. Jünemann and Al-Shukri [407] compared trospium 20 mg twice daily with tolterodine 2 mg twice daily in a placebo-controlled double-blind study on 232 patients with urodynamically proven DO, urgency incontinence without demonstrable DO, or mixed incontinence. Trospium reduced the frequency of micturition, which was the primary endpoint, more than tolterodine and placebo, and also reduced the number of incontinence episodes more than the comparators. Dry mouth was comparable in the trospium and tolterodine groups (7 and 9 %, respectively).

Halaska et al. [341] studied the tolerability and efficacy of trospium chloride in doses of 20 mg twice daily for long-term therapy in patients with urgency syndrome. The trial comprised a total of 358 patients with urgency syndrome or urgency incontinence. After randomization in the ratio of 3:1, participants were treated continuously for 52 weeks with either trospium chloride (20 mg twice daily) or oxybutynin (5 mg twice daily).

Urodynamic measurements were performed at the beginning, and at 26 and 52 weeks to determine the maximal cystometric bladder capacity. Analysis of the micturition diary clearly indicated a reduction of the micturition frequency, incontinence frequency, and a reduction of the number of urgency episodes in both treatment groups. Mean maximum cystometric bladder capacity increased during treatment with trospium chloride by 92 mL after 26 weeks and 115 mL after 52 weeks ($P=0.001$). Further comparison with oxybutynin did not reveal any statistically significant differences in urodynamic variables between the drugs. Adverse events occurred in 65 % of the patients treated with trospium and 77 % of those treated with oxybutynin. The main symptom encountered in both treatment groups was dryness of the mouth. An overall assessment for each of the drugs revealed a comparable efficacy level and a better benefit-risk ratio for trospium than for oxybutynin due to better tolerability.

Zinner et al. [846] treated 523 patients with symptoms associated with OABs and urgency incontinence with 20 mg trospium twice daily or placebo in a 12-week, multicenter, parallel, double-blind, placebo-controlled trial. Dual primary endpoints were change in average number of toilet voids and change in urgency incontinent episodes per 24 h. Secondary efficacy variables were change in average of volume per void, voiding urgency severity, urinations during day and night, time to onset of action, and change in Incontinence Impact Questionnaire. By week 12, trospium significantly decreased average frequency of toilet voids per 24 h (-2.37) and urgency incontinent episodes 59 % compared to placebo (-1.29; 44 %). It significantly increased average volume per void (32 mL; placebo: 7.7) mL and decreased average urgency severity and daytime frequency. All effects occurred by week 1 and all were sustained throughout the study. Nocturnal frequency decreased significantly by week 4 (-0.43; placebo: 0.17) and Incontinence Impact Questionnaire scores improved at week 12. Trospium was well tolerated. The most common side effects were dry mouth (21.8 %; placebo 6.5 %), constipation (9.5 %; placebo 3.8 %), and headache (6.5 %; placebo 4.6 %). In a large

US multicenter trial with the same design, and including 658 patients with OABs, Rudy et al. [653] confirmed the data by Zinner et al. [846], both with respect to efficacy and adverse effects.

Dose escalation seems to improve therapeutic efficacy. In a 12-week, randomized, double-blind, phase IIIb study including 1,658 patients with urinary frequency plus urgency incontinence received trospium chloride 15 mg TID ($n=828$) or 2.5 mg oxybutynin hydrochloride TID ($n=830$). After 4 weeks, daily doses were doubled and not readjusted in 29.2 % (242/828) of patients in the trospium group, and in 23.3 % (193/830) in the oxybuytnin group, until the end of treatment. At study end, there were no relevant differences between the "dose adjustment" subgroups and the respective "no dose adjustment" subgroups (trospium: $P=0.249$; oxybutynin: $P=0.349$). After dose escalation, worsening of dry mouth was higher in both dose-adjusted subgroups compared to the respective "no dose adjustment" subgroups ($P<0.001$). Worsening of dry mouth was lower in the trospium groups than in the oxybutynin groups [97].

An extended release formulation of trospium allowing once daily dosing has been introduced [700] and its effects tested in controlled trials [141, 235, 504, 671, 672, 719, 845]. These studies demonstrated similar efficacy as found with previous formulations, but include experiences in, e.g., elderly patients (>75 years), obese patients, and in patients who use multiple concomitant medications. The most frequent side effects were dry mouth (12.9 %; placebo 4.6) and constipation (7.5 %; placebo 1.8) [235].

Intravesical application of trospium may be an interesting alternative. Fröhlich et al. [288] performed a randomized, single-blind, placebo-controlled, mono-centre clinical trial in 84 patients with urgency or urgency incontinence. Compared to placebo, intravesical trospium produced a significant increase in maximum bladder capacity and a decrease of detrusor pressure accompanied by an increase of residual urine. There was an improvement in uninhibited bladder contractions. No adverse events were reported. Interestingly, intravesical trospium does not seem to be absorbed [800], thus offering an opportunity for treatment with minimal systemic antimuscuscarinic effects.

Assessment. Trospium has a well-documented effect in OABs/DO, and tolerability and safety seem acceptable (Table 13.1).

Antimuscarinics with "Mixed" Action

Some drugs used for treatment of the OABs/DO have been shown to have more than one mechanism of action. They all have a more or less pronounced antimuscarinic effect and, in addition, an often poorly defined "direct" action on bladder muscle. For several of these drugs, the antimuscarinic effects can be demonstrated at much lower drug concentrations than the direct action, which may involve blockade of voltage-operated Ca^{2+} channels. Most probably, the clinical effects of these drugs can be explained mainly by an antimuscarinic action. Among the drugs with mixed actions was terodiline, which was withdrawn from the market because it was suspected to cause polymorphic ventricular tachycardia (torsade de pointes) in some patients [185, 723].

Oxybutynin Chloride

Oxybutynin is a tertiary amine that is well absorbed and undergoes extensive upper gastrointestinal and first-pass hepatic metabolism via the cytochrome P-450 system (CYP3A4) into multiple metabolites. The primary metabolite, N-desethyloxybutynin (DEO), has pharmacological properties similar to the parent compound [799], but occurs in much higher concentrations after oral administration [377]. It has been implicated as the major cause of the troublesome side effect of dry mouth associated with the administration of oxybutynin. It seems reasonable to assume that the effect of oral oxybutynin to a large extent is exerted by the metabolite. The occurrence of an active metabolite may also explain the lack of correlation between plasma concentration of oxybutynin itself and side effects in geriatric patients reported by Ouslander et al. [607]. The plasma half-life of the oxybutynin is

approximately 2 h, but with wide interindividual variation [242, 377].

Oxybutynin has several pharmacological effects in vitro, some of which seem difficult to relate to its effectiveness in the treatment of DO. It has both an antimuscarinic and a direct muscle relaxant effect, and in addition, local anesthetic actions. The latter effect may be of importance when the drug is administered intravesically, but probably plays no role when it is given orally. In vitro, oxybutynin was 500 times weaker as a smooth muscle relaxant than as an antimuscarinic agent [411]. Most probably, when given systemically, oxybutynin acts mainly as an antimuscarinic drug. Oxybutynin has a high affinity for muscarinic receptors in human bladder tissue and effectively blocks carbachol-induced contractions [581, 799]. The drug was shown to have slightly higher affinity for muscarinic M_1 and M_3 receptors than for M_2 receptors [580, 592], but the clinical significance of this is unclear.

The immediate release (IR) form of oxybutynin (OXY-IR) is recognized for its efficacy and most of the newer anti-muscarinic agents have been compared to it once efficacy over placebo has been determined. In general, the new formulations of oxybutynin and other antimuscarinic agents offer patients efficacy roughly equivalent to that of OXY-IR, and the advantage of the newer formulations lies in improved dosing schedules and side effect profile [62, 224, 227]. An extended release oxybutynin (OXY-ER) once daily oral formulation and an oxybutynin transdermal delivery system (OXY-TDS) are available. OXY-TDS offers a twice-weekly dosing regimen and the potential for improved patient compliance and tolerability. Some of the available formulations of oybutynin were overviewed by McCrery and Appell [538].

Immediate-release oxybutynin (OXY-IR). Several controlled studies have shown that OXY-IR is effective in controlling DO, including neurogenic DO [38, 827]. The recommended oral dose of the IR form is 5 mg three times daily or four times daily, even if lower doses have been used. Thüroff et al. [761] summarized 15 randomized controlled studies on a total of 476 patients treated with oxybutynin. The mean decrease in incontinence was recorded as 52 % and the mean reduction in frequency per 24 h was 33 % (data on placebo not presented). The overall "subjective improvement" rate was reported as 74 % (range 61–100 %). The mean percent of patients reporting an adverse effect was 70 (range 17–93 %). Oxybutynin, 7.5–15 mg/day, significantly improved quality of life of patients suffering from overactive bladder in a large open multi-center trial. In this study, patients' compliance was 97 % and side effects, mainly dry mouth, were reported by only 8 % of the patients [20]. In nursing home residents ($n=75$), Ouslander et al. [608] found that oxybutynin did not add to the clinical effectiveness of prompted voiding in a placebo-controlled, double-blind, cross-over trial. On the other hand, in another controlled trial in elderly subjects ($n=57$), oxybutynin with bladder training was found to be superior to bladder training alone [741].

Several open studies in patients with spinal cord injuries have suggested that oxybutynin, given orally or intravesically, can be of therapeutic benefit [449, 740].

The therapeutic effect of OXY-IR on DO is associated with a high incidence of side effects (up to 80 % with oral administration). These are typically antimuscarinic in nature (dry mouth, constipation, drowsiness, blurred vision) and are often dose-limiting [73, 239, 404, 405]. The effects on the ECG of oxybutynin were studied in elderly patients with urinary incontinence (Hussain et al., 1998); no changes were found. It cannot be excluded that the commonly recommended dose 5 mg×3 is unnecessarily high in some patients, and that a starting dose of 2.5 mg×2 with following dose-titration would reduce the number of adverse effects [20].

Extended release oxybutynin (OXY-ER). This formulation was developed to decrease liver metabolite formation of DEO with the presumption that it would result in decreased side effects, especially dry mouth, and improve patient compliance with remaining on oxybutynin therapy (see [65]). The formulation utilizes an osmotic system to release the drug at a controlled rate over 24 h

distally primarily into the large intestine where absorption is not subject to first-pass metabolism in the liver. This reduction in metabolism is meant to improve the rate of dry mouth complaints when compared to OXY-IR. DEO is still formed through the hepatic cytochrome P-450 enzymes, but clinical trials have indeed demonstrated improved dry mouth rates compared with OXY-IR [61]. Salivary output studies have also been interesting. Two hours after administration of OXY-IR or TOLT-IR, salivary production decreased markedly and then gradually returned to normal. With OXY-ER, however, salivary output was maintained at predose levels throughout the day [135].

The effects of OXY-ER have been well documented [695]. In the OBJECT study [62], the efficacy and tolerability of 10 mg OXY-ER was compared to a twice daily 2 mg dose of TOLT-IR. OXY-ER was statistically more effective than the TOLT-IR in weekly urgency incontinence episodes (OXY-ER from 25.6 to 6.1 %; TOLT-IR 24.1 to 7.8), total incontinence (OXY-ER from 28.6 to 7.1 %; TOLT-IR 27.0 to 9.3), and frequency (OXY-ER from 91.8 to 67.1 %; TOLT-IR 91.6 to 71.5) and both medications were equally well tolerated. The basic study was repeated as the OPERA study [224] with the difference that this study was a direct comparison of the two extended-release forms, OXY-ER (10 mg) and TOLT-ER (4 mg), and the results were quite different. In this study there was no significant difference in efficacy for the primary endpoint of urgency incontinence; however, TOLT-ER had a statistically lower incidence of dry mouth. OXY-ER was only statistically better at 10 mg than TOLT-ER 4 mg in the reduction of the rate of urinary frequency. These studies made it clear that in comparative studies IR entities of one drug should no longer be compared with ER entities of the other.

Greater reductions in urgency and total incontinence have been reported in patients treated in dose-escalation studies with OXY-ER. In two randomized studies, the efficacy and tolerability of OXY-ER were compared with OXY-IR. In the 1999 study [23], 105 patients with urgency or mixed incontinence were randomized to receive 5–30 mg OXY-ER once daily or 5 mg of OXY-IR 1–4 times/day. Dose titrations began at 5 mg and the dose was increased every 4–7 days until one of three endpoints was achieved. These were (1) the patient reported no urgency incontinence during the final 2 days of the dosing period; (2) the maximum tolerable dose was reached; the maximum allowable dose (30 mg for OXY-ER or 20 mg for OXY-IR) was reached. The mean percentage reduction in weekly urgency and total incontinence episodes was statistically similar between OXY-ER and OXY-IR, but dry mouth was reported statistically more often with OXY-IR. In the 2000 study [789], 226 patients were randomized between OXY-ER and OXY-IR with weekly increments of 5 mg daily up to 20 mg daily. As in the 1999 study, OXY-ER again achieved a >80 % reduction in urgency and total incontinence episodes and a significant percentage of patients became dry. A negative aspect of these studies is that there were no naïve patients included, as all patients were known responders to oxybutynin. Similar efficacy results have been achieved, however, with OXY-ER in a treatment-naïve population [313].

In an RCT comparing different daily doses of oxybutynin (5, 10 and 15 mg), Corcos et al. [187] found a significant dose–response relationship for both urgency incontinence episodes and dry mouth. The greatest satisfaction was with 15 mg oxybutynin/day.

In a multicenter, prospective, observational, flexible-dosing Korean study, Yoo et al. [832] investigate the prescription pattern and dose distribution of OXY-ER in patients with the OAB syndrome in actual clinical practice. The dosage for each patient was adjusted after discussions of efficacy and tolerability between doctor and patient, over a 12-week treatment period. Efficacy was measured by administering the Primary OAB Symptom Questionnaire (POSQ) before and after treatment. Patients were also administered; the patient perception of treatment benefit (PPTB) questionnaire is at the end of the study. Of the 809 patients enrolled, 590 (73.2 %) continued to take study medication for 12 weeks. Most patients were prescribed 5–10 mg/day oxybutynin ER as both starting and maintenance doses, with a dose escalation rate of only 14.9 %. All OAB symptoms evaluated by the POSQ were

improved; 94.1 % of patients reported benefits from treatment and 89.3 % were satisfied.

Transdermal oxybutynin (OXY-TDS). Transdermal delivery also alters oxybutynin metabolism reducing DEO production to an even greater extent than OXY-ER. A study [201] comparing OXY-TDS with OXY-IR demonstrated a statistically equivalent reduction in daily incontinent episodes (from 7.3 to 2.3: 66 % for OXY-TDS, and 7.4 to 2.6: 72 % for OXY-IR), but much less dry mouth (38 % for OXY-TDS and 94 % for OXY-IR). In another study [227] the 3.9-mg daily dose patch significantly (vs. placebo) reduced the mean number of daily incontinence episodes (from 4.7 to 1.9; placebo from 5.0 to 2.9), while reducing average daily urinary frequency confirmed by an increased average voided volume (from 165 to 198 mL; placebo from 175 to 182 mL). Furthermore, dry mouth rate was similar to placebo (7 % vs. 8.3 %). In a third study [229, 234] OXY-TDS was compared not only to placebo but to TOLT-ER. Both drugs equivalently and significantly reduced daily incontinence episodes and increased the average voided volume, but TOLT-ER was associated with a significantly higher rate of antimuscarinic adverse events. The primary adverse event for OXY-TDS was application site reaction pruritis in 14 % and erythema in 8.3 % with nearly 9 % feeling that the reactions were severe enough to withdraw from the study, despite the lack of systemic problems.

The pharmacokinetics and adverse effect dynamics of OXY-TDS (3.9 mg/day) and OXY-ER (10 mg/day) were compared in healthy subjects in a randomized, 2-way crossover study [61]. Multiple blood and saliva samples were collected and pharmacokinetic parameters and total salivary output were assessed. OXY-TDS administration resulted in greater systemic availability and minimal metabolism to DEO compared to OXY-ER which resulted in greater salivary output in OXY-TDS patients and less dry mouth symptomatology than when taking OXY-ER.

Dmochowski et al. [231] analyzing the combined results of two RCTs concluded that transdermal oxybutynin was shown to be efficacious and well tolerated. The most common systemic side effect was dry mouth (7.0 % vs. placebo 5.3 %). Application site erythema occurred in 7 % and pruritus in 16.1 %. Also Cartwright and Cardozo [129], reviewing published and presented data, concluded that transdermal oxybutynin has a good balance between efficacy and tolerability with a rate of systemic antimuscarinic side effects lower that with oral antimuscarinics—however, this benefit was offset by the rate of local skin reaction. The reviews of Sahai et al. [663] and Staskin and Salvatore [718] largely confirmed these conclusions, which also have been supported by further studies [130].

Oxybutynin topical gel. Given the efficacy and tolerability of the transdermal application, limited only by skin site reactions, a gel formulation was developed. Oxybutynin topical gel (OTG) was approved by the US FDA in January 2009. OTG is applied once daily to the abdomen, thigh, shoulder, or upper arm area [715]. The 1 g application dose delivers approximately 4 mg of drug to the circulation with stable plasma concentrations and a "favorable" DEO metabolite: oxybutynin ratio believed to minimizing antimuscarinic side effects [717]. In a multicenter RCT, 789 patients (89 % women) with urgency-predominant incontinence were assigned to OTG or placebo once daily for 12 weeks [715]. The mean number of urgency episodes, as recorded by 3-day voiding diary, was reduced by 3.0 episodes/day vs. 2.5 in the placebo arm ($P < 0.0001$). Urinary frequency decreased by 2.7 episodes/day and voided volume increased by 21 mL (vs. 2.0 episodes ($P = 0.0017$) and 3.8 mL ($P = 0.0018$), respectively, in the placebo group). Dry mouth was reported in 6.9 % of the treatment group vs. 2.8 % of the placebo group. Skin reaction at the application site was reported in 5.4 % of the treatment group vs. 1.0 % in the placebo arm. It was felt that improved skin tolerability of the gel over the OXY transdermal patch delivery system was secondary to lack of adhesive and skin occlusion. The gel dries rapidly upon application and leaves no residue; person-to-person transference via skin contact is largely eliminated if clothing is worn over the application site [230]. The evolution of the transdermal gel allows greater patient

tolerability and improved compliance. This was confirmed by Sand et al. [669, 670] showing that in 704 women with OABs, OTG significantly reduced the number (mean ± standard deviation) of daily incontinence episodes (OTG, -3.0 ± 2.8 episodes; placebo, -2.5 ± 3.0 episodes), reduced urinary frequency, increased voided volume, and improved select health-related quality-of-life domains vs. placebo. Dry mouth was the only drug-related adverse event significantly more common with OTG (7.4 %) than with placebo (2.8 %).

Other administration forms. Rectal administration [180] was reported to have fewer adverse effects than the conventional tablets.

Administered intravesically, oxybutynin has in several studies been demonstrated to increase bladder capacity and produce clinical improvement with few side effects, both in neurogenic and in other types of DO, and both in children and adults [264, 298, 335, 499], although adverse effects may occur [428, 611].

Effects on cognition. Several studies have documented the possibility that oxybutynin may have negative effects on cognitive functions, particularly in the elderly population but also in children (see, e.g., [432, 433, 456]). This factor should be taken into consideration when prescribing the drug.

Assessment. Oxybutynin has a well-documented efficacy in the treatment of OABsDO (Table 13.1). Despite the adverse effect profile, it is still an established therapeutic option.

Propiverine Hydrochloride

Several aspects of the preclinical, pharmacokinetic, and clinical effects of propiverine have been reviewed by Madersbacher and Mürz [506]. The drug is rapidly absorbed (t_{max} 2 h), but has a high first pass metabolism, and its biological availability is about 50 %. Propiverine is an inducer of hepatic cytochrome P450 enzymes in rats in doses about 100-times above the therapeutic doses in man [801]. Several active metabolites are formed which quantitatively and qualitatively differ from the mother compound [347, 568, 733, 820, 843]. Most probably these metabolites contribute to the clinical effects of the drug, but their individual contributions have not been clarified [549]. The half-life of propiverine itself is about 11–14 h. An extended release preparation was shown to be effective [409, 535]. Oral absorption of propiverine is site-dependent and influenced by dosage form and circadiantime-dependent elimination processes [535].

Propiverine has combined antimuscarinic and calcium antagonistic actions [343, 766]. The importance of the calcium antagonistic component for the drug's clinical effects has not been established. Propiverine has no selectivity for muscarinic receptor subtypes. The effects of propiverine on cardiac ion channels and action potentials were investigated by Christ et al. [170]. Propiverine blocked in a concentration-dependent manner HERG channels expressed in HEK293 cells, as well as native I(Kr) current in ventricular myocytes of guinea pig. However, action potential duration was not prolonged in guinea-pig and human ventricular tissue, and the investigators concluded that their results did not provide evidence for an enhanced cardiovascular safety risk with the drug.

Propiverine has been shown to have beneficial effects in patients with DO in several investigations. Thüroff et al. [761] collected nine randomized studies on a total of 230 patients and found a 17 % reduction in micturitions per 24 h, a 64 mL increase in bladder capacity, and a 77 % (range 33–80 %) subjective improvement. Side effects were found in 14 % (range 8–42 %). In patients with neurogenic DO, controlled clinical trials have demonstrated propiverine's superiority over placebo [726]. Propiverine also increased bladder capacity and decreased maximum detrusor contractions. Controlled trials comparing propiverine, flavoxate, and placebo [807], and propiverine, oxybutynin and placebo [505, 808] have confirmed the efficacy of propiverine and suggested that the drug may have equal efficacy and fewer side effects than oxybutynin. In a comparative RCT including 131 patients with neurogenic DO, propiverine and oxybutynin were compared [727]. The drugs were found to be equally effective in

increasing bladder capacity and lowering bladder pressure. Propiverine caused a significantly lower frequency of dry mouth than oxybutynin.

Also in children and adolescents with neurogenic DO, propiverine was found to be effective [328, 680], with a low incidence rate of adverse events: <1.5 % [328]. A randomized, double-blind, placebo-controlled trial with parallel-group design in children aged 5–10 year was performed by Marschall-Kehrel et al. [524]. Of 171 randomized children, 87 were treated with propiverine and 84 with placebo. Decrease in voiding frequency per day was the primary efficacy parameter; secondary endpoints included voided volume and incontinence episodes. There was a significant decrease in voiding frequency episodes for propiverine vs. placebo. Superiority could also be demonstrated for voided volume and incontinence episodes per day. Propiverine was well-tolerated: 23 % of side effects were reported for propiverine and 20 % for placebo.

In a randomized, double-blind, multicenter clinical trial, patients with idiopathic DO were treated with 15 mg propiverine twice daily or 2 mg TOLT-IR twice daily over a period of 28 days [408]. The maximum cystometric capacity was determined at baseline and after 4 weeks of therapy. The difference of both values was used as the primary endpoint. Secondary endpoints were voided volume per micturition, evaluation of efficacy (by the investigator), tolerability, post-void residual urine, and quality of life. It was found that the mean maximum cystometric capacity increased significantly ($p < 0.01$) in both groups. The volume at first urgency and the frequency/volume chart parameters also showed relevant improvements during treatment. The most common adverse event, dry mouth, occurred in 20 patients in the propiverine group and in 19 patients in the tolterodine group. The scores for the quality of life improved comparably in both groups.

Madersbacher et al. [505] compared the tolerability and efficacy of propiverine (15 mg three times daily) oxybutynin (5 mg twice daily) and placebo in 366 patients with urgency and urgency incontinence in a randomized, double-blind placebo-controlled clinical trial. Urodynamic efficacy of propiverine was judged similar to that of oxybutynin, but the incidence of dry mouth and the severity of dry mouth were judged less with propiverine than with oxybutynin. Dorschner et al. [241] investigated in a double-blind, multicenter, placebo-controlled, randomized study the efficacy and cardiac safety of propiverine in 98 elderly patients (mean age 68 years), suffering from urgency, urgency incontinence, or mixed urgency-stress incontinence. After a 2-week placebo run-in period, the patients received propiverine (15 mg three times daily) or placebo (three times daily) for 4 weeks. Propiverine caused a significant reduction of the micturition frequency (from 8.7 to 6.5) and a significant decrease in episodes of incontinence (from 0.9 to 0.3 per day). The incidence of adverse events was very low (2 % dryness of the mouth under propiverine—2 out of 49 patients). Resting and ambulatory ECGs indicated no significant changes. The cardiac safety of propiverine was further studied by Donath et al. [236] in two comprehensively designed mono-centric ECG studies (including 24 healthy females, followed by a second study on 24 male patients with CHD and a pathological Pardee-Q-wave in the ECG). Both studies were placebo-controlled and compared the effects of single (30 mg s.i.d.) and multiple dosing (15 mg TID) of propiverine hydrochloride in a crossover design over 6 and 13 days, respectively. They were performed to investigate the influence of propiverine hydrochloride and its main metabolite propiverine-N-oxide on cardiac function with regard to QTc prolongation, QTc dispersion, and T-wave shape. No negative effects on cardiac safety could be demonstrated.

Abrams et al. [3] compared the effects of propiverine and oxybutynin on ambulatory urodynamic monitoring (AUM) parameters, safety, and tolerability in OABs patients. Patients ($n = 77$) received two of the following treatments during two 2-week periods: propiverine 20 mg once daily, propiverine 15 mg three times daily, oxybutynin 5 mg three times daily, and placebo. They found that oxybutynin 15 mg was more effective than propiverine 20 mg in reducing symptomatic and asymptomatic involuntary detrusor contractions in ambulatory patients.

Oxybutynin had a higher rate of dry mouth, and propiverine had a more pronounced effect on gastrointestinal, cardiovascular, and visual function.

Yamaguchi et al. [824] performed a multicenter, 12-week, double-blind phase III trial in Japanese men and women with OABs (1,593 patients were randomized and 1,584 were treated), comparing solifenacin 5 or 10 mg, propiverine 20 mg, and placebo. Changes at endpoint in number of voids/24 h, urgency, incontinence, urgency incontinence and nocturia episodes, volume voided/void, restoration of continence and quality of life (QoL) were examined. It was found that at endpoint, there were greater reductions in mean (SD) voids/24 h with all drug regimens than with placebo. All active treatments improved the volume voided and QoL vs. placebo; solifenacin 10 mg reduced nocturia episodes and significantly improved urgency episodes and volume voided vs. propiverine 20 mg, and solifenacin 5 mg caused less dry mouth. Solifenacin 10 mg caused more dry mouth and constipation than propiverine 20 mg. Wada et al. [793] performed a prospective nonrandomized crossover study of female OABs patients, assigned alternately to treatment with propiverine (20 mg) for 8 weeks then solifenacin (5 mg) for 8 weeks or solifenacin for 8 weeks then propiverine for 8 weeks. At baseline, eighth week and 16th week symptoms were assessed using OABSS. Of the 121 patients enrolled, 83 were analyzed. Both drugs were effective. Urgency was further improved after switching from propiverine to solifenacin, but not after switching from solifenacin to propiverine. Solifenacin was better tolerated than propiverine.

In another multicenter, prospective, parallel, double-blind, placebo-controlled trial, Lee et al. [482] studied the effects of 30 mg propiverine/day in 264 OABs patients (mean age 52.2 years), 221 of whom had efficacy data available from baseline and at least one on-treatment visit with >75 compliance. The study was focused on improving urgency. Overall, among patients treated with propiverine, 39 % rated their treatment as providing "much benefit," compared with 15 % in the placebo group. Adverse events reported by 32 (22.5 %) and 10 (12.7 %) patients in the propiverine and placebo group were all tolerable.

Masumori et al. [530] examined prospectively the efficacy and safety of propiverine in patients with OABs who poorly responded to previous treatment with solifenacin, tolterodine, or imidafenacin. Of 73 patients enrolled (29 males and 44 females, median age 71 years), 52 completed the protocol treatment. The OABSS was significantly improved by propiverine treatment. The scores of OAB symptoms (nighttime frequency, urgency and urge incontinence) except daytime frequency also improved significantly. No increase in PVR was observed. The most frequent adverse event was dry mouth (13.7 %), followed by constipation (6.8 %).

In a non-controlled study in patients with wet OABs the efficacy of propiverine on symptoms and quality of life was confirmed [463].

Assessment. Propiverine has a documented beneficial effect in the treatment of OABs/DO (Table 13.1) and seems to have an acceptable side effect profile.

Flavoxate Hydrochloride

Flavoxate is often discussed as a drug with mixed actions; however, its main mechanism of action may not be antimuscarinic. Flavoxate is well absorbed, and oral bioavailability appeared to be close to 100 % [334]. The drug is extensively metabolized and plasma half-life was found to be 3.5 h [692]. Its main metabolite (3-methylflavone-8-carboxylic acid, MFCA) has been shown to have low pharmacological activity [111, 132]. The main mechanism of flavoxate's effect on smooth muscle has not been established. The drug has been found to possess a moderate calcium antagonistic activity, to have the ability to inhibit PDE, and to have local anesthetic properties; no antimuscarinic effect was found [333]. Uckert et al. [776], on the other hand, found that in strips of human bladder, the potency of flavoxate to reverse contraction induced by muscarinic receptor stimulation and by electrical field stimulation was comparable, It has been suggested that pertussis toxin-sensitive G-proteins in the brain are involved in the flavoxate-induced suppression of the micturition reflex, since intracerebroventricularly or intrathecally administered flavoxate abolished isovolumetric rhythmic bladder contractions in anesthetized rats [603].

The clinical effects of flavoxate in patients with DO and frequency, urgency, and incontinence have been studied in both open and controlled investigations, but with varying rates of success [654]. Stanton [714] compared emepronium bromide and flavoxate in a double-blind, cross-over study of patients with detrusor overactivity and reported improvement rates of 83 % and 66 % after flavoxate or emepronium bromide, respectively, both administered as 200 mg three times daily. In another double-blind, cross-over study comparing flavoxate 1,200 mg/day with that of oxybutynin 15 mg daily in 41 women with idiopathic motor or sensory urgency, and utilizing both clinical and urodynamic criteria, Milani et al. [552] found both drugs effective. No difference in efficacy was found between them, but flavoxate had fewer and milder side effects. Other investigators, comparing the effects of flavoxate with those of placebo, have not been able to show any beneficial effect of flavoxate at dosages up to 400 mg three times daily [104, 157, 198]. In general, few side effects have been reported during treatment with flavoxate. On the other hand, its efficacy, compared to other therapeutic alternatives, is not well documented (Table 13.1).

Assessment. No RCTs seem to have been performed with flavoxate during the last decade. The scarcity of documented clinical efficacy should be considered before using the drug.

References

1. Abrams P, Amarenco G, Bakke A, et al. Tamsulosin: efficacy and safety in patients with neurogenic lower urinary tract dysfunction due to suprasacral spinal cord injury. J Urol. 2003;170(4 Pt 1):1242.
2. Abrams P, Andersson KE. Muscarinic receptor antagonists for overactive bladder. BJU Int. 2007;100(5):987.
3. Abrams P, Cardozo L, Chapple C, et al. Comparison of the efficacy, safety, and tolerability of propiverine and oxybutynin for the treatment of overactive bladder syndrome. Int J Urol. 2006;13(6):692.
4. Abrams P, Cardozo L, Fall M, et al. The standardisation of terminology of lower urinary tract function:

report from the Standardisation Sub-committee of the International Continence Society. Neurourol Urodyn. 2002;21(2):167.

5. Abrams P, Kaplan S, De Koning Gans HJ, Millard R. Safety and tolerability of tolterodine for the treatment of overactive bladder in men with bladder outlet obstruction. J Urol. 2006;175(3 Pt 1):999–1004.

6. Abrams P, Kelleher C, Huels J, et al. Clinical relevance of health-related quality of life outcomes with darifenacin. BJU Int. 2008;102(2):208.

7. Abrams P, Kelleher C, Staskin D, et al. Combination treatment with mirabegron and solifenacin in patients with overactive bladder (OAB)—efficacy results from a phase 2 study (Symphony). J Urol. 2013;189(4 Suppl):e803.

8. Abrams P, Swift S. Solifenacin is effective for the treatment of OAB dry patients: a pooled analysis. Eur Urol. 2005;48(3):483.

9. Agency for Healthcare Policy and Research. Urinary Incontinence Guideline Panel. Urinary incontinence in adults: clinical practice guideline (AHCPR publication #92-0038). Rockville, MD: US Department of Health and Human Services; 1992.

10. Ahmad I, Krishna NS, Small DR, et al. Aetiology and management of acute female urinary retention. Br J Med Surg Urol. 2009;2:27–33.

11. Aizawa N, Homma Y, Igawa Y. Effects of mirabegron, a novel β3-adrenoceptor agonist, on primary bladder afferent activity and bladder microcontractions in rats compared with the effects of oxybutynin. Eur Urol. 2012;62(6):1165–73.

12. Akbar M, Abel R, Seyler TM, et al. Repeated botulinum-A toxin injections in the treatment of myelodysplastic children and patients with spinal cord injuries with neurogenic bladder dysfunction. BJU Int. 2007;100(3):639.

13. Al-Badr A, Ross S, Soroka D, et al. What is the available evidence for hormone replacement therapy in women with stress urinary incontinence? J Obstet Gynecol Can. 2003;25(7):567.

14. Alhasso A, Glazener CMA, Pickard R, N'Dow J. Adrenergic drugs for urinary incontinence in adults (Review). Cochrane Database Syst Rev. 2005;(3):CD001842. doi:10.1022/14651858. Reprinted in The Cochrane Library 2008, Issue 2.

15. Alhasso A, Glazener CMA, Pickard R, et al. Adrenergic drugs for urinary incontinence in adults. Cochrane Database Syst Rev. 2003;(2): CD001842.

16. Allousi S, Laval K-U, Eckert R. Trospium chloride (Spasmolyt) in patients with motor urge syndrome (detrusor instability): a double-blind, randomised, multicentre, placebo-controlled study. J Clin Res. 1998;1:439.

17. Alloussi SH, Mürtz G, Gitzhofer S, et al. Failure of monotherapy in primary monosymptomatic enuresis: a combined desmopressin and propiverine treatment regimen improves efficacy outcomes. BJU Int. 2009;103(12):1706–12.

18. Alloussi SH, Mürtz G, Lang C, et al. Desmopressin treatment regimens in monosymptomatic and non-monosymptomatic enuresis: a review from a clinical perspective. J Pediatr Urol. 2011;7(1):10–20.

19. Al-Zahrani AA, Gajewski JB. Association of symptoms with urodynamic findings in men with overactive bladder syndrome. BJU Int. 2012;110(11 Pt C):E891–5.

20. Amarenco G, Marquis P, McCarthy C, et al. Qualité de vie des femmes souffrant d'mpériosité mictionnelle avec ou sans fuites: étude prospective aprés traitement par oxybutinine (1701 cas). Presse Med. 1998;27:5.

21. Amend B, Hennenlotter J, Schäfer T, et al. Effective treatment of neurogenic detrusor dysfunction by combined high-dosed antimuscarinics without increased side-effects. Eur Urol. 2008;53(5):1021–8.

22. Anders RJ, Wang E, Radhakrishnan J, et al. Overflow urinary incontinence due to carbamazepine. J Urol. 1985;134:758.

23. Anderson RU, Mobley D, Blank B, et al. Once-daily controlled versus immediate-release oxybutynin chloride for urge urinary incontinence. OROS Oxybutynin Study Group. J Urol. 1999;161:1809.

24. Andersson K-E. Pharmacology of lower urinary tract smooth muscles and penile erectile tissues. Pharmacol Rev. 1993;45:253.

25. Andersson K-E. Pathways for relaxation of detrusor smooth muscle. In: Baskin LS, Hayward SW, editors. Advances in bladder research. New York, NY: Kluwer Academic/Plenum; 1999. p. 241.

26. Andersson KE. Bladder activation: afferent mechanisms. Urology. 2002;59(5 Suppl 1):43.

27. Andersson K-E. Potential benefits of muscarinic M3 receptor selectivity. Eur Urol Suppl. 2002;1(4):23.

28. Andersson K-E. Alpha-adrenoceptors and benign prostatic hyperplasia: basic principles for treatment with alpha-adrenoceptor antagonists. World J Urol. 2002;19(6):390.

29. Andersson KE. Antimuscarinics for treatment of overactive bladder. Lancet Neurol. 2004;3(1):46.

30. Andersson KE. Treatment-resistant detrusor overactivity—underlying pharmacology and potential mechanisms. Int J Clin Pract Suppl. 2006;151:8–16.

31. Andersson KE. LUTS treatment: future treatment options. Neurourol Urodyn. 2007;26(6 Suppl): 934–47.

32. Andersson KE. Muscarinic acetylcholine receptors in the urinary tract. Handb Exp Pharmacol. 2011;202:319–44.

33. Andersson KE. Antimuscarinic mechanisms and the overactive detrusor: an update. Eur Urol. 2011;59(3):377–86.

34. Andersson KE. Drugs and future candidates. Can Urol Assoc J. 2011;5(5 Suppl 2):S131–3.

35. Andersson KE, Appell R, Cardozo LD, et al. The pharmacological treatment of urinary incontinence. BJU Int. 1999;84(9):923.

36. Andersson KE, Arner A. Urinary bladder contraction and relaxation: physiology and pathophysiology. Physiol Rev. 2004;84(3):935–86.

37. Andersson KE, Campeau L, Olshansky B. Cardiac effects of muscarinic receptor antagonists used for

voiding dysfunction. Br J Clin Pharm. 2011;72:186–96.

38. Andersson K-E, Chapple CR. Oxybutynin and the overactive bladder. World J Urol. 2001;19(5):319.

39. Andersson K-E, Chapple CR, Cardozo L, et al. Pharmacological treatment of urinary incontinence. In: Abrams P, Cardozo L, Khoury S, Wein A, editors. Incontinence, 4th international consultation on incontinence. Plymouth: Plymbridge Distributors Ltd.; 2009. p. 633.

40. Andersson K-E, Chapple CR, Cardozo L, et al. Pharmacological treatment of urinary incontinence. In: Abrams P, Cardozo L, Khoury S, Wein A, editors. Incontinence 5th international consultation on incontinence. Vienna: ICUD-EAU; 2013. p. 623–728.

41. Andersson KE, de Groat WC, McVary KT, et al. Tadalafil for the treatment of lower urinary tract symptoms secondary to benign prostatic hyperplasia: pathophysiology and mechanism(s) of action. Neurourol Urodyn. 2011;30(3):292–301.

42. Andersson K-E, Fullhase C, Soler R. Urothelial effects of oral antimuscarinic agents. Curr Urol Rep. 2008;9(6):459.

43. Andersson KE, Gratzke C. Pharmacology of alpha1-adrenoceptor antagonists in the lower urinary tract and central nervous system. Nat Clin Pract Urol. 2007;4(7):368–78.

44. Andersson KE, Gratzke C, Hedlund P. The role of the transient receptor potential (TRP) superfamily of cation-selective channels in the management of the overactive bladder. BJU Int. 2010;106(8):1114–27.

45. Andersson KE, Martin N, Nitti V. Selective β3-adrenoceptor agonists in the treatment of overactive bladder. J Urol. 2013;190(4):1173–80.

46. Andersson K-E, Michel MC. Urinary tract. Handbook of experimental pharmacology. Berlin: Springer; 2011.

47. Andersson KE, Olshansky B. Treating patients with overactive bladder syndrome with antimuscarinics: heart rate considerations. BJU Int. 2007;100:1007.

48. Andersson KE, Pehrson R. CNS involvement in overactive bladder: pathophysiology and opportunities for pharmacological intervention. Drugs. 2003;63(23):2595.

49. Andersson K-E, Persson K. The L-arginine/nitric oxide pathway and non-adrenergic, non-cholinergic relaxation of the lower urinary tract. Gen Pharmacol. 1993;24:833.

50. Andersson KE, Sarawate C, Kahler KH, et al. Cardiovascular morbidity, heart rates and use of anti-muscarinics in patients with overactive bladder. BJU Int. 2010;106(2):268–74.

51. Andersson K-E, Uckert S, Stief C, et al. Phosphodiesterases (PDEs) and PDE inhibitors for treatment of LUTS. Neurourol Urodyn. 1997;26(6 Suppl):928.

52. Andersson K-E, Wein AJ. Pharmacology of the lower urinary tract—basis for current and future

treatments of urinary incontinence. Pharmacol Rev. 2004;56(4):581.

53. Andersson K, Wein A. Pharmacologic management of lower urinary tract storage and emptying failure. In: Wein A, Kavoussi L, Novick A, Partin A, Peters C, editors. Campbell-Walsh urology. Philadelphia, PA: Elsevier Saunders; 2012. p. 1967–2002.

54. Andrews MD, Fish P, Blagg J, et al. Pyrimido [4,5-d] azepines as potent and selective 5-HT2C receptor agonists: design, synthesis and evaluation of PF-3246799 as a treatment for urinary incontinence. Bioorg Med Chem Lett. 2011;21(9):2715–20.

55. Aoki KR. Review of a proposed mechanism for the antinociceptive action of botulinum toxin type A. Neurotoxicology. 2005;26(5):785.

56. Aoki K, Hirayama A, Tanaka N, et al. A higher level of prostaglandin E2 in the urinary bladder in young boys and boys with lower urinary tract obstruction. Biomed Res. 2009;30(6):343–7.

57. Apostolidis A, Brady CM, Yiangou Y, et al. Capsaicin receptor TRPV1 in urothelium of neurogenic human bladders and effect of intravesical resiniferatoxin. Urology. 2005;65(2):400–5.

58. Apostolidis A, Gonzales GE, Fowler CJ. Effect of intravesical Resiniferatoxin (RTX) on lower urinary tract symptoms, urodynamic parameters, and quality of life of patients with urodynamic increased bladder sensation. Eur Urol. 2006;50(6):1299.

59. Apostolidis A, Kirana PS, Chiu G, et al. Gender and age differences in the perception of bother and health care seeking for lower urinary tract symptoms: results from the hospitalised and outpatients' profile and expectations study. Eur Urol. 2009;56(6): 937–47.

60. Apostolidis A, Popat R, Yiangou Y, et al. Decreased sensory receptors P2X3 and TRPV1 in suburothelial nerve fibers following intradetrusor injections of botulinum toxin for human detrusor overactivity. J Urol. 2005;174(3):977.

61. Appell RA, Chancellor MB, Zobrist RH, et al. Pharmacokinetics, metabolism, and saliva output during transdermal and extended-release oral oxybutynin administration in healthy subjects. Mayo Clin Proc. 2003;78(6):696.

62. Appell RA, Sand P, Dmochowski R, et al. Overactive bladder: judging effective control and treatment study group. Prospective randomized controlled trial of extended-release oxybutynin chloride and tolterodine tartrate in the treatment of overactive bladder: results of the OBJECT Study. Mayo Clin Proc. 2001;76(4):358.

63. Araki I. TRP channels in urinary bladder mechano-sensation. Adv Exp Med Biol. 2011;704:861–79.

64. Araki I, Du S, Kobayashi H, et al. Roles of mechano-sensitive ion channels in bladder sensory transduction and overactive bladder. Int J Urol. 2008;15(8): 681–7.

65. Arisco AM, Brantly EK, Kraus SR. Oxybutynin extended release for the management of overactive

bladder: a clinical review. Drug Des Devel Ther. 2009;3:151–61.

66. Asplund R, Sundberg B, Bengtsson P. Oral desmopressin for nocturnal polyuria in elderly subjects: a double-blind, placebo-controlled randomized exploratory study. BJU Int. 1999;83:591.

67. Athanasopoulos A, Cruz F. The medical treatment of overactive bladder, including current and future treatments. Expert Opin Pharmacother. 2011;12(7):1041–55.

68. Athanasopoulos A, Gyftopoulos K, Giannitsas K, et al. Combination treatment with an alpha-blocker plus an anticholinergic for bladder outlet obstruction: a prospective, randomized, controlled study. J Urol. 2003;169:2253.

69. Austin PF, Ferguson G, Yan Y, et al. Combination therapy with desmopressin and an anticholinergic medication for nonresponders to desmopressin for monosymptomatic nocturnal enuresis: a randomized, double-blind, placebo-controlled trial. Pediatrics. 2008;122(5):1027–32.

70. Avelino A, Charrua A, Frias B, Cruz CD, Boudes M, de Ridder D, Cruz F. TRP channels in bladder function. Acta Physiol (Oxf). 2013;207(1):110–22.

71. Avelino A, Cruz F. TRPV1 (vanilloid receptor) in the urinary tract: expression, function and clinical applications. Naunyn Schmiedebergs Arch Pharmacol. 2006;373(4):287–99.

72. Bae JH, Oh MM, Shim KS, et al. The effects of long-term administration of oral desmopressin on the baseline secretion of antidiuretic hormone and serum sodium concentration for the treatment of nocturia: a circadian study. J Urol. 2007;178(1):200.

73. Baigrie RJ, Kelleher JP, Fawcett DP, et al. Oxybutynin: is it safe? Br J Urol. 1988;62:319.

74. Baldessarini KJ. Drugs in the treatment of psychiatric disorders. In: Gilman AG, Goodman LS, Gilman A, editors. The pharmacological basis of therapeutics. 7th ed. New York: McMillan; 1985. p. 387.

75. Baldo A, Berger TH, Kofler M, et al. The influence of intrathecal baclofen on detrusor function. A urodynamic study. NeuroUrol Urodyn. 2000;19:444 (abstract 53).

76. Banakhar MA, Al-Shaiji TF, Hassouna MM. Pathophysiology of overactive bladder. Int Urogynecol J. 2012;23(8):975–82.

77. Barendrecht MM, Oelke M, Laguna MP, et al. Is the use of parasympathomimetics for treating an underactive urinary bladder evidence-based? BJU Int. 2007;99:749.

78. Basra RK, Wagg A, Chapple C, et al. A review of adherence to drug therapy in patients with overactive bladder. BJU Int. 2008;102:774–9.

79. Bayliss M, Wu C, Newgreen D, et al. A quantitative study of atropine-resistant contractile responses in human detrusor smooth muscle, from stable, unstable and obstructed bladders. J Urol. 1999;162:1833.

80. Bechara A, Romano S, Casabe A, et al. Comparative efficacy assessment of tamsulosin vs. tamsulosin plus tadalafil in the treatment of LUTS/BPH. Pilot study. J Sex Med. 2008;5:2170–8.

81. Beckmann-Knopp S, Rietbrock S, Weyhenmeyer R, et al. Inhibitory effects of trospium chloride on cytochrome P450 enzymes in human liver microsomes. Pharmacol Toxicol. 1999;6:299.

82. Beermann B, Hellstrom K, Rosen A. On the metabolism of propantheline in man. Clin Pharmacol Ther. 1972;13(2):212.

83. Behr-Roussel D, Oger S, Caisey S, et al. Vardenafil decreases bladder afferent nerve activity in unanesthetized, decerebrate, spinal cord-injured rats. Eur Urol. 2010;59:272–9.

84. Bent A, Gousse A, Hendrix S. Duloxetine compared with placebo for the treatment of women with urinary incontinence. Neurourol Urodyn. 2008;27(3):212–21.

85. Bent S, Tiedt TN, Odden MC, et al. The relative safety of ephedra compared with other herbal products. Ann Intern Med. 2003;138(6):468.

86. Berridge MJ. Smooth muscle cell calcium activation mechanisms. J Physiol. 2008;586(Pt 21):5047–61.

87. Bharucha AE, Seide B, Guan Z, et al. Effect of tolterodine on gastrointestinal transit and bowel habits in healthy subjects. Neurogastroenterol Motil. 2008;20(6):643.

88. Biers SM, Reynard JM, Brading AF. The effects of a new selective beta3-adrenoceptor agonist (GW427353) on spontaneous activity and detrusor relaxation in human bladder. BJU Int. 2006;98(6):1310.

89. Bigger JT, Giardina EG, Perel JM, et al. Cardiac antiarrhythmic effect of imipramine hydrochloride. N Engl J Med. 1977;296:206.

90. Birder L, Andersson KE. Urothelial signaling. Physiol Rev. 2013;93(2):653–80.

91. Birder LA, de Groat WC. Mechanisms of disease: involvement of the urothelium in bladder dysfunction. Nat Clin Pract Urol. 2007;4(1):46–54.

92. Birder LA, Kanai AJ, de Groat WC, et al. Vanilloid receptor expression suggests a sensory role for urinary bladder epithelial cells. Proc Natl Acad Sci USA. 2001;98(23):13396–401.

93. Birder LA, Nakamura Y, Kiss S, et al. Altered urinary bladder function in mice lacking the vanilloid receptor TRPV1. Nat Neurosci. 2002;5(9):856–60.

94. Blaivas JG, Labib KB, Michalik J, et al. Cystometric response to propantheline in detrusor hyperreflexia: therapeutic implications. J Urol. 1980;124:259.

95. Blue DR, Daniels DV, Gever JR, et al. Pharmacological characteristics of Ro 115-1240, a selective? 1A-1L-adrenoceptor partial agonist: a potential therapy for stress urinary incontinence. BJU Int. 2004;93(1):162.

96. Blyweert W, Van Der Aa F, De Ridder D. Cannabinoid therapy in detrusor overactivity: local versus systemic effect in a spinalised rat model. Neurourol Urodyn. 2003;22:379–80.

97. Bödeker RH, Madersbacher H, Neumeister C, Zellner M. Dose escalation improves therapeutic outcome: post hoc analysis of data from a 12-week, multicentre, double-blind, parallel-group trial of

trospium chloride in patients with urinary urge incontinence. BMC Urol. 2010;10:15.

98. Bolduc S, Moore K, Nadeau G, et al. Prospective open label study of solifenacin for overactive bladder in children. J Urol. 2010;184(4 Suppl):1668–73.

99. Bosch RJLH, Griffiths DJ, Blom JHM, et al. Treatment of benign prostatic hyperplasia by androgen deprivation: effects on prostate size and urodynamic parameters. J Urol. 1989;141:68.

100. Bosch JL, Weiss JP. The prevalence and causes of nocturia. J Urol. 2010;184(2):440–6.

101. Brady CM, Apostolidis AN, Harper M, et al. Parallel changes in bladder suburothelial vanilloid receptor TRPV1 and pan-neuronal marker PGP9.5 immunoreactivity in patients with neurogenic detrusor overactivity after intravesical resiniferatoxin treatment. BJU Int. 2004;93(6):770.

102. Brady CM, DasGupta R, Dalton C, et al. An open-label pilot study of cannabis-based extracts for bladder dysfunction in advanced multiple sclerosis. Mult Scler. 2004;10:425–33.

103. Brennan PE, Whitlock GA, Ho DK, et al. Discovery of a novel azepine series of potent and selective 5-HT2C agonists as potential treatments for urinary incontinence. Bioorg Med Chem Lett. 2009;19:4999–5003.

104. Briggs KS, Castleden CM, Asher MJ. The effect of flavoxate on uninhibited detrusor contractions and urinary incontinence in the elderly. J Urol. 1980;123:665.

105. Brubaker L, FitzGerald MP. Nocturnal polyuria and nocturia relief in patients treated with solifenacin for overactive bladder symptoms. Int Urogynecol J Pelvic Floor Dysfunct. 2007;18(7):737.

106. Brynne N, Dalen P, Alvan G, et al. Influence of CYP2D6 polymorphism on the pharmacokinetics and pharmacodynamics of tolterodine. Clin Pharmacol Ther. 1998;63:529.

107. Brynne N, Stahl MMS, Hallén B, et al. Pharmacokinetics and pharmacodynamics of tolterodine in man: a new drug for the treatment of urinary bladder overactivity. Int J Clin Pharmacol Ther. 1997;35:287.

108. Buckley BS, Lapitan MC. Drugs for treatment of urinary retention after surgery in adults. Cochrane Database Syst Rev. 2010;(10):CD008023.

109. Bump RC, Voss S, Beardsworth A, et al. Long-term efficacy of duloxetine in women with stress urinary incontinence. Br J Urol Int. 2008;102:214.

110. Bushman W, Steers WD, Meythaler JM. Voiding dysfunction in patients with spastic paraplegia: urodynamic evaluation and response to continuous intrathecal baclofen. Neurourol Urodyn. 1993;12(2):163.

111. Caine M, Gin S, Pietra C, et al. Antispasmodic effects of flavoxate, MFCA, and REC 15/2053 on smooth muscle of human prostate and urinary bladder. Urology. 1991;37(4):390.

112. Callegari E, Malhotra B, Bungay PJ, et al. A comprehensive non-clinical evaluation of the CNS penetration potential of antimuscarinic agents for the treatment of overactive bladder. Br J Clin Pharmacol. 2011;72:235–46.

113. Cameron AP, Clemens JQ, Latini JM, McGuire EJ. Combination drug therapy improves compliance of the neurogenic bladder. J Urol. 2009;182(3):1062–7.

114. Campbell N, Perkins A, Hui S, et al. Association between prescribing of anticholinergic medications and incident delirium: a cohort study. J Am Geriatr Soc. 2011;59 Suppl 2:S277–81.

115. Cannon A, Carter PG, McConnell AA, et al. Desmopressin in the treatment of nocturnal polyuria in the male. BJU Int. 1999;84:20.

116. Cao DS, Yu SQ, Premkumar LS. Modulation of transient receptor potential Vanilloid 4-mediated membrane currents and synaptic transmission by protein kinase C. Mol Pain. 2009;5:5.

117. Capo' JP, Lucente V, Forero-Schwanhaeuser S, He W. Efficacy and tolerability of solifenacin in patients aged ≥65 years with overactive bladder: post-hoc analysis of 2 open-label studies. Postgrad Med. 2011;123(1):94–104.

118. Carbone A, Palleschi G, Conte A, et al. Gabapentin treatment of neurogenic overactive bladder. Clin Neuropharmacol. 2006;29(4):206.

119. Cardozo LD, Bachmann G, McClish D, et al. Meta-analysis of oestrogen therapy in the management of urogenital atrophy in postmenopausal women: second report of the Hormones and Urogenital Therapy Committee. Obstet Gynaecol. 1998;92:722–7.

120. Cardozo L, Castro-Diaz D, Gittelman M, et al. Reductions in overactive bladder-related incontinence from pooled analysis of phase III trials evaluating treatment with solifenacin. Int Urogynecol J Pelvic Floor Dysfunct. 2006;17(5):512.

121. Cardozo L, Chapple CR, Toozs-Hobson P, et al. Efficacy of trospium chloride in patients with detrusor instability: a placebo-controlled, randomized, double-blind, multicentre clinical trial. BJU Int. 2000;85(6):659.

122. Cardozo L, Dixon A. Increased warning time with darifenacin: a new concept in the management of urinary urgency. J Urol. 2005;173(4):1214.

123. Cardozo L, Drutz HP, Baygari SK, et al. Pharmacological treatment of women awaiting surgery for stress urinary incontinence. Obstet Gynecol. 2004;104(3):511–9.

124. Cardozo L, Lisec M, Millard R, et al. Randomized, double-blind placebo controlled trial of the once daily antimuscarinic agent solifenacin succinate in patients with overactive bladder. J Urol. 2004;172(5 Pt 1):1919.

125. Cardozo L, Lose G, McClish D, et al. A systematic review of the effects of estrogens for symptoms suggestive of overactive bladder. Acta Obstetr Gynaecol Scand. 2004;83:892.

126. Cardozo LD, Stanton SL. A comparison between bromocriptine and indomethacin in the treatment of detrusor instability. J Urol. 1980;123:39.

127. Cardozo LD, Stanton SL, Robinson H, et al. Evaluation on flurbiprofen in detrusor instability. Br Med J. 1980;280:281.

128. Caremel R, Oger-Roussel S, Behr-Roussel D, et al. Nitric oxide/cyclic guanosine monophosphate signalling mediates an inhibitory action on sensory pathways of the micturition reflex in the rat. Eur Urol. 2010;58:616–25.

129. Cartwright R, Cardozo L. Transdermal oxybutynin: sticking to the facts. Eur Urol. 2007;51(4):907.

130. Cartwright R, Srikrishna S, Cardozo L, Robinson D. Patient-selected goals in overactive bladder: a placebo controlled randomized double-blind trial of transdermaloxybutynin for the treatment of urgency and urge incontinence. BJU Int. 2011;107(1):70–6.

131. Catterall WA, Striessnig J, Snutch TP, et al. International Union of Pharmacology. XL. Compendium of voltage-gated ion channels: calcium channels. Pharmacol Rev. 2003;55:579.

132. Cazzulani P, Pietra C, Abbiati GA, et al. Pharmacological activities of the main metabolite of flavoxate 3-methylflavone-8-carboxylic acid. Arzneimittelforschung. 1988;38(3):379.

133. Cerruto MA, Asimakopoulos AD, Artibani W, et al. Insight into new potential targets for the treatment of overactive bladder and detrusor overactivity. Urol Int. 2012;89(1):1–8.

134. Chai TC, Gray ML, Steers WD. The incidence of a positive ice water test in bladder outlet obstructed patients: evidence for bladder neural plasticity. J Urol. 1998;160(1):34.

135. Chancellor MB, Appell RA, Sathyan G, et al. A comparison of the effects on saliva output of oxybutynin chloride and tolterodine tartrate. Clin Ther. 2001;23(5):753.

136. Chancellor MB, Atan A, Rivas DA, et al. Beneficial effect of intranasal desmopressin for men with benign prostatic hyperplasia and nocturia: preliminary results. Tech Urol. 1999;5:191.

137. Chancellor MB, Erhard MJ, Hirsch IH, Stass Jr WE. Prospective evaluation of terazosin for the treatment of autonomic dysreflexia. J Urol. 1994;151(1):111–3.

138. Chancellor MB, Fowler CJ, Apostolidis A, et al. Drug insight: biological effects of botulinum toxin A in the lower urinary tract. Nat Clin Pract Urol. 2008;5(6):319.

139. Chancellor MB, Kaufman J. Case for pharmacotherapy development for underactive bladder. J Urol. 2008;72(5):966–7.

140. Chancellor MB, Kianifard F, Beamer E, et al. A comparison of the efficacy of darifenacin alone vs. darifenacin plus a Behavioural Modification Programme upon the symptoms of overactive bladder. Int J Clin Pract. 2008;62(4):606.

141. Chancellor MB, Oefelein MG, Vasavada S. Obesity is associated with a more severe overactive bladder disease state that is effectively treated with once-daily administration of trospium chloride extended release. Neurourol Urodyn. 2010;29(4):551–4.

142. Chancellor MB, Staskin DR, Kay GG, et al. Blood-brain barrier permeation and efflux exclusion of anticholinergics used in the treatment of overactive bladder. Drugs Aging. 2012;29(4):259–73.

143. Chang SC, Lin AT, Chen KK, Chang LS. Multifactorial nature of male nocturia. Urology. 2006;67(3):541–4.

144. Chapple CR, Abrams P, Andersson K-E, et al. Randomised, double-blind, placebo-controlled phase ii study to investigate the efficacy and safety of the EP-1 receptor antagonist, ONO-8539, in Idiopathic overactive bladder. J Urol. 2014;191(1):253–60.

145. Chapple CR, Amarenco G, López Aramburu MA, on behalf of the BLOSSOM Investigator Group. A proof-of-concept study: mirabegron, a new therapy for overactive bladder. Neurourol Urodyn. 2013;32(8):1116–22.

146. Chapple CR, Arano P, Bosch JL, et al. Solifenacin appears effective and well tolerated in patients with symptomatic idiopathic detrusor overactivity in a placebo- and tolterodine-controlled phase 2 dose-finding study. BJU Int. 2004;93(1):71.

147. Chapple CR, Cardozo L, Steers WD, et al. Solifenacin significantly improves all symptoms of overactive bladder syndrome. Int J Clin Pract. 2006;60(8):959.

148. Chapple C, DuBeau C, Ebinger U, et al. Long-term darifenacin treatment for overactive bladder in patients aged 65 years and older: analysis of results from a 2-year, open-label extension study. Curr Med Res Opin. 2007;23(11):2697.

149. Chapple CR, Dvorak V, Radziszewski P, et al., on behalf of the Dragon Investigator Group. A phase II dose-ranging study of mirabegron in patients with overactive bladder. Int Urogynecol J. 2013;24:1447–58.

150. Chapple CR, Fianu-Jonsson A, Indig M, et al., STAR study group. Treatment outcomes in the STAR study: a subanalysis of solifenacin 5 mg and tolterodine ER 4 mg. Eur Urol. 2007;52(4):1195.

151. Chapple CR, Kaplan SA, Mitcheson D, et al. Randomized double-blind, active-controlled phase 3 study to assess 12-month safety and efficacy of mirabegron, a β(3)-adrenoceptor agonist, in overactive bladder. Eur Urol. 2013;63(2):296–305.

152. Chapple C, Khullar V, Gabriel Z, et al. The effects of antimuscarinic treatments in overactive bladder: a systematic review and meta-analysis. Eur Urol. 2005;48:5.

153. Chapple CR, Khullar V, Gabriel Z, et al. The effects of antimuscarinic treatments in overactive bladder: an update of a systematic review and meta-analysis. Eur Urol. 2008;54(3):543.

154. Chapple CR, Martinez-Garcia R, Selvaggi L, et al. A comparison of the efficacy and tolerability of solifenacin succinate and extended release tolterodine at treating overactive bladder syndrome: results of the STAR trial. Eur Urol. 2005;48(3):464.

155. Chapple C, Milsom I. Urinary incontinence and pelvic prolapse: epidemiology and pathophysiology. In: Wein A, Kavoussi L, Novick A, Partin A, Peters C, editors. Campbell-Walsh urology. Philadelphia, PA: Elsevier Saunders; 2012. p. 1871–908.

156. Chapple CR, Montorsi F, Tammela TLJ, et al., on behalf of the European Silodosin Study Group. Silodosin therapy for lower urinary tract symptoms in men with suspected benign prostatic hyperplasia: results of an international, randomized, double-blind, placebo- and active-controlled clinical trial performed in Europe. Eur Urol. 2011;59(3):342–52.

157. Chapple CR, Parkhouse H, Gardener C, et al. Double-blind, placebo-controlled, cross-over study of flavoxate in the treatment of idiopathic detrusor instability. Br J Urol. 1990;66:491.

158. Chapple C, Patel A. Botulinum toxin—new mechanisms, new therapeutic directions? Eur Urol. 2006;49(4):606–8.

159. Chapple CR, Patroneva A, Raines SR. Effect of an ATP-sensitive potassium channel opener in subjects with overactive bladder: a randomized, double-blind, placebo-controlled study (ZD0947IL/0004). Eur Urol. 2006;49:879.

160. Chapple CR, Rechberger T, Al-Shukri S, et al., YM-905 Study Group. Randomized, double-blind placebo- and tolterodine-controlled trial of the once-daily antimuscarinic agent solifenacin in patients with symptomatic overactive bladder. BJU Int. 2004;93(3):303.

161. Chapple C, Steers W, Norton P, et al. A pooled analysis of three phase III studies to investigate the efficacy, tolerability and safety of darifenacin, a muscarinic M3 selective receptor antagonist, in the treatment of overactive bladder. BJU Int. 2005;95(7):993.

162. Chapple CR, Van Kerrebroeck PE, Jünemann KP, et al. Comparison of fesoterodine and tolterodine in patients with overactive bladder. BJU Int. 2008;102(9):1128–32.

163. Chapple C, Van Kerrebroeck P, Tubaro A, et al. Clinical efficacy, safety, and tolerability of once-daily fesoterodine in subjects with overactive bladder. Eur Urol. 2007;52(4):1204.

164. Charrua A, Cruz CD, Cruz F, Avelino A. Transient receptor potential vanilloid subfamily 1 is essential for the generation of noxious bladder input and bladder overactivity in cystitis. J Urol. 2007;177(4):1537–41.

165. Charrua A, Cruz CD, Narayanan S, et al. GRC-6211, a new oral specific TRPV1 antagonist, decreases bladder overactivity and noxious bladder input in cystitis animal models. J Urol. 2009;181(1):379–86.

166. Charrua A, Reguenga C, Cordeiro JM, et al. Functional transient receptor potential vanilloid 1 is expressed in human urothelial cells. J Urol. 2009;182(6):2944–50.

167. Choo MS, Doo CK, Lee KS. Satisfaction with tolterodine: assessing symptom-specific patient-reported goal achievement in the treatment of overactive bladder in female patients (STARGATE study). Int J Clin Pract. 2008;62(2):191.

168. Christ GJ, Andersson KE. Rho-kinase and effects of Rho-kinase inhibition on the lower urinary tract. Neurourol Urodyn. 2007;26(6 Suppl):948–54.

169. Christ GJ, Day NS, Day M, et al. Bladder injection of "naked" hSlo/pcDNA3 ameliorates detrusor hyperactivity in obstructed rats in vivo. Am J Physiol Regul Integr Comp Physiol. 2001;281(5): R1699–709.

170. Christ T, Wettwer E, Wuest M, et al. Electrophysiological profile of propiverine–relationship to cardiac risk. Naunyn Schmiedebergs Arch Pharmacol. 2008;376(6):431–40.

171. Chuang YC, Thomas CA, Tyagi S, et al. Human urine with solifenacin intake but not tolterodine or darifenacin intake blocks detrusor overactivity. Int Urogynecol J Pelvic Floor Dysfunct. 2008;19(10): 1353.

172. Chung DE, Te AE, Staskin DR, Kaplan SA. Efficacy and safety of tolterodine extended release and dutasteride in male overactive bladder patients with prostates >30 grams. Urology. 2010;75(5):1144–8.

173. Chutka DS, Takahashi PY. Urinary incontinence in the elderly. Drug treatment options. Drugs. 1998;56:587.

174. Clemett D, Jarvis B. Tolterodine: a review of its use in the treatment of overactive bladder. Drugs Aging. 2001;18(4):277.

175. Cody JD, Richardson K, Moehrer B, et al. Oestrogen therapy for urinary incontinence in post-menopausal women. Cochrane Database Syst Rev. 2009;(4):CD001405. doi:10.1002/14651858. CD001405.pub2.

176. Coelho A, Cruz F, Cruz CD, Avelino A. Spread of OnabotulinumtoxinA after bladder injection. Experimental study using the distribution of cleaved SNAP-25 as the marker of the toxin action. Eur Urol. 2012;61(6):1178–84.

177. Coelho A, Cruz F, Cruz CD, Avelino A. Effect of onabotulinumtoxinA on intramural parasympathetic ganglia: an experimental study in the guinea pig bladder. J Urol. 2012;187(3):1121–6.

178. Coelho A, Dinis P, Pinto R, Gorgal T, et al. Distribution of the high-affinity binding site and intracellular target of botulinum toxin type A in the human bladder. Eur Urol. 2010;57(5):884–90.

179. Collado Serra A, Rubio-Briones J, Puvol Payás M, et al. Postprostatectomy established stress urinary incontinence treated with duloxetine. Urology. 2011;78(2):261–6.

180. Collas D, Malone-Lee JG. The pharmacokinetic properties of rectal oxybutynin—a possible alternative to intravesical administration. Neurourol Urodyn. 1997;16:346.

181. Colli E, Digesu GA, Olivieri L. Overactive bladder treatments in early phase clinical trials. Expert Opin Investig Drugs. 2007;16(7):999–1007.

182. Colli E, Rigatti P, Montorsi F, et al. BXL628, a novel vitamin D3 analog arrests prostate growth in patients with benign prostatic hyperplasia: a randomized clinical trial. Eur Urol. 2006;49(1):82.
183. Colli E, Tankó LB. Gonadotropin-releasing hormone antagonists: from basic science to the clinic in patients with benign prostatic hyperplasia and lower urinary tract symptoms. UroToday Int J. 2010;3(5). doi:10.3834/uij.1944-5784.2010.10.14.
184. Conlon K, Christy C, Westbrook S, et al. Pharmacological properties of 2-((R-5-chloro-4-methoxymethylindan-1-yl)-1H-imidazole (PF-3774076), a novel and selective alpha1A-adrenergic partial agonist, in in vitro and in vivo models of urethral function. J Pharmacol Exp Ther. 2009;330(3):892–901.
185. Connolly MJ, Astridge PS, White EG, Morley CA, Cowan JC. Torsades de pointes ventricular tachycardia and terodiline. Lancet. 1991;338(8763):344.
186. Copas PM, Bukovsky A, Asubyr B, et al. Estrogen, progesterone and androgen receptor expression in levator ani muscle and fascia. J Womens Health Gend Based Med. 2001;10(8):785.
187. Corcos J, Casey R, Patrick A, et al. A double-blind randomized dose-response study comparing daily doses of 5, 10 and 15 mg controlled-release oxybutynin: balancing efficacy with severity of dry mouth. BJU Int. 2006;97(3):520.
188. Cornu J-N, Merlet B, Ciofu C, et al. Duloxetine for mild to moderate postprostatectomy incontinence: preliminary results of a randomized, placebo-controlled trial. Eur Urol. 2011;59(1):148–54.
189. Covenas R, Martin F, Belda M, et al. Mapping of neurokinin-like immunoreactivity in the human brainstem. BMC Neurosci. 2003;4(1):3.
190. Coyne KS, Elinoff V, Gordon DA, et al. Relationships between improvements in symptoms and patient assessments of bladder condition, symptom bother and health-related quality of life in patients with overactive bladder treated with tolterodine. Int J Clin Pract. 2008;62(6):925.
191. Crescioli C, Ferruzzi P, Caporali A, et al. Inhibition of spontaneous and androgen-induced prostate growth by a nonhypercalcemic calcitriol analog. Endocrinology. 2003;144(7):3046.
192. Crescioli C, Ferruzzi P, Caporali A, et al. Inhibition of prostate cell growth by BXL-628, a calcitriol analogue selected for a phase II clinical trial in patients with benign prostate hyperplasia. Eur J Endocrinol. 2004;150(4):591.
193. Crescioli C, Morelli A, Adorini L, et al. Human bladder as a novel target for vitamin D receptor ligands. J Clin Endocrinol Metab. 2005;90(2):962–72.
194. Crescioli C, Villari D, Forti G, et al. Des (1-3) IGF-I-stimulated growth of human stromal BPH cells is inhibited by a vitamin D3 analogue. Mol Cell Endocrinol. 2002;198(1–2):69–75.
195. Cruz F, Guimarães M, Silva C, et al. Suppression of bladder hyperreflexia by intravesical resiniferatoxin. Lancet. 1997;350(9078):640.
196. Cruz F, Herschorn S, Aliotta P, et al. Efficacy and safety of onabotulinumtoxinA in patients with urinary incontinence due to neurogenic detrusor overactivity: a randomised, double-blind, placebo-controlled trial. Eur Urol. 2011;60(4):742–50.
197. Cvetkovic RS, Plosker GL. Desmopressin in adults with nocturia. Drugs. 2005;65:99.
198. Dahm TL, Ostri P, Kristensen JK, et al. Flavoxate treatment of micturition disorders accompanying benign prostatic hypertrophy: a double-blind placebo-controlled multicenter investigation. Urol Int. 1955;55:205.
199. Das A, Chancellor MB, Watanabe T, et al. Intravesical capsaicin in neurologic impaired patients with detrusor hyperreflexia. J Spinal Cord Med. 1996;19(3):190.
200. Dasgupta R, Fowler CJ. The management of female voiding dysfunction: Fowler's syndrome-a contemporary update. Curr Opin Urol. 2003;13:293–9.
201. Davila GW, Daugherty CA, Sanders SW. A short-term, multicenter, randomized double-blind dose titration study of the efficacy and anticholinergic side effects of transdermal compared to immediate release oral oxybutynin treatment of patients with urge urinary incontinence. J Urol. 2001;166(1):140.
202. de Groat WC. A neurologic basis for the overactive bladder. Urology. 1997;50(6A Suppl):36–52.
203. de Groat WC, Yoshimura N. Pharmacology of the lower urinary tract. Annu Rev Pharmacol Toxicol. 2001;41:691.
204. De Guchtenaere A, Van Herzeele C, Raes A, et al. Oral lyophylizate formulation of desmopressin: superior pharmacodynamics compared to tablet due to low food interaction. J Urol. 2011;185(6):2308–13.
205. De Guchtenaere A, Vande Walle C, Van Sintjan P, et al. Desmopressin resistant nocturnal polyuria may benefit from furosemide therapy administered in the morning. J Urol. 2007;178:2635.
206. De Laet K, De Wachter S, Wyndaele JJ. Systemic oxybutynin decreases afferent activity of the pelvic nerve of the rat: new insights into the working mechanism of antimuscarinics. Neurourol Urodyn. 2006;25(2):156.
207. de Mey C, Mateva L, Krastev Z, et al. Effects of hepatic dysfunction on the single-dose pharmacokinetics of fesoterodine. J Clin Pharmacol. 2011;51(3):397–405.
208. de Paiva A, Meunier FA, Molgó J, et al. Functional repair of motor endplates after botulinum neurotoxin type A poisoning: biphasic switch of synaptic activity between nerve sprouts and their parent terminals. Proc Natl Acad Sci USA. 1999;96(6):3200–5.
209. De Ridder D, Chandiramani V, Dasgupta P, et al. Intravesical capsaicin as a treatment for refractory detrusor hyperreflexia: a dual center study with long-term followup. J Urol. 1997;158(6):2087.
210. de Sèze M, Gallien P, Denys P, et al. Intravesical glucidic capsaicin versus glucidic solvent in neurogenic

detrusor overactivity: a double blind controlled randomized study. Neurourol Urodyn. 2006;25(7):752.

211. de Sèze M, Wiart L, Joseph PA, et al. Capsaicin and neurogenic detrusor hyperreflexia: a double-blind placebo-controlled study in 20 patients with spinal cord lesions. Neurourol Urodyn. 1998;17(5):513.

212. Deaney C, Glickman S, Gluck T, et al. Intravesical atropine suppression of detrusor hyperreflexia in multiple sclerosis. J Neurol Neurosurg Psychiatry. 1998;65:957.

213. Debruyne F, Gres AA, Arustamov DL. Placebo-controlled dose-ranging phase 2 study of subcutaneously administered LHRH antagonist cetrorelix in patients with symptomatic benign prostatic hyperplasia. Eur Urol. 2008;54(1):170.

214. Del Popolo G, Filocamo MT, Li Marzi V, et al. Neurogenic detrusor overactivity treated with English botulinum toxin a: 8-year experience of one single centre. Eur Urol. 2008;53(5):1013.

215. DeLancey JOL. The pathophysiology of stress urinary incontinence in women and its implications for surgical treatment. World J Urol. 1997;15:268.

216. Dell'utri C, Digesu GA, Bhide A, Khullar V. Fesoterodine in randomised clinical trials: an updated systematic clinical review of efficacy and safety. Int Urogynecol J. 2012;23(10):1337–44.

217. Denmeade SR, Egerdie B, Steinhoff G, et al. Phase 1 and 2 studies demonstrate the safety and efficacy of intraprostatic injection of PRX302 for the targeted treatment of lower urinary tract symptoms secondary to benign prostatic hyperplasia. Eur Urol. 2011;59(5):747–54.

218. Denys P, Le Normand L, Ghout I, et al., VESITOX study group in France. Efficacy and safety of low doses of onabotulinumtoxinA for the treatment of refractory idiopathic overactive bladder: a multicentre, double-blind, randomised, placebo-controlled dose-ranging study. Eur Urol. 2012;61(3):520–9.

219. Diefenbach K, Jaeger K, Wollny A, et al. Effect of tolterodine on sleep structure modulated by CYP2D6 genotype. Sleep Med. 2008;9(5):579.

220. Digesu GA, Khullar V, Cardozo L, Salvatore S. Overactive bladder symptoms: do we need urodynamics? Neurourol Urodyn. 2003;22(2):105.

221. Dinis P, Charrua A, Avelino A, Cruz F. Intravesical resiniferatoxin decreases spinal c-fos expression and increases bladder volume to reflex micturition in rats with chronic inflamed urinary bladders. BJU Int. 2004;94(1):153–7.

222. Dinis P, Charrua A, Avelino A, et al. The distribution of sensory fibers immunoreactive for the TRPV1 (capsaicin) receptor in the human prostate. Eur Urol. 2005;48(1):162–7.

223. Diokno AC. Medical management of urinary incontinence. Gastroenterology. 2004;126(1 Suppl 1):S77–81.

224. Diokno AC, Appell RA, Sand PK, et al. Prospective, randomized, double-blind study of the efficacy and tolerability of the extended-release formulations of oxybutynin and tolterodine for overactive bladder:

results of the OPERA trial. Mayo Clin Proc. 2003;78(6):687.

225. Dmochowski R, Abrams P, Marschall-Kehrel D, et al. Efficacy and tolerability of tolterodine extended release in male and female patients with overactive bladder. Eur Urol. 2007;51(4):1054.

226. Dmochowski R, Chapple C, Nitti VW, et al. Efficacy and safety of onabotulinumtoxinA for idiopathic overactive bladder: a double-blind, placebo controlled, randomized, dose ranging trial. J Urol. 2010;184(6):2416–22.

227. Dmochowski RR, Davila GW, Zinner NR, et al. Efficacy and safety of transdermal oxybutynin in patients with urge and mixed urinary incontinence. J Urol. 2002;168(2):580.

228. Dmochowski R, Kreder K, MacDiarmid S, et al. The clinical efficacy of tolterodine extended-release is maintained for 24 h in patients with overactive bladder. BJU Int. 2007;100(1):107.

229. Dmochowski RR, Miklos JR, Norton PA, et al. Duloxetine vs. placebo in the treatment of North American women with stress urinary incontinence. J Urol. 2003;170:1259.

230. Dmochowski RR, Newman DK, Sand PK, et al. Pharmacokinetics of oxybutynin chloride topical gel: effects of application site, baths, sunscreen and person-to-person transference. Clin Drug Investig. 2011;31(8):559–71.

231. Dmochowski RR, Nitti V, Staskin D, et al. Transdermal oxybutynin in the treatment of adults with overactive bladder: combined results of two randomized clinical trials. World J Urol. 2005;23(4):263.

232. Dmochowski RR, Peters KM, Morrow JD, et al. Randomized, double-blind, placebo-controlled trial of flexible-dose fesoterodine in subjects with overactive bladder. Urology. 2010;75(1):62–8.

233. Dmochowski R, Roehrborn C, Klise S, et al. Urodynamic effects of once daily tadalafil in men with lower urinary tract symptoms secondary to clinical benign prostatic hyperplasia: a randomized, placebo controlled 12-week clinical trial. J Urol. 2010;183:1092–7.

234. Dmochowski RR, Sand PK, Zinner NR, et al. Comparative efficacy and safety of transdermal oxybutynin and oral tolterodine versus placebo in previously treated patients with urge and mixed urinary incontinence. Urology. 2003;62(2):237.

235. Dmochowski RR, Sand PK, Zinner NR, et al. Trospium 60 mg once daily (QD) for overactive bladder syndrome: results from a placebo-controlled interventional study. Urology. 2008;71(3):449.

236. Donath F, Braeter M, Feustel C. The influence of propiverine hydrochloride on cardiac repolarization in healthy women and cardiac male patients. Int J Clin Pharmacol Ther. 2011;49(6):353–65.

237. Dong M, Yeh F, Tepp WH, et al. SV2 is the protein receptor for botulinum neurotoxin A. Science. 2006;312(5773):592.

238. Donker P, Van der Sluis C. Action of beta adrenergic blocking agents on the urethral pressure profile. Urol Int. 1976;31:6.

239. Donnellan CA, Fook L, McDonald P, et al. Oxybutynin and cognitive dysfunction. BMJ. 1997;315:1363.

240. Doroshyenko O, Jetter A, Odenthal KP, et al. Clinical pharmacokinetics of trospium chloride. Clin Pharmacokinet. 2005;44(7):701.

241. Dorschner W, Stolzenburg JU, Griebenow R, et al. Efficacy and cardiac safety of propiverine in elderly patients—a double-blind, placebo-controlled clinical study. Eur Urol. 2000;37:702.

242. Douchamps J, Derenne F, Stockis A, et al. The pharmacokinetics of oxybutynin in man. Eur J Clin Pharmacol. 1988;35:515.

243. Downie JW, Karmazyn M. Mechanical trauma to bladder epithelium liberates prostanoids which modulate neurotransmission in rabbit detrusor muscle. J Pharmacol Exp Ther. 1984;230:445.

244. Dowson C, Sahai A, Watkins J, et al. The safety and efficacy of botulinum toxin-A in the management of bladder oversensitivity: a randomised double-blind placebo-controlled trial. Int J Clin Pract. 2011;65(6):698–704.

245. Dowson C, Watkins J, Khan MS, et al. Repeated botulinum toxin type a injections for refractory overactive bladder: medium-term outcomes, safety profile, and discontinuation rates. Eur Urol. 2012;61(4):834–9.

246. Duckett J, Aggarwal I, Patil A. Duloxetine treatment for women awaiting continence surgery. Int Urogynecol J Pelvic Floor Dysfunct. 2006;17(6): 563–5.

247. Duthie JB, Vincent M, Herbison GP, Wilson DI, Wilson D. Botulinum toxin injections for adults with overactive bladder syndrome. Cochrane Database Syst Rev. 2011;(12):CD005493.

248. Dwyer P, Kelleher C, Young J, et al. Long-term benefits of darifenacin treatment for patient quality of life: results from a 2-year extension study. Neurourol Urodyn. 2008;27(6):540.

249. Dwyer PL, Teele JS. Prazosin: a neglected cause of genuine stress incontinence. Obstet Gynecol. 1992;79:117.

250. Eckford SD, Carter PG, Jackson SR, et al. An open, in-patient incremental safety and efficacy study of desmopressin in women with multiple sclerosis and nocturia. Br J Urol. 1995;76:459.

251. Eckford SD, Swami KS, Jackson SR, et al. Desmopressin in the treatment of nocturia and enuresis in patients with multiple sclerosis. Br J Urol. 1994;74:733.

252. Edwards JL. Diagnosis and management of benign prostatic hyperplasia. Am Fam Physician. 2008;77:1403–10.

253. Ekström B, Andersson K-E, Mattiasson A. Urodynamic effects of intravesical instillation of atropine and phentolamine in patients with detrusor hyperactivity. J Urol. 1992;149:155.

254. Elhilali MM, Pommerville P, Yocum RC, et al. Prospective, randomized, double-blind, vehicle controlled, multicenter phase IIb clinical trial of the pore forming protein PRX302 for targeted treatment of symptomatic benign prostatic hyperplasia. J Urol. 2013;189(4):1421–6.

255. Elinoff V, Bavendam T, Glasser DB, et al. Symptom-specific efficacy of tolterodine extended release in patients with overactive bladder: the IMPACT trial. Int J Clin Pract. 2006;60(6):745.

256. Eltink C, Lee J, Schaddelee M, et al. Single dose pharmacokinetics and absolute bioavailability of mirabegron, a β3-adrenoceptor agonist for treatment of overactive bladder. Int J Clin Pharmacol Ther. 2012;50(11):838–50.

257. Emberton M, Cornel EB, Bassi PF, et al. Benign prostatic hyperplasia as a progressive disease: a guide to the risk factors and options for medical management. Int J Clin Pract. 2008;62:1076–86.

258. Emberton M, Fitzpatrick J. The Reten-World survey of the management of acute urinary retention: preliminary results. BJU Int. 2008;101 Suppl 3:27–32.

259. Endo RM, Girao MJ, Sartori MG, et al. Effect of estrogen-progestogen hormonal replacement therapy on periurethral and bladder vessels. Int Urogynecol J Pelvic Floor Dysfunct. 2000;11(2):120.

260. Enskat R, Deaney CN, Glickman S. Systemic effects of intravesical atropine sulphate. BJU Int. 2001;87:613.

261. Eri LM, Tveter KJ. A prospective, placebo-controlled study of the luteinizing hormone-releasing hormone agonist leuprolide as treatment for patients with benign prostatic hyperplasia. J Urol. 1993;150:359.

262. Everaerts W, Gevaert T, Nilius B, De Ridder D. On the origin of bladder sensing: Tr(i)ps in urology. Neurourol Urodyn. 2008;27(4):264–73.

263. Everaerts W, Zhen X, Ghosh D, et al. Inhibition of the cation channel TRPV4 improves bladder function in mice and rats with cyclophosphamide-induced cystitis. Proc Natl Acad Sci U S A. 2010;107(44):19084–9.

264. Fader M, Glickman S, Haggar V, et al. Intravesical atropine compared to oral oxybutynin for neurogenic detrusor overactivity: a double-blind, randomized crossover trial. J Urol. 2007;177(1):208.

265. Falconer C, Ekman-Ordeberg G, Blomgren B, et al. Paraurethral connective tissue in stress incontinent women after menopause. Acta Obstet Gynaecol Scand. 1998;77(1):95.

266. Fantl JA, Bump RC, Robinson D, et al. Efficacy of estrogen supplementation in the treatment of urinary incontinence. Obstet Gynaecol. 1996;88:745.

267. Fantl JA, Cardozo L, McClish DK. Estrogen therapy in the management of urinary incontinence in postmenopausal women: a meta-analysis. First report of the Hormones and Urogenital Therapy Committee. Obstet Gynaecol. 1994;83:12.

268. Fellenius E, Hedberg R, Holmberg E, et al. Functional and metabolic effects of terbutaline and

propranolol in fast and slow contracting skeletal muscle in vitro. Acta Physiol Scand. 1980;109:89.

269. Fibbi B, Morelli A, Vignozzi L, et al. Characterization of phosphodiesterase type 5 expression and functional activity in the human male lower urinary tract. J Sex Med. 2009;7:59–69.

270. Filocamo MT, LiMarzi V, Del Popoilo G, et al. Pharmacologic treatment in postprostatectomy stress urinary incontinence. Eur Urol. 2007;51:1559.

271. Finney SM, Andersson KE, Gillespie JI, Stewart LH. Antimuscarinic drugs in detrusor overactivity and the overactive bladder syndrome: motor or sensory actions? BJU Int. 2006;98(3):503.

272. Fitzpatrick JM, Desgrandchamps F, Adjali K, Gomez Guerra L, Hong SJ, El Khalid S, Ratana-Olarn K, Reten-World Study Group. Management of acute urinary retention: a worldwide survey of 6074 men with benign prostatic hyperplasia. BJU Int. 2012;109(1):88–95.

273. Fitzpatrick J, Kirby R. Management of acute urinary retention. BJU Int. 2006;97 Suppl 2:16–20.

274. Foote J, Glavind K, Kralidis G, et al. Treatment of overactive bladder in the older patient: pooled analysis of three phase III studies of darifenacin, an M3 selective receptor antagonist. Eur Urol. 2005;48(3):471.

275. Fowler CJ, Auerbach S, Ginsberg D, et al. OnabotulinumtoxinA improves health-related quality of life in patients with urinary incontinence due to idiopathic overactive bladder: a 36-week, double-blind, placebo-controlled, randomized, dose-ranging trial. Eur Urol. 2012;62(1):148–57.

276. Fowler CJ, Beck RO, Gerrard S, et al. Intravesical capsaicin for the treatment of detrusor hyperreflexia. J Neurol Neurosurg Psychiatry. 1994;57:169.

277. Fowler CJ, Griffiths D, de Groat WC. The neural control of micturition. Nat Rev Neurosci. 2008;9(6):453–66.

278. Fowler CJ, Jewkes D, McDonald WI, et al. Intravesical capsaicin for neurogenic bladder dysfunction. Lancet. 1992;339(8803):1239.

279. Fraser MO, Chancellor MB. Neural control of the urethra and development of pharmacotherapy for stress urinary incontinence. BJU Int. 2003;91(8):743.

280. Frazier EP, Mathy MJ, Peters SL, et al. Does cyclic AMP mediate rat urinary bladder relaxation by isoproterenol? J Pharmacol Exp Ther. 2005;313(1):260.

281. Frazier EP, Peters SLM, Braverman AS, et al. Signal transduction underlying control of urinary bladder smooth muscle tone by muscarinic receptors and β-adrenoceptors. Naunyn Schmiedebergs Arch Pharmacol. 2008;377:449.

282. Fredrikson S. Nasal spray desmopressin in treatment of bladder dysfunction in patients with multiple sclerosis. Acta Neurol Scand. 1996;94:31.

283. Freeman RM, Adekanmi O, Waterfield MR, et al. The effect of cannabis on urge incontinence in patients with multiple sclerosis: a multicentre, randomised placebocontrolled trial (CAMS-LUTS). Int Urogynecol J Pelvic Floor Dysfunct. 2006;17:636–41.

284. Freeman R, Hill S, Millard R, et al., Tolterodine Study Group. Reduced perception of urgency in treatment of overactive bladder with extended-release tolterodine. Obstet Gynecol. 2003;102(3):605.

285. Frenkl TL, Zhu H, Reiss T, et al. A multicenter, double-blind, randomized, placebo controlled trial of a neurokinin-1 receptor antagonist for overactive bladder. J Urol. 2010;184(2):616–22.

286. Frew R, Lundy PM. A role for Q type Ca2+ channels in neurotransmission in the rat urinary bladder. Br J Pharmacol. 1995;116:1595.

287. Frias B, Charrua A, Avelino A, et al. Transient receptor potential vanilloid 1 mediates nerve growth factor-induced bladder hyperactivity and noxious input. BJU Int. 2012;110(8 Pt B):E422–8.

288. Fröhlich G, Burmeister S, Wiedemann A, et al. Intravesical instillation of trospium chloride, oxybutynin and verapamil for relaxation of the bladder detrusor muscle. A placebo controlled, randomized clinical test. Arzneimittelforschung. 1998;48(5):486 (German).

289. Fu X, Rezapour M, Wu X, et al. Expression of estrogen receptor alpha and beta in anterior vaginal walls of genuine stress incontinence women. Int Urogynaecol J Pelivc Floor Dysfunct. 2003;14(4):276.

290. Fujimura T, Tamura K, Tsutsumi T, et al. Expression and possible functional role of the beta3-adrenoceptor in human and rat detrusor muscle. J Urol. 1999;161(2):680.

291. Furuta A, Naruoka T, Suzuki Y, et al. α2-Adrenoceptor as a new target for stress urinary incontinence. Low Urin Tract Symptoms. 2009;1:526–9.

292. Fusgen I, Hauri D. Trospium chloride: an effective option for medical treatment of bladder overactivity. Int J Clin Pharmacol Ther. 2000;38(5):223.

293. Gacci M, Vittori G, Tosi N, et al. A randomised, placebo-controlled study to assess safety and efficacy of vardenafil 10 mg and tamsulosin 0,4 mg versus tamsulosin 0.4 mg alone in the treatment of lower urinary tract symptoms secondary to benign prostatic hyperplasia. J Sex Med. 2012;9(6):1624–33.

294. Garely AD, Kaufman JM, Sand PK, et al. Symptom bother and health-related quality of life outcomes following solifenacin treatment for overactive bladder: the VESIcare Open-Label Trial (VOLT). Clin Ther. 2006;28(11):1935.

295. Gebhardt J, Richard D, Barrett T. Expression of estrogen receptor isoforms alpha and beta messenger RNA in vaginal tissue of premenopausal and postmenopausal women. Am J Obstet Gynaecol. 2001;185:1325.

296. Gee NS, Brown JP, Dissanayake VU, et al. The novel anticonvulsant drug, gabapentin (Neurontin), binds to the alpha2delta subunit of a calcium channel. J Biol Chem. 1996;271(10):5768.

297. Geirsson G, Fall M, Sullivan L. Clinical and urodynamic effects of intravesical capsaicin treatment in patients with chronic traumatic spinal detrusor hyperreflexia. J Urol. 1995;154(5):1825.

298. George J, Tharion G, Richar J, et al. The effectiveness of intravesical oxybutynin, propantheline, and capsaicin in the management of neuropathic bladder following spinal cord injury. ScientificWorld J. 2007;7:1683.

299. Gevaert T, Vriens J, Segal A, et al. Deletion of the transient receptor potential cation channel TRPV4 impairs murine bladder voiding. J Clin Invest. 2007;117(11):3453–62.

300. Ghoneim GM, Van Leeuwen JS, Elser DM, et al. A randomized controlled trial of duloxetine alone, pelvic floor muscle training alone, combined treatment, and no treatment in women with stress urinary incontinence. J Urol. 2005;173:1647.

301. Giannantoni A, Conte A, Farfariello V, Proietti S, et al. Onabotulinumtoxin-A intradetrusorial injections modulate bladder expression of NGF, TrkA, p75 and TRPV1 in patients with detrusor overactivity. Pharmacol Res. 2013;68(1):118–24.

302. Giannantoni A, Di Stasi SM, Nardicchi V, et al. Botulinum-A toxin injections into the detrusor muscle decrease nerve growth factor bladder tissue levels in patients with neurogenic detrusor overactivity. J Urol. 2006;175(6):2341.

303. Giardina EG, Bigger Jr JT, Glassman AH, et al. The electrocardiographic and antiarrhythmic effects of imipramine hydrochloride at therapeutic plasma concentrations. Circulation. 1979;60:1045.

304. Giembycz MA. Life after PDE4: overcoming adverse events with dual-specificity phosphodiesterase inhibitors. Curr Opin Pharmacol. 2005;5(3):238.

305. Gilja I, Radej M, Kovacic M, et al. Conservative treatment of female stress incontinence with imipramine. J Urol. 1984;132:909.

306. Gillespie JL. Phosphodiesterase-linked inhibition of nonmicturition activity in the isolated bladder. BJU Int. 2004;93(9):1325.

307. Gillespie JI, Drake MJ. The actions of sodium nitroprusside and the phosphodiesterase inhibitor dipyridamole on phasic activity in the isolated guinea-pig bladder. BJU Int. 2004;93:851–8.

308. Gillman P. Tricyclic antidepressant pharmacology and therapeutic drug interactions updated. Br J Pharmacol. 2007;151(6):737–48.

309. Giuliano F, Übert S, Maggi M, et al. The mechanism of action of phosphodiesterase type 5 inhibitors in the treatment of lower urinary tract symptoms related to benign prostatic hyperplasia. Eur Urol. 2013;63(3):506–16.

310. Glazener CMA, Evans JHC. Desmopressin for nocturnal enuresis in children. Cochrane Database Syst Rev. 2002;(3):CD002112.

311. Glazener CM, Evans JH, Peto RE. Tricyclic and related drugs for nocturnal enuresis in children. Cochrane Database Syst Rev. 2003;(3):CD002117.

312. Gleason DM, Reilly SA, Bottacini MR, et al. The urethral continence zone and its relation to stress incontinence. J Urol. 1974;112:81.

313. Gleason DM, Susset J, White C, et al. Evaluation of a new once-daily formulation of oxybutynin the treatment of urinary urge incontinence. The Ditropan XL Study Group. Urology. 1999;54:420.

314. Glickman S, Tsokkos N, Shah PJ. Intravesical atropine and suppression of detrusor hypercontractility in the neuropathic bladder. A preliminary study. Paraplegia. 1995;33:36.

315. Goessl C, Knispel HH, Fiedler U, et al. Urodynamic effects of oral oxybutynin chloride in children with myelomeningocele and detrusor hyperreflexia. Urology. 1998;51(1):94–8.

316. Gomes CM, Castro Filho JE, Rejowski RF, et al. Experience with different botulinum toxins for the treatment of refractory neurogenic detrusor overactivity. Int Braz J Urol. 2010;36(1):66–74.

317. Gomes T, Juurlink DN, Mamdani MM. Comparative adherence to oxybutynin or tolterodine among older patients. Eur J Clin Pharmacol. 2012;68(1):97–9.

318. Gopalakrishnan M, Shieh C-C. Potassium channel subtypes as molecular targets for overactive bladder and other urological disorders. Expert Opin Ther Targets. 2004;8:437.

319. Gotoh M, Kamihira O, Kinikawa T, et al. Comparison of α1A-selective adrenoceptor antagonist, tamsulosin, and α1D-selective adrenoceptor antagonist, naftopidil, for efficacy and safety in the treatment of benign prostatic hyperplasia: a randomized controlled trial. BJU Int. 2005;96(4):581–6.

320. Grady D, Brown JS, Vittinghoff E, et al. Postmenopausal hormones and incontinence: the Heart and Estrogen/Progestin Replacement Study. Obstet Gynaecol. 2001;97:116.

321. Gratzke C, Streng T, Park A, et al. Distribution and function of cannabinoid receptors 1 and 2 in the rat, monkey and human bladder. J Urol. 2009;181: 1939–48.

322. Gratzke C, Streng T, Stief CG, et al. Effects of cannabinor, a novel selective cannabinoid 2 receptor agonist, on bladder function in normal rats. Eur Urol. 2010;57(6):1093–100.

323. Gratzke C, Streng T, Stief CG, et al. Cannabinor, a selective cannabinoid-2 receptor agonist, improves bladder emptying in rats with partial urethral obstruction. J Urol. 2011;185:731–6.

324. Green SA, Alon A, Ianus J, et al. Efficacy and safety of a neurokinin-1 receptor antagonist in postmenopausal women with overactive bladder with urge urinary incontinence. J Urol. 2006;176(6 Pt 1):2535.

325. Griffiths D. Imaging bladder sensations. Neurourol Urodyn. 2007;26(6 Suppl):899.

326. Griffiths DJ. Use of functional imaging to monitor central control of voiding in humans. Handb Exp Pharmacol. 2011;202:81–97.

327. Griffiths D, Tadic SD. Bladder control, urgency, and urge incontinence: evidence from functional brain imaging. Neurourol Urodyn. 2008;27(6):466.

328. Grigoleit U, Mürtz G, Laschke S, et al. Efficacy, tolerability and safety of propiverine hydrochloride in children and adolescents with congenital or traumatic neurogenic detrusor overactivity–a retrospective study. Eur Urol. 2006;49(6):1114.

329. Grodstein F, Lifford K, Resnick NM, Curham GC. Postmenopausal hormone therapy and risk of developing urinary incontinence. Obstet Gynaecol. 2004;103(2):254.

330. Grond S, Sablotzki A. Clinical pharmacology of tramadol. Clin Pharmacokinet. 2004;43(13):879.

331. Gu B, Fraser MO, Thor KB, et al. Induction of bladder sphincter dyssynergia by κ-2 opioid receptor agonists in the female rat. J Urol. 2004;171:472.

332. Gu BJ, Ishizuka O, Igawa Y, et al. Role of supraspinal tachykinins for micturition in conscious rats with and without bladder outlet obstruction. Naunyn Schmiedebergs Arch Pharmacol. 2000;361(5):543.

333. Guarneri L, Robinson E, Testa R. A review of flavoxate: pharmacology and mechanism of action. Drugs Today. 1994;30:91.

334. Guay DR. Clinical pharmacokinetics of drugs used to treat urge incontinence. Clin Pharmacokinet. 2003;42(14):1243.

335. Guerra LA, Moher D, Sampson M, et al. Intravesical oxybutynin for children with poorly compliant neurogenic bladder: a systematic review. J Urol. 2008;180(3):1091.

336. Gutman GA, Chandy KG, Adelman JP, et al. International Union of Pharmacology. XLI. Compendium of voltage-gated ion channels: potassium channels. Pharmacol Rev. 2003;55:583.

337. Haab F, Cardozo L, Chapple C, et al., Solifenacin Study Group. Long-term open-label solifenacin treatment associated with persistence with therapy in patients with overactive bladder syndrome. Eur Urol. 2005;47(3):376.

338. Haab F, Corcos J, Siami P, et al. Long-term treatment with darifenacin for overactive bladder: results of a 2-year, open-label extension study. BJU Int. 2006;98(5):1025.

339. Haab F, Stewart L, Dwyer P. Darifenacin, an M3 selective receptor antagonist, is an effective and well-tolerated once-daily treatment for overactive bladder. Eur Urol. 2004;45(4):420.

340. Haferkamp A, Schurch B, Reitz A, et al. Lack of ultrastructural detrusor changes following endoscopic injection of botulinum toxin type a in overactive neurogenic bladder. Eur Urol. 2004;46(6):784.

341. Halaska M, Ralph G, Wiedemann A, et al. Controlled, double-blind, multicentre clinical trial to investigate long-term tolerability and efficacy of trospium chloride in patients with detrusor instability. World J Urol. 2003;20(6):392.

342. Hampel C, Gillitzer R, Pahernik S, et al. Medikamentöse Therapie der weiblichen Harninkontinenz. Urologe A. 2005;44:244.

343. Haruno A. Inhibitory effects of propiverine hydrochloride on the agonist-induced or spontaneous contractions of various isolated muscle preparations. Arzneimittelforschung. 1992;42:815.

344. Hashim H, Abrams P. Do symptoms of overactive bladder predict urodynamics detrusor overactivity? Neurourol Urodyn. 2004;23(5/6):484.

345. Hashim H, Abrams P. Pharmacologic management of women with mixed urinary incontinence. Drugs. 2006;66(5):591.

346. Hashim H, Malmberg L, Graugaard-Jensen C, et al. Desmopressin, as a "designer-drug," in the treatment of overactive bladder syndrome. Neurourol Urodyn. 2009;28(1):40–6.

347. Haustein KO, Huller G. On the pharmacokinetics and metabolism of propiverine in man. Eur J Drug Metab Pharmacokinet. 1988;13(2):81.

348. Helfand BT, Evans RM, McVary KT. A comparison of the frequencies of medical therapies for overactive bladder in men and women: analysis of more than 7.2 million aging patients. Eur Urol. 2010;57(4):586–91.

349. Hendrix SL, Cochrane BB, Nygaard IE, et al. Effects of estrogen with and without progestin on urinary incontinence. JAMA. 2005;293(8):935.

350. Hendrix SL, McNeeley SG. Effect of selective estrogen receptor modulators on reproductive tissues other than endometrium. Ann N Y Acad Sci. 2001;949:243.

351. Henriksson L, Andersson K-E, Ulmsten U. The urethral pressure profiles in continent and stress incontinent women. Scand J Urol Nephrol. 1979;13:5.

352. Herbison P, Hay-Smith J, Ellis G, et al. Effectiveness of anticholinergic drugs compared with placebo in the treatment of overactive bladder: systematic review. Br Med J. 2003;326:841.

353. Herschorn S, Barkin J, Castro-Diaz D, et al. A phase III, randomized, double-blind, parallel-group, placebo-controlled, multicentre study to assess the efficacy and safety of the β3-adrenoceptor agonist, mirabegron in patients with symptoms of overactive bladder. Urology. 2013;82(2):313–20.

354. Herschorn S, Gajewski J, Ethans K, et al. Efficacy of botulinum toxin A injection for neurogenic detrusor overactivity and urinary incontinence: a randomized, double-blind trial. J Urol. 2011;185(6):2229–35.

355. Herschorn S, Gajewski J, Schulz J, Corcos J. A population-based study of urinary symptoms and incontinence: the Canadian Urinary Bladder Survey. BJU Int. 2008;101(1):52.

356. Herschorn S, Pommerville P, Stothers L, Egerdie B, Gajewski J, Carlson K, Radomski S, Drutz H, Schulz J, Barkin J, Hirshberg E, Corcos J. Tolerability of solifenacin and oxybutynin immediate release in older (>65 years) and younger (≤65 years) patients with overactive bladder: sub-analysis from a Canadian, randomized, double-blind study. Curr Med Res Opin. 2011;27(2):375–82.

357. Herschorn S, Swift S, Guan Z, et al. Comparison of fesoterodine and tolterodine extended release for the treatment of overactive bladder: a head-to-head placebo-controlled trial. BJU Int. 2010;105(1):58–66.

358. Hextall A. Oestrogens and lower urinary tract function. Maturitas. 2000;36:83.

359. Hextall A, Bidmead J, Cardozo L, et al. The impact of the menstrual cycle on urinary symptoms and the

results of urodynamic investigation. BJOG. 2001;108(11):1193.

360. Hicks A, McCafferty GP, Riedel E, et al. GW427353 (solabegron), a novel, selective beta3-adrenergic receptor agonist, evokes bladder relaxation and increases micturition reflex threshold in the dog. J Pharmacol Exp Ther. 2007;323(1):202.

361. Hill S, Khullar V, Wyndaele JJ, et al. Dose response with darifenacin, a novel once-daily M3 selective receptor antagonist for the treatment of overactive bladder: results of a fixed dose study. Int Urogynecol J Pelvic Floor Dysfunct. 2006;17(3):239.

362. Hills CJ, Winter SA, Balfour JA. Tolterodine. Drugs. 1998;55:813.

363. Hilton P, Hertogs K, Stanton SL. The use of desmopressin (DDAVP) for nocturia in women with multiple sclerosis. J Neurol Neurosurg Psychiatry. 1983;46:854.

364. Hilton P, Stanton SL. The use of desmopressin (DDAVP) in nocturnal urinary frequency in the female. Br J Urol. 1982;54:252.

365. Hoebeke P, De Pooter J, De Caestecker K, et al. Solifenacin for therapy resistant overactive bladder. J Urol. 2009;182(4 Suppl):2040–4.

366. Hoebeke PB, Vande Walle J. The pharmacology of paediatric incontinence. BJU Int. 2000;86(5): 581–9.

367. Höfner K, Burkart M, Jacob G, et al. Safety and efficacy of tolterodine extended release in men with overactive bladder symptoms and presumed nonobstructive benign prostatic hyperplasia. World J Urol. 2007;25(6):627.

368. Holmes DM, Montz FJ, Stanton SL. Oxybutinin versus propantheline in the management of detrusor instability. A patient regulated variable dose trial. Br J Obstet Gynaecol. 1989;96:607.

369. Holstege G. Micturition and the soul. J Comp Neurol. 2005;493(1):15–20.

370. Homma Y, Yamaguchi O. Long-term safety, tolerability, and efficacy of the novel anti-muscarinic agent imidafenacin in Japanese patients with overactive bladder. Int J Urol. 2008;15(11):986–91.

371. Homma Y, Yamaguchi T, Yamaguchi O. A randomized, double-blind, placebo-controlled phase II dose-finding study of the novel anti-muscarinic agentimidafenacin in Japanese patients with overactive bladder. Int J Urol. 2008;15(9):809–15.

372. Hoverd PA, Fowler CJ. Desmopressin in the treatment of daytime urinary frequency in patients with multiple sclerosis. J Neurol Neurosurg Psychiatry. 1998;65:778.

373. Howe BB, Halterman TJ, Yochim CL, et al. Zeneca ZD6169: a novel KATP channel opener with in vivo selectivity for urinary bladder. J Pharmacol Exp Ther. 1995;274:884.

374. Hsiao SM, Chang TC, Wu WY, Chen CH, Yu HJ, Lin HH. Comparisons of urodynamic effects, therapeutic efficacy and safety of solifenacinversus tolterodine for female overactive bladder syndrome. J Obstet Gynaecol Res. 2011;37(8):1084–91.

375. Hu S, Kim HS. Modulation of ATP sensitive and large-conductance Ca2+-activated K+ channels by Zeneca ZD6169 in guinea pig bladder smooth muscle cells. J Pharmacol Exp Ther. 1997;280:38.

376. Hudman D, Elliott RA, Norman RI. K(ATP) channels mediate the beta(2)-adrenoceptor agonist-induced relaxation of rat detrusor muscle. Eur J Pharmacol. 2000;397(1):169.

377. Hughes KM, Lang JCT, Lazare R, et al. Measurement of oxybutynin and its N-desethyl metabolite in plasma, and its application to pharmacokinetic studies in young, elderly and frail elderly volunteers. Xenobiotica. 1992;22:859.

378. Humeau Y, Doussau F, Grant NJ, et al. How botulinum and tetanus neurotoxins block neurotransmitter release. Biochimie. 2000;82(5):427.

379. Hunsballe JM, Djurhuus JC. Clinical options for imipramine in the management of urinary incontinence. Urol Res. 2001;29:118.

380. Hurley DJ, Turner CL, Yalcin I, et al. Duloxetine for the treatment of stress urinary incontinence: an integrated analysis of safety. Eur J Obstet Gynecol Reprod Biol. 2006;125:120.

381. Hussain RM, Hartigan-Go K, Thomas SHL, et al. Effect of oxybutynin on the QTc interval in elderly patients with urinary incontinence. Br J Clin Pharmacol. 1994;37:485P.

382. Hyman MJ, Groutz A, Blaivas JG. Detrusor instability in men: correlation of lower urinary tract symptoms with urodynamic findings. J Urol. 2001;166(2):550.

383. Igawa Y, Aizawa N, Homma Y. Beta3-adrenoceptor agonists: possible role in the treatment of overactive bladder. Korean J Urol. 2010;51(12):811–8.

384. Igawa Y, Michel MC. Pharmacological profile of β3-adrenoceptor agonists in clinical development for the treatment of overactive bladder syndrome. Naunyn Schmiedebergs Arch Pharmacol. 2013;386(3):177–83.

385. Igawa Y, Yamazaki Y, Takeda H, et al. Functional and molecular biological evidence for a possible beta3-adrenoceptor in the human detrusor muscle. Br J Pharmacol. 1999;126(3):819.

386. Igawa Y, Yamazaki Y, Takeda H, et al. Relaxant effects of isoproterenol and selective beta3-adrenoceptor agonists on normal, low compliant and hyperreflexic human bladders. J Urol. 2001;165(1):240.

387. Iijima K, De Wachter S, Wyndaele JJ. Effects of the M3 receptor selective muscarinic antagonist darifenacin on bladder afferent activity of the rat pelvic nerve. Eur Urol. 2007;52(3):842.

388. Ikeda Y, Zabbarova IV, Birder LA, et al. Botulinum neurotoxin serotype A suppresses neurotransmitter release from afferent as well as efferent nerves in the urinary bladder. Eur Urol. 2012;62(6):1157–64.

389. Ikemoto I, Kiyota H, Ohishi Y, et al. Usefulness of tamsulosin hydrochloride and naftopidil in patients with urinary disturbances caused by benign prostatic hyperplasia: a comparative, randomized, two-drug crossover study. Int J Urol. 2003;10(11):587–94.

390. Insel PA, Tang C-M, Hahntow I, et al. Impact of GPCRs in clinical medicine: genetic variants and drug targets. Biochim Biophys Acta. 2007;1768:994.

391. Irwin DE, Abrams P, Milsom I, et al., EPIC Study Group. Understanding the elements of overactive bladder: questions raised by the EPIC study. BJU Int. 2008;101(11):1381-7.

392. Irwin DE, Milsom I, Hunskaar S, et al. Population-based survey of urinary incontinence, overactive bladder, and other lower urinary tract symptoms in five countries: results of the EPIC study. Eur Urol. 2006;50(6):1306.

393. Ishiko O, Hirai K, Sumi T, et al. Hormone replacement therapy plus pelvic floor muscle exercise for postmenopausal stress incontinence. A randomized controlled trial. J Reprod Med. 2001;46:213.

394. Ishiko O, Ushiroyama T, Saji F, et al. Beta(2)-adrenergic agonists and pelvic floor exercises for female stress incontinence. Int J Gynaecol Obstet. 2000;71:39.

395. Ishizuka O, Igawa Y, Lecci A, et al. Role of intrathecal tachykinins for micturition in unanaesthetized rats with and without bladder outlet obstruction. Br J Pharmacol. 1994;113(1):111.

396. Ishizuka O, Igawa Y, Nishizawa O, et al. Role of supraspinal tachykinins for volume- and L-dopa-induced bladder activity in normal conscious rats. Neurourol Urodyn. 2000;19(1):101.

397. Ishizuka O, Mattiasson A, Andersson KE. Effects of neurokinin receptor antagonists on L-dopa induced bladder hyperactivity in normal conscious rats. J Urol. 1995;154(4):1548.

398. Jackson S, Shepherd A, Abrams P. The effect of oestradiol on objective urinary leakage in postmenopausal stress incontinence: a double blind placebo controlled trial. Neurourol Urodyn. 1996;15:322.

399. Janssen DA, Hoenderop JG, Jansen KC, et al. The mechanoreceptor TRPV4 is localized in adherence junctions of the human bladder urothelium: a morphological study. J Urol. 2011;186(3):1121-7.

400. Jeremy JY, Tsang V, Mikhailidis DP, et al. Eicosanoid synthesis by human urinary bladder mucosa: pathological implications. Br J Urol. 1987;59:36.

401. Ji RR, Samad TA, Jin SX, et al. p38 MAPK activation by NGF in primary sensory neurons after inflammation increases TRPV1 levels and maintains heat hyperalgesia. Neuron. 2002;36(1):57-68.

402. Johnson II TM, Miller M, Tang T, et al. Oral ddAVP for nighttime urinary incontinence in characterized nursing home residents: a pilot study. J Am Med Dir Assoc. 2006;7:6.

403. Jones RL, Giembycz MA, Woodward DF. Prostanoid receptor antagonists: development strategies and therapeutic applications. Br J Pharmacol. 2009;158:104-45.

404. Jonville AP, Dutertre JP, Autret E, Barbellion M. [Adverse effects of oxybutynin chloride (Ditropan). Evaluation of the official survey of Regional Pharmacovigilance Centers]. Therapie. 1992;47(5):389-92.

405. Jonville AP, Dutertre JP, Autret E, et al. Effets indésirables du chlorure d'oxybutynine (Ditropan®). Therapie. 1992;47:389.

406. Jugus MJ, Jaworski JP, Patra PB, et al. Dual modulation of urinary bladder activity and urine flow by prostanoid EP3 receptors in the conscious rat. Br J Pharmacol. 2009;158:372-81.

407. Jünemann KP, Al-Shukri S. Efficacy and tolerability of trospium chloride and tolterodine in 234 patients with urge-syndrome: a double-blind, placebo-controlled multicentre clinical trial. Neurourol Urodyn. 2000;19:488.

408. Jünemann KP, Halaska M, Rittstein T, et al. Propiverine versus tolterodine: efficacy and tolerability in patients with overactive bladder. Eur Urol. 2005;48(3):478.

409. Jünemann KP, Hessdörfer E, Unamba-Oparah I, et al. Propiverine hydrochloride immediate and extended release: comparison of efficacy and tolerability in patients with overactive bladder. Urol Int. 2006;77(4):334.

410. Juul KV, Klein BM, Sandstrom R, et al. Gender difference in antidiuretic response to desmopressin. Am J Physiol Renal Physiol. 2011;300:F1116-22.

411. Kachur JF, Peterson JS, Carter JP, et al. R and S enantiomers of oxybutynin: pharmacological effects in guinea pig bladder and intestine. J Pharmacol Exp Ther. 1988;247:867.

412. Kaidoh K, Igawa Y, Takeda H, et al. Effects of selective beta2 and beta3-adrenoceptor agonists on detrusor hyperreflexia in conscious cerebral infarcted rats. J Urol. 2002;168(3):1247.

413. Kaiho Y, Nishiguchi J, Kwon DD, et al. The effects of a type 4 phosphodiesterase inhibitor and the muscarinic cholinergic antagonist tolterodine tartrate on detrusor overactivity in female rats with bladder outlet obstruction. BJU Int. 2008;101(5):615.

414. Kaisary AV. Beta adrenoceptor blockade in the treatment of female stress urinary incontinence. J Urol (Paris). 1984;90:351.

415. Kalejaiye O, Speakman MJ. Management of acute and chronic retention in men. Eur Urol. 2009;8(Suppl):523-9.

416. Kamo I, Chancellor MB, De Groat WC, et al. Differential effects of activation of peripheral and spinal tachykinin neurokinin3 receptors on the micturition reflex in rats. J Urol. 2005;174:776.

417. Kanagarajah P, Ayyathurai R, Caruso DJ, et al. Role of botulinum toxin-A in refractory idiopathic overactive bladder patients without detrusor overactivity. Int Urol Nephrol. 2012;44(1):91-7.

418. Kanayama N, Kanari C, Masuda Y, et al. Drug-drug interactions in the metabolism of imidafenacin: role of the human cytochrome P450 enzymes and UDP-glucuronic acid transferases, and potential of imidafenacin to inhibit human cytochrome P450 enzymes. Xenobiotica. 2007;37(2):139-54.

419. Kang IS, Sung ZH, et al. The efficacy and safety of combination therapy with alpha-blocker and low-dose propiverine hydrochloride for benign prostatic

hyperplasia accompanied by overactive bladder symptoms. Korean J Urol. 2009;50:1078–82.

420. Kanie S, Otsuka A, Yoshikawa S, et al. Pharmacological effect of TRK-380, a novel selective human β3-adrenoceptor agonist, on mammalian detrusor strips. Urology. 2012;79(3):744.e1-7.

421. Kaplan SA, Goldfischer ER, Steers WD, et al. Solifenacin treatment in men with overactive bladder: effects on symptoms and patient-reported outcomes. Aging Male. 2010;13(2):100–7.

422. Kaplan SA, Gonzalez RR, Te AE. Combination of alfuzosin and sildenafil is superior to monotherapy in treating lower urinary tract symptoms and erectile dysfunction. Eur Urol. 2007;51:1717–23.

423. Kaplan SA, Roehrborn CG, Chancellor M, et al. Extended-release tolterodine with or without tamsulosin in men with lower urinary tract symptoms and overactive bladder: effects on urinary symptoms assessed by the International Prostate Symptom Score. BJU Int. 2008;102(9):1133–9.

424. Kaplan SA, Roehrborn CG, Rovner ES, et al. Tolterodine and tamsulosin for treatment of men with lower urinary tract symptoms and overactive bladder: a randomized controlled trial. JAMA. 2006;296(19):2319.

425. Kaplan SA, Schneider T, Foote JE, et al. Superior efficacy of fesoterodine over tolterodine extended release with rapid onset: a prospective, head-to-head, placebo-controlled trial. BJU Int. 2011;107(9):1432–40.

426. Kaplan SA, Walmsley K, Te AE. Tolterodine extended release attenuates lower urinary tract symptoms in men with benign prostatic hyperplasia. J Urol. 2008;179(5 Suppl):S82.

427. Karsenty G, Denys P, Amarenco G, et al. Botulinum toxin A (Botox) intradetrusor injections in adults with neurogenic detrusor overactivity/neurogenic overactive bladder: a systematic literature review. Eur Urol. 2008;53(2):275.

428. Kasabian NG, Vlachiotis JD, Lais A, et al. The use of intravesical oxybutynin chloride in patients with detrusor hypertonicity and detrusor hyperreflexia. J Urol. 1994;151:944.

429. Katofiasc MA, Nissen J, Audia JE, et al. Comparison of the effects of serotonin selective norepinephrine selective, and dual serotonin and norepinephrine reuptake inhibitors on lower urinary tract function in cats. Life Sci. 2002;71(11):1227.

430. Kavia R, De Ridder D, Constantinescu S, et al. Randomised controlled trial of Sativex to treat detrusor overactivity in multiple sclerosis. Mult Scler. 2010;16:1349–59.

431. Kawabe K, Yoshida M, Homma Y, Silodosin Clinical Study Group. Silodosin, a new alpha1A-adrenoceptor-selective antagonist for treating benign prostatic hyperplasia: results of a phase III randomized, placebo-controlled, double-blind study in Japanese men. BJU Int. 2006;98(5):1019–24.

432. Kay G, Crook T, Rekeda L, et al. Differential effects of the antimuscarinic agents darifenacin and oxybu-

tynin ER on memory in older subjects. Eur Urol. 2006;50(2):317.

433. Kay GG, Ebinger U. Preserving cognitive function for patients with overactive bladder: evidence for a differential effect with darifenacin. Int J Clin Pract. 2008;62(11):1792–800.

434. Kay GG, Wesnes KA. Pharmacodynamic effects of darifenacin, a muscarinic M selective receptor antagonist for the treatment of overactive bladder, in healthy volunteers. BJU Int. 2005;96(7):1055.

435. Keane DP, Sims TJ, Abrams P, et al. Analysis of collagen status in premenopausal nulliparous women with genuine stress incontinence. Br J Obstet Gynaecol. 1997;104(9):994.

436. Kelleher CJ, Cardozo L, Chapple CR, Haab F, Ridder AM. Improved quality of life in patients with overactive bladder symptoms treated with solifenacin. BJU Int. 2005;95:81–5.

437. Kelleher C, Cardozo L, Kobashi K, et al. Solifenacin: as effective in mixed urinary incontinence as in urge urinary incontinence. Int Urogynecol J Pelvic Floor Dysfunct. 2006;17(4):382.

438. Kelleher CJ, Dmochowski RR, Berriman S, et al. Sustained improvement in patient-reported outcomes during long-term fesoterodine treatment for overactive bladder symptoms: pooled analysis of two open-label extension studies. BJU Int. 2012;110(3):392–400.

439. Kelleher CJ, Tubaro A, Wang JT, et al. Impact of fesoterodine on quality of life: pooled data from two randomized trials. BJU Int. 2008;102(1):56.

440. Kennedy C, Tasker PN, Gallacher G, et al. Identification of atropine- and P2X1 receptor antagonist-resistant, neurogenic contractions of the urinary bladder. J Neurosci. 2007;27(4):845.

441. Kerbusch T, Wahlby U, Milligan PA, Karlsson MO. Population pharmacokinetic modelling of darifenacin and its hydroxylated metabolite using pooled data, incorporating saturable first-pass metabolism, CYP2D6 genotype and formulation-dependent bioavailability. Br J Clin Pharmacol. 2003;56(6):639.

442. Kernan WN, Viscoli CM, Brass LM, et al. Phenylpropanolamine and the risk of hemorrhagic stroke. N Engl J Med. 2000;343(25):1826.

443. Kessler TM, Bachmann LM, Minder C, et al. Adverse event assessment of antimuscarinics for treating overactive bladder: a network meta-analytic approach. PLoS One. 2011;6(2):e16718.

444. Kessler TM, Studer UE, Burkhard FC. The effect of terazosin on functional bladder outlet obstruction in women: a pilot study. J Urol. 2006;176(4 Pt 1):1487.

445. Khera M, Somogyi GT, Kiss S, et al. Botulinum toxin A inhibits ATP release from bladder urothelium after chronic spinal cord injury. Neurochem Int. 2004;45(7):987.

446. Khullar V, Amarenco G, Angulo JC, Cambronero J, Høye K, Milsom I, Radziszewski P, Rechberger T, Boerrigter P, Drogendijk T, Wooning M, Chapple C. Efficacy and tolerability of mirabegron, a β(3)-adrenoceptor agonist, in patients with overactive

bladder: results from a randomised European-Australian phase 3 trial. Eur Urol. 2013;63(2):283–95.

447. Khullar V, Foote J, Seifu Y, Egermark M. Time-to-effect with darifenacin in overactive bladder: a pooled analysis. Int Urogynecol J. 2011;22(12):1573–80.

448. Khullar V, Rovner ES, Dmochowski R, et al. Fesoterodine dose response in subjects with overactive bladder syndrome. Urology. 2008;71(5):839.

449. Kim YH, Bird ET, Priebe M, et al. The role of oxybutynin in spinal cord injured patients with indwelling catheters. J Urol. 1996;158:2083.

450. Kim YT, Kwon DD, Kim J, et al. Gabapentin for overactive bladder and nocturia after anticholinergic failure. Int Braz J Urol. 2004;30(4):275.

451. Kim YS, Sainz RD. Beta adrenergic agonists and hypertrophy of skeletal muscles. Life Sci. 1992;50:397.

452. Kim Y, Yoshimura N, Masuda H, et al. Intravesical instillation of human urine after oral administration of trospium, tolterodine and oxybutynin in a rat model of detrusor overactivity. BJU Int. 2006;97:400.

453. Kinn AC, Larsson PO. Desmopressin: a new principle for symptomatic treatment of urgency and incontinence in patients with multiple sclerosis. Scand J Urol Nephrol. 1990;24:109.

454. Kishimoto T, Morita T, Okamiya Y, et al. Effect of clenbuterol on contractile response in periurethral striated muscle of rabbits. Tohoku J Exp Med. 1991;165(3):243.

455. Kitagawa Y, Kuribayashi M, Narimoto K, Kawaguchi S, Yaegashi H, Namiki M. Immediate effect on overactive bladder symptoms following administration of imidafenacin. Urol Int. 2011;86(3):330–3.

456. Klausner AP, Steers WD. Antimuscarinics for the treatment of overactive bladder: a review of central nervous system effects. Curr Urol Rep. 2007;8(6):441.

457. Klutke CG, Burgio KL, Wyman JF, et al. Combined effects of behavioral intervention and tolterodine in patients dissatisfied with overactive bladder medication. J Urol. 2009;181(6):2599–607.

458. Kobayashi F, Yageta Y, Yamazaki T, et al. Pharmacological effects of imidafenacin (KRP-197/ONO-8025), a new bladder selective anti-cholinergic agent, in rats. Comparison of effects on urinary bladder capacity and contraction, salivary secretion and performance in the Morris water maze task. Arzneimittelforschung. 2007;57(3):147–54.

459. Koelbl H, Nitti V, Baessler K, et al. Pathophysiology of urinary incontinence, faecal incontinence and pelvic organ prolapse. In: Abrams P, Cardozo L, Khoury S, Wein A, editors. Incontinence. 21st ed. Paris: Health Publication; 2009. p. 255–330.

460. Kojima Y, Sasaki S, Imura M, et al. Correlation between expression of alpha-adrenoceptor subtype mRNA and severity of lower urinary tract symptoms or bladder outlet obstruction in benign prostatic hyperplasia patients. BJU Int. 2011;107:438–42.

461. Kojima Y, Sasaki S, Kubota Y, et al. Expression of alpha1-adrenoceptor subtype mRNA as a predictor of the efficacy of subtype selective alpha1-adrenoceptor antagonists in the management of benign prostatic hyperplasia. J Urol. 2008;179(3):1040–6.

462. Kok ET, Schouten BW, Bohnen AM, et al. Risk factors for lower urinary tract symptoms suggestive of benign prostatic hyperplasia in a community based population of healthy aging men: the Krimpen Study. J Urol. 2009;181:710–6.

463. Komatsu T, Gotoh M, Funahashi Y, et al. Efficacy of propiverine in improving symptoms and quality of life in female patients with wet overactive bladder. Low Urin Tract Symptoms. 2009;1:22–4.

464. Krauwinkel W, van Dijk J, Schaddelee M, et al. Pharmacokinetic properties of mirabegron, a β3-adrenoceptor agonist: results from two phase I, randomized, multiple-dose studies in healthy young and elderly men and women. Clin Ther. 2012;34(10):2144–60.

465. Kuipers M, Tran D, Krauwinkel W, et al. Absolute bioavailability of YM905 in healthy male volunteers. A single-dose randomized, two-period crossover study. Presented at the 32nd International Continence Society Annual Meeting, Heidelberg, Germany; August 2002.

466. Kullmann FA, Shah MA, Birder LA, de Groat WC. Functional TRP and ASIC-like channels in cultured urothelial cells from the rat. Am J Physiol Renal Physiol. 2009;296(4):F892–901.

467. Kuo HC. Effectiveness of intravesical resiniferatoxin in treating detrusor hyper-reflexia and external sphincter dyssynergia in patients with chronic spinal cord lesions. BJU Int. 2003;92(6):597.

468. Kuo HC. Clinical effects of suburothelial injection of botulinum A toxin on patients with nonneurogenic detrusor overactivity refractory to anticholinergics. Urology. 2005;66(1):94.

469. Kuo HC. Multiple intravesical instillation of low-dose resiniferatoxin is effective in the treatment of detrusor overactivity refractory to anticholinergics. BJU Int. 2005;95(7):1023.

470. Kuo HC. Comparison of effectiveness of detrusor, suburothelial and bladder base injections of botulinum toxin a for idiopathic detrusor overactivity. J Urol. 2007;178(4 Pt 1):1359.

471. Kuo HC, Liao CH, Chung SD. Adverse events of intravesical botulinum toxin a injections for idiopathic detrusor overactivity: risk factors and influence on treatment outcome. Eur Urol. 2010;58(6):919–26.

472. Kuo HC, Liu HT, Yang WC. Therapeutic effect of multiple resiniferatoxin intravesical instillations in patients with refractory detrusor overactivity: a randomized, double-blind, placebo controlled study. J Urol. 2006;176(2):641.

473. Kupelian V, Fitzgerald MP, Kaplan SA, Norgaard JP, Chiu GR, Rosen RC. Association of nocturia and mortality. Results from the third national health and

nutrition examination survey. J Urol. 2011;185(2):571–7.

474. Kupelian V, Wei J, O'Leary M, Norgaard JP, Rosen R, McKinlay J. Nocturia and quality of life: results from the Boston Area Community Health Survey. Eur Urol. 2012;61(1):78–84.

475. Lazzeri M, Beneforti P, Turini D, et al. Urodynamic effects of intravesical resiniferatoxin in humans: preliminary results in stable and unstable detrusor. J Urol. 1997;158(6):2093.

476. Lazzeri M, Spinelli M, Beneforti P, et al. Intravesical resiniferatoxin for the treatment of detrusor hyperreflexia refractory to capsaicin in patients with chronic spinal cord diseases. Scand J Urol Nephrol. 1998;32(5):331.

477. Lecci A, Maggi CA. Tachykinins as modulators of the micturition reflex in the central and peripheral nervous system. Regul Pept. 2001;101(1–3):1–18.

478. Lee T, Andersson K-E, Streng T, Hedlund P. Simultaneous registration of intraabdominal and intravesical pressures during cystometry in conscious rats—effects of bladder outlet obstruction and intravesical PGE2. Neurourol Urodyn. 2008;27:88–95.

479. Lee KS, Choo MS, Kim DY, et al. Combination treatment with propiverine hydrochloride plus doxazosin controlled release gastrointestinal therapeutic system formulation for overactive bladder and coexisting benign prostatic obstruction: a prospective, randomized, controlled multicenter study. J Urol. 2005;174(4 Pt 1):1334.

480. Lee SH, Chung BH, Kim SJ, et al. Initial combined treatment with anticholinergics and α-blockers for men with lower urinary tract symptoms related to BPH and overactive bladder: a prospective, randomized, multi-center, double-blind, placebo-controlled study. Prostate Cancer Prostatic Dis. 2011;14(4):320–5.

481. Lee JY, Kim HW, Lee SJ, et al. Comparison of doxazosin with or without tolterodine in men with symptomatic bladder outlet obstruction and an overactive bladder. BJU Int. 2004;94(6):817.

482. Lee KS, Lee HW, Choo MS, et al. Urinary urgency outcomes after propiverine treatment for an overactive bladder: the 'Propiverine study on overactive bladder including urgency data'. BJU Int. 2010;105(11):1565–70.

483. Lee KS, Lee HW, Han DH. Does anticholinergic medication have a role in treating men with overactive bladder and benign prostatic hyperplasia? Naunyn Schmiedebergs Arch Pharmacol. 2008;377(4–6):491.

484. Leon LA, Hoffman BE, Gardner SD, et al. Effects of the beta 3-adrenergic receptor agonist disodium 5-[(2R)-2-[[(2R)-2-(3-chlorophenyl)-2-hydroxyethyl]amino]propyl]-1,3-benzodioxole-2,2-dicarboxylate (CL-316243) on bladder micturition reflex in spontaneously hypertensive rats. J Pharmacol Exp Ther. 2008;326(1):178.

485. Lepor H, Hill LA. Silodosin for the treatment of benign prostatic hyperplasia: pharmacology and cardiovascular tolerability. Pharmacotherapy. 2010;30(12):1303–12.

486. Lepor H, Kazzazi A, Djavan B. α-Blockers for benign prostatic hyperplasia: the new era. Curr Opin Urol. 2012;22(1):7–15.

487. Leslie CA, Pavlakis AJ, Wheeler Jr JS, et al. Release of arachidonate cascade products by the rabbit bladder: neurophysiological significance? J Urol. 1984;132:376.

488. Leung FP, Yung LM, Yao X, et al. Store-operated calcium entry in vascular smooth muscle. Br J Pharmacol. 2008;153(5):846–57.

489. Liguori G, Trombetta C, De Giorgi G, et al. Efficacy and safety of combined oral therapy with tadalafil and alfuzosin: an integrated approach to the management of patients with lower urinary tract symptoms and erectile dysfunction. Preliminary report. J Sex Med. 2009;6:544–52.

490. Lin HH, Sheu BC, Lo MC, et al. Comparison of treatment outcomes for imipramine for female genuine stress incontinence. Br J Obstet Gynaecol. 1999;106:1089.

491. Lipton RB, Kolodner K, Wesnes K. Assessment of cognitive function of the elderly population: effects of darifenacin. J Urol. 2005;173(2):493.

492. Liu HT, Chancellor MB, Kuo HC. Urinary nerve growth factor levels are elevated in patients with detrusor overactivity and decreased in responders to detrusor botulinum toxin-A injection. Eur Urol. 2009;56(4):700–6.

493. Liu HT, Kuo HC. Increased expression of transient receptor potential vanilloid subfamily 1 in the bladder predicts the response to intravesical instillations of resiniferatoxin in patients with refractory idiopathic detrusor overactivity. BJU Int. 2007;100(5):1086.

494. Liu L, Mansfield KJ, Kristiana I, et al. The molecular basis of urgency: regional difference of vanilloid receptor expression in the human urinary bladder. Neurourol Urodyn. 2007;26(3):433–8.

495. Longhurst PA, Briscoe JA, Rosenberg DJ, et al. The role of cyclic nucleotides in guinea-pig bladder contractility. Br J Pharmacol. 1997;121(8):1665.

496. Lose G, Jorgensen L, Thunedborg P. Doxepin in the treatment of female detrusor overactivity: a randomized double-blind crossover study. J Urol. 1989;142:1024.

497. Lose G, Lalos O, Freeman RM, et al. Efficacy of desmopressin (Minirin) in the treatment of nocturia: a double-blind placebo-controlled study in women. Am J Obstet Gynecol. 2003;189:1106.

498. Lose G, Mattiasson A, Walter S, et al. Clinical experience with desmopressin for long-term treatment of nocturia. J Urol. 2004;172:1021.

499. Lose G, Norgaard JP. Intravesical oxybutynin for treating incontinence resulting from an overactive detrusor. BJU Int. 2001;87:767.

500. Low BY, Liong ML, Yuen KH, et al. Terazosin therapy for patients with female lower urinary tract symptoms: a randomized, double-blind, placebo controlled trial. J Urol. 2008;179(4):1461.

501. Lowenstein L, Kenton K, Mueller ER, et al. Solifenacin objectively decreases urinary sensation in women with overactive bladder syndrome. Int Urol Nephrol. 2012;44(2):425–9.

502. Lucioni A, Bales GT, Lotan TL, et al. Botulinum toxin type A inhibits sensory neuropeptide release in rat bladder models of acute injury and chronic inflammation. BJU Int. 2008;101(3):366.

503. Luo D, Liu L, Han P, Wei Q, Shen H. Solifenacin for overactive bladder: a systematic review and meta-analysis. Int Urogynecol J. 2012;23(8):983–91. doi:10.1007/s00192-011-1641-7.

504. MacDiarmid SA, Ellsworth PI, Ginsberg DA, et al. Safety and efficacy of once-daily trospium chloride extended-release in male patients with overactive bladder. Urology. 2011;77(1):24–9.

505. Madersbacher H, Halaska M, Voigt R, et al. A placebo-controlled, multicentre study comparing the tolerability and efficacy of propiverine and oxybutynin in patients with urgency and urge incontinence. BJU Int. 1999;84:646.

506. Madersbacher H, Mürz G. Efficacy, tolerability and safety profile of propiverine in the treatment of the overactive bladder (non-neurogenic and neurogenic). World J Urol. 2001;19:324.

507. Madersbacher H, Stohrer M, Richter R, et al. Trospium chloride versus oxybutynin: a randomized, double-blind, multicentre trial in the treatment of detrusor hyper-reflexia. Br J Urol. 1995;75(4):452.

508. Madhuvrata P, Cody JD, Ellis G, et al. Which anticholinergic drug for overactive bladder symptoms in adults. Cochrane Database Syst Rev. 2012;(1):CD005429.

509. Maggi CA, Borsini F, Lecci A, et al. The effect of acute and chronic administration of imipramine on spinal and supraspinal micturition reflexes in rats. J Pharmacol Exp Ther. 1989;248:278.

510. Malhotra B, Gandelman K, Sachse R, Wood N. Assessment of the effects of renal impairment on the pharmacokinetic profile of fesoterodine. J Clin Pharmacol. 2009;49(4):477–82.

511. Malhotra B, Gandelman K, Sachse R, et al. The design and development of fesoterodine as a prodrug of 5-hydroxymethyl tolterodine (5-HMT), the active metabolite of tolterodine. Curr Med Chem. 2009;16(33):4481–9.

512. Malhotra BK, Glue P, Sweeney K, et al. Thorough QT study with recommended and supratherapeutic doses of tolterodine. Clin Pharmacol Ther. 2007;81(3):377.

513. Malhotra B, Guan Z, Wood N, Gandelman K. Pharmacokinetic profile of fesoterodine. Int J Clin Pharmacol Ther. 2008;46(11):556–63.

514. Malhotra B, Sachse R, Wood N. Influence of food on the pharmacokinetic profile of fesoterodine. Int J Clin Pharmacol Ther. 2009;47(6):384–90.

515. Malhotra B, Wood N, Sachse R, Gandelman K. Thorough QT study of the effect of fesoterodine on cardiac repolarization. Int J Clin Pharmacol Ther. 2010;48(5):309–18.

516. Malik M, van Gelderen EM, Lee JH, et al. Proarrhythmic safety of repeat doses of mirabegron in healthy subjects: a randomized, double-blind, placebo-, and active-controlled thorough QT study. Clin Pharmacol Ther. 2012;92(6):696.

517. Maneuf YP, Gonzalez MI, Sutton KS, et al. Cellular and molecular action of the putative GABA-mimetic, gabapentin. Cell Mol Life Sci. 2003;60(4):742.

518. Mangera A, Andersson KE, Apostolidis A, et al. Contemporary management of lower urinary tract disease with botulinum toxin A: a systematic review of botox (onabotulinumtoxinA) and dysport (abobotulinumtoxinA). Eur Urol. 2011;60(4):784–95.

519. Maniscalco M, Singh-Franco D, Wolowich WR, et al. Solifenacin succinate for the treatment of symptoms of overactive bladder. Clin Ther. 2006;28(9):1247.

520. Marencak J, Cossons NH, Darekar A, Mills IW. Investigation of the clinical efficacy and safety of pregabalin alone or combined with tolterodine in female subjects with idiopathic overactive bladder. Neurourol Urodyn. 2011 Jan;30(1):75–82.

521. Mariappan P, Ballantyne Z, N'Dow JMO, et al. Serotonin and noradrenaline reuptake inhibitors (SNRI) for stress urinary incontinence in adults (review). Cochrane Database Syst Rev. 2005;(3):CD 004742. Also published in The Cochrane Library 2007, issue 3.

522. Marks LS, Gittelman MC, Hill LA, Volinn W, Hoel G. Rapid efficacy of the highly selective a1A-adrenoceptor antagonist silodosin in men with signs and symptoms of benign prostatic hyperplasia: pooled results of 2 phase 3 studies. J Urol. 2009;181:2634–40.

523. Marks LS, Gittelman MC, Hill LA, Volinn W, Hoel G. Silodosin in the treatment of the signs and symptoms of benign prostatic hyperplasia: a 9-month, open-label extension study. Urology. 2009;6:1318–22.

524. Marschall-Kehrel D, Feustel C, Persson de Geeter C, et al. Treatment with propiverine in children suffering from nonneurogenic overactive bladder and urinary incontinence: results of a randomized placebo-controlled phase 3 clinical trial. Eur Urol. 2009;55(3):729–36.

525. Martin SW, Radley SC, Chess-Williams R, et al. Relaxant effects of potassium-channel openers on normal and hyper-reflexic detrusor muscle. Br J Urol. 1997;80:405.

526. Martin MR, Schiff AA. Fluphenazine/nortriptyline in the irritative bladder syndrome: a double-blind placebo-controlled study. Br J Urol. 1984;56:178.

527. Martínez-García R, Abadías M, Araño P, et al. Cizolirtine citrate, an effective treatment for symptomatic patients with urinary incontinence second-

ary to overactive bladder: a pilot dose-finding study. Eur Urol. 2009;56(1):184–90.

528. Maruyama O, Kawachi Y, Hanazawa K, et al. Naftopidil monotherapy vs naftopidil and an anticholinergic agent combined therapy for storage symptoms associated with benign prostatic hyperplasia: A prospective randomized controlled study. Int J Urol. 2006;13(10):1280–5.

529. Massaro AM, Lenz KL. Aprepitant: a novel antiemetic for chemotherapy-induced nausea and vomiting. Ann Pharmacother. 2005;39(1):77.

530. Masumori N, Miyamoto S, Tsukamoto T, et al. The efficacy and safety of propiverine hydrochloride in patients with overactive bladder symptoms who poorly responded to previous anticholinergic agents. Adv Urol. 2011;2011:714978.

531. Matsukawa Y, Gotoh M, Komatsu T, et al. Efficacy of silodosin for relieving benign prostatic obstruction: prospective pressure flow study. J Urol. 2009;182:2831–5.

532. Matthiesen TB, Rittig S, Norgaard JP, et al. Nocturnal polyuria and natriuresis in male patients with nocturia and lower urinary tract symptoms. J Urol. 1996;156:1292.

533. Mattiasson A, Abrams P, van Kerrebroeck P, et al. Efficacy of desmopressin in the treatment of nocturia: a double-blind placebo-controlled study in men. BJU Int. 2002;89:855.

534. Mattiasson A, Blaakaer J, Hoye K, et al., Tolterodine Scandinavian Study Group. Simplified bladder training augments the effectiveness of tolterodine in patients with an overactive bladder. BJU Int. 2003;91(1):54.

535. May K, Westphal K, Giessmann T, et al. Disposition and antimuscarinic effects of the urinary bladder spasmolytics propiverine: influence of dosage forms and circadian-time rhythms. J Clin Pharmacol. 2008;48(5):570.

536. McCafferty GP, Misajet BA, Laping NJ, et al. Enhanced bladder capacity and reduced prostaglandin E2-mediated bladder hyperactivity in EP3 receptor knockout mice. Am J Physiol Renal Physiol. 2008;295:F507–14.

537. McConnell JD, Roehrborn CG, Bautista OM et al., Medical Therapy of Prostatic Symptoms (MTOPS) Research Group. The long-term effect of doxazosin, finasteride, and combination therapy on the clinical progression of benign prostatic hyperplasia. N Engl J Med. 2003;349(25):2387.

538. McCrery RJ, Appell RA. Oxybutynin: an overview of the available formulations. Ther Clin Risk Manag. 2006;2(1):19.

539. McGuire EJ, Savastano JA. Urodynamics and management of the neuropathic bladder in spinal cord injury patients. J Am Paraplegia Soc. 1985;8(2):28–32.

540. McNeill SA, Hargreave TB. Alfuzosin once daily facilitates return to voiding in patients in acute urinary retention. J Urol. 2004;171:2316.

541. McNeill SA, Hargreave TB, Roehrborn CG. Alfuzosin 10 mg once daily in the management of acute urinary retention: results of a double-blind placebo-controlled study. Urology. 2005;65:83.

542. McVary KT, Monnig W, Camps Jr JL, et al. Sildenafil citrate improves erectile function and urinary symptoms in men with erectile dysfunction and lower urinary tract symptoms associated with benign prostatic hyperplasia: a randomized, double-blind trial. J Urol. 2007;177(3):1071.

543. McVary KT, Roehrborn CG, Avins AL, et al. Update on AUA guideline on the management of benign prostatic hyperplasia. J Urol. 2011;185:1793–803.

544. McVary KT, Roehrborn CG, Kaminetsky JC, et al. Tadalafil relieves lower urinary tract symptoms secondary to benign prostatic hyperplasia. J Urol. 2007;177(4):1401.

545. Menarini M, Del Popolo G, Di Benedetto P, et al. Trospium chloride in patients with neurogenic detrusor overactivity: is dose titration of benefit to the patients? Int J Clin Pharmacol Ther. 2006;44(12):623.

546. Meng J, Wang J, Lawrence G, et al. Synaptobrevin I mediates exocytosis of CGRP from sensory neurons and inhibition by botulinum toxins reflects their antinociceptive potential. J Cell Sci. 2007;120(Pt 16):2864.

547. Merriam FV, Wang ZY, Guerios SD, Bjorling DE. Cannabinoid receptor2 is increased in acutely and chronically inflamed bladder of rats. Neurosci Lett. 2008;445:130–4.

548. Michel MC. Fesoterodine: a novel muscarinic receptor antagonist for the treatment of overactive bladder syndrome. Expert Opin Pharmacother. 2008;9(10):1787.

549. Michel MC, Hegde SS. Treatment of the overactive bladder syndrome with muscarinic receptor antagonists: a matter of metabolites? Naunyn Schmiedebergs Arch Pharmacol. 2006;374(2):79.

550. Michel MC, Vrydag W. Alpha1-, alpha2- and beta-adrenoceptors in the urinary bladder, urethra and prostate. Br J Pharmacol. 2006;147 Suppl 2:S88.

551. Michel MC, Wetterauer U, Vogel M, et al. Cardiovascular safety and overall tolerability of solifenacin in routine clinical use: a 12-week, open-label, post-marketing surveillance study. Drug Saf. 2008;31(6):505.

552. Milani R, Scalambrino S, Milia R, et al. Double-blind crossover comparison of flavoxate and oxybutynin in women affected by urinary urge syndrome. Int Urogynecol J. 1993;4:3.

553. Millard RJ, Asia Pacific Tolterodine Study Group. Clinical efficacy of tolterodine with or without a simplified pelvic floor exercise regimen. Neurourol Urodyn. 2004;23(1):48.

554. Millard RJ, Moore K, Rencken R, et al. Duloxetine versus placebo in the treatment of stress urinary incontinence: a four continent randomized clinical trial. BJU Int. 2004;93:311.

555. Miller DW, Hinton M, Chen F. Evaluation of drug efflux transporter liabilities of darifenacin in cell culture models of the blood-brain and blood-ocular barriers. Neurourol Urodyn. 2011;30(8):1633–8.

556. Mirabegron prescribing information. http://www.us.astellas.com/docs/myrbetriq-full-pi.pdf

557. Miyazato M, Sasatomi K, Hiragata S, et al. GABA receptor activation in the lumbosacral spinal cord decreases detrusor overactivity in spinal cord injured rats. J Urol. 2008;179(3):1178–83.

558. Moehrer B, Hextall A, Jackson S. Oestrogens for urinary incontinence in women. Cochrane Database Syst Rev. 2003;(2):CD001405. Review. Update in: Cochrane Database Syst Rev. 2009;(4):CD001405.

559. Morelli A, Filippi S, Comeglio P, et al. Acute vardenafil administration improves bladder oxygenation in spontaneously hypertensive rats. J Sex Med. 2009;7:107–20.

560. Morelli A, Filippi S, Sandner P, et al. Vardenafil modulates bladder contractility through cGMP-mediated inhibition of RhoA/Rho kinase signaling pathway in spontaneously hypertensive rats. J Sex Med. 2009;6:1594–608.

561. Morelli A, Sarchielli E, Comeglio P, et al. Phosphodiesterase type 5 expression in human and rat lower urinary tract tissues and the effect of tadalafil on prostate gland oxygenation in spontaneously hypertensive rats. J Sex Med. 2011;8:2746–60.

562. Morelli A, Vignozzi L, Filippi S, et al. BXL-628, a vitamin D receptor agonist effective in benign prostatic hyperplasia treatment, prevents RhoA activation and inhibits RhoA/Rho kinase signaling in rat and human bladder. Prostate. 2007;67(3):234.

563. Morenilla-Palao C, Planells-Cases R, García-Sanz N, et al. Regulated exocytosis contributes to protein kinase C potentiation of vanilloid receptor activity. Biol Chem. 2004;279(24):25665.

564. Morganroth J, Lepor H, Hill LA, et al. Effects of the selective a1A-adrenoceptor antagonist silodosin on ECGs of healthy men in a randomized, double blind, placebo-moxifloxacin-controlled study. Clin Pharmacol Ther. 2010;87:609–13.

565. Morita T, Ando M, Kihara K, et al. Effects of prostaglandins E1, E2 and F2alpha on contractility and cAMP and cGMP contents in lower urinary tract smooth muscle. Urol Int. 1994;52:200.

566. Morita T, Iizuka H, Iwata T, et al. Function and distribution of beta3-adrenoceptors in rat, rabbit and human urinary bladder and external urethral sphincter. J Smooth Muscle Res. 2000;36(1):21.

567. Mostwin J, Bourcier A, Haab F, et al. Pathophysiology of urinary incontinence, fecal incontinence and pelvic organ prolapse. In: Abrams P, Cardozo L, Khoury S, Wein A, editors. Incontinence. Plymouth, UK: Health Publications; 2005. p. 423.

568. Muller C, Siegmund W, Huupponen R, et al. Kinetics of propiverine as assessed by radioreceptor assay in poor and extensive metabolizers of debrisoquine. Eur J Drug Metab Pharmacokinet. 1993;18(3):265.

569. Murakami S, Chapple CR, Akino H, et al. The role of the urothelium in mediating bladder responses to isoprenaline. BJU Int. 2007;99(3):669.

570. Murakami S, Yoshida M, Iwashita H, et al. Pharmacological effects of KRP-197 on the human isolated urinary bladder. Urol Int. 2003;71(3):290–8.

571. Muskat Y, Bukovsky I, Schneider D, et al. The use of scopolamine in the treatment of detrusor instability. J Urol. 1996;156:1989.

572. Musselman DM, Ford AP, Gennevois DJ, et al. A randomized crossover study to evaluate Ro 115-1240, a selective alpha 1 A/1L-adrenoceptor partial agonist in women with stress urinary incontinence. BJU Int. 2004;93(1):78.

573. Naglie G, Radomski SB, Brymer C, et al. A randomized, double-blind, placebo controlled crossover trial of nimodipine in older persons with detrusor instability and urge incontinence. J Urol. 2002;167:586.

574. Nakagawa H, Niu K, Hozawa A, et al. Impact of nocturia on bone fractures and mortality in older people: a Japanese longitudinal cohort study. J Urol. 2010;184:1413–8.

575. Natalin R, Reis LO, Alpendre C, et al. Triple therapy in refractory detrusor overactivity: a preliminary study. World J Urol. 2009;28:79–85.

576. Neveus T, Tullus K. Tolterodine and imipramine in refractory enuresis: a placebo-controlled crossover study. Pediatr Nephrol. 2008;23:263.

577. Ney P, Pandita RK, Newgreen DT, et al. Pharmacological characterization of a novel investigational antimuscarinic drug, fesoterodine, in vitro and in vivo. BJU Int. 2008;101(8):1036.

578. Nilvebrant L, Andersson K-E, Gillberg PG. Tolterodine—a new bladder-selective antimuscarinic agent. Eur J Pharmacol. 1997;327(2–3):195.

579. Nilvebrant L, Gillberg PG, Sparf B. Antimuscarinic potency and bladder selectivity of PNU-200577, a major metabolite of tolterodine. Pharmacol Toxicol. 1997;81(4):16.

580. Nilvebrant L, Sparf B. Dicyclomine, benzhexol and oxybutynin distinguish between subclasses of muscarinic binding sites. Eur J Pharmacol. 1986;123:133.

581. Nilvebrant L, Sparf B. Receptor binding profiles of some selective muscarinic antagonists. Eur J Pharmacol. 1988;151(1):83–96.

582. Nishiguchi J, Kwon DD, Kaiho Y, et al. Suppression of detrusor overactivity in rats with bladder outlet obstruction by a type 4 phosphodiesterase inhibitor. BJU Int. 2007;99(3):680.

583. Nitti VW. Botulinum toxin for the treatment of idiopathic and neurogenic overactive bladder: state of the art. Rev Urol. 2006;8(4):198.

584. Nitti VW, Auerbach S, Martin N, et al. Results of a randomized phase III trial of mirabegron in patients with overactive bladder. J Urol. 2013;189(4):1388–95.

585. Nitti VW, Dmochowski R, Herschorn S, Sand P, Thompson C, Nardo C, Yan X, Haag-Molkenteller C, EMBARK Study Group. OnabotulinumtoxinA

for the treatment of patients with overactive bladder and urinary incontinence: results of a phase 3, randomized, placebo controlled trial. J Urol. 2013;189(6):2186–93.

586. Nitti VW, Dmochowski R, Sand PK, et al. Efficacy, safety and tolerability of fesoterodine for overactive bladder syndrome. J Urol. 2007;178(6):2488–94.

587. Nitti VW, Rosenberg S, Mitcheson DH, et al. Urodynamics and safety of the β 3-adrenoceptor agonist, mirabegron, in males with lower urinary tract symptoms and bladder outlet obstruction. J Urol. 2013;190(4):1320–7.

588. Nitti VW, Rovner ES, Bavendam T. Response to fesoterodine in patients with an overactive bladder and urgency urinary incontinence is independent of the urodynamic finding of detrusor overactivity. BJU Int. 2010;105(9):1268–75.

589. Noel S, Claeys S, Hamaide A. Acquired urinary incontinence in the bitch: update and perspectives from human medicine. Part 1: the bladder component, pathophysiology and medical treatment. Vet J. 2010;186:10–7.

590. Noguchi M, Eguchi Y, Ichiki J, et al. Therapeutic efficacy of clenbuterol for urinary incontinence after radical prostatectomy. Int J Urol. 1997;4:480.

591. Nomiya M, Yamaguchi O. A quantitative analysis of mRNA expression of alpha 1 and beta-adrenoceptor subtypes and their functional roles in human normal and obstructed bladders. J Urol. 2003;170(2 Pt 1):649.

592. Norhona-Blob L, Kachur JF. Enantiomers of oxybutynin: in vitro pharmacological characterization at M1, M2 and M3 muscarinic receptors and in vivo effects on urinary bladder contraction, mydriasis and salivary secretion in guinea pigs. J Pharmacol Exp Ther. 1991;256:562.

593. Norton PA, Zinner NR, Yalcin I, et al. Duloxetine versus placebo in the treatment of stress urinary incontinence. Am J Obstet Gynecol. 2002;187:40.

594. Novara G, Galfano A, Secco S, et al. Systematic review and meta-analysis of randomized controlled trials with antimuscarinic drugs for overactive bladder. Eur Urol. 2008;54(4):740–63.

595. O'Reilly BA, Kosaka AH, Knight GF, Chang TK, Ford AP, Rymer JM, Popert R, Burnstock G, McMahon SB. P2X receptors and their role in female idiopathic detrusor instability. J Urol. 2002;167(1):157–64.

596. Ochs GA. Intrathecal baclofen. Baillieres Clin Neurol. 1993;2(1):73–86.

597. Oelke M, Bachmann A, Descazeaud A, et al. EAU guidelines on the treatment and follow-up of non-neurogenic male lower urinary tract symptoms including benign prostatic obstruction. Eur Urol. 2013;64(1):118–40.

598. Oger S, Behr-Roussel D, Gorny D, et al. Combination of alfuzosin and tadalafil exerts in vitro an additive relaxant effect on human corpus cavernosum. J Sex Med. 2008;5:935–45.

599. Oger S, Behr-Roussel D, Gorny D, et al. Signalling pathways involved in sildenafil-induced relaxation of human bladder dome smooth muscle. Br J Pharmacol. 2010;160:1135–43.

600. Ohlstein EH, Michel MC, Von Keitz A. The beta-3 adrenoceptor agonist solabegron is safe and effective for improving symptoms of overactive bladder. Eur Urol. 2012;11(Suppl):e685.

601. Ohmori S, Miura M, Toriumi C, et al. Absorption, metabolism, and excretion of [14C]imidafenacin, a new compound for treatment of overactive bladder, after oral administration to healthy male subjects. Drug Metab Dispos. 2007;35(9):1624–33.

602. Ohno T, Nakade S, Nakayama K, et al. Absolute bioavailability of imidafenacin after oral administration to healthy subjects. Br J Clin Pharmacol. 2008;65(2):197–202.

603. Oka M, Kimura Y, Itoh Y, et al. Brain pertussis toxin-sensitive G proteins are involved in the flavoxate hydrochloride-induced suppression of the micturition reflex in rats. Brain Res. 1996;727(1–2):91.

604. Olshansky B, Ebinger U, Brum J, et al. Differential pharmacological effects of antimuscarinic drugs on heart rate: a randomized, placebo-controlled, double-blind, crossover study with tolterodine and darifenacin in healthy participants >=50 years. J Cardiovasc Pharmacol Ther. 2008;13(4):241–51.

605. Otsuka A, Shinbo H, Matsumoto R, et al. Expression and functional role of beta-adrenoceptors in the human urinary bladder urothelium. Naunyn Schmiedebergs Arch Pharmacol. 2008;377(4–6):473.

606. Ouslander JG. Management of overactive bladder. N Engl J Med. 2004;350:786.

607. Ouslander JG, Blaustein J, Connor A, et al. Pharmacokinetics and clinical effects of oxybutynin in geriatric patients. J Urol. 1988;140:47.

608. Ouslander JG, Schnelle JF, Uman G, et al. Does oxybutynin add to the effectiveness of prompted voiding for urinary incontinence among nursing home residents? A placebo-controlled trial. J Am Geriatr Soc. 1995;43:610.

609. Palea S, Artibani W, Ostardo E, et al. Evidence for purinergic neurotransmission in human urinary bladder affected by interstitial cystitis. J Urol. 1993;150(6):2007.

610. Palmer J. Report of a double-blind crossover study of flurbiprofen and placebo in detrusor instability. J Int Med Res. 1983;11 Suppl 2:11.

611. Palmer LS, Zebold K, Firlit CF, et al. Complications of intravesical oxybutynin chloride therapy in the pediatric myelomeningocele population. J Urol. 1997;157:638.

612. Parker-Autry CY, Burgio KL, Richter HE. Vitamin D status: a review with implications for the pelvic floor. Int Urogynecol J. 2012;23(11):1517–26.

613. Patel AK, Patterson JM, Chapple CR. Botulinum toxin injections for neurogenic and idiopathic detrusor overactivity: a critical analysis of results. Eur Urol. 2006;50(4):684.

614. Pehrson R, Andersson KE. Effects of tiagabine, a gamma-aminobutyric acid re-uptake inhibitor, on normal rat bladder function. J Urol. 2002;167(5):2241.

615. Pehrson R, Andersson KE. Tramadol inhibits rat detrusor overactivity caused by dopamine receptor stimulation. J Urol. 2003;170(1):272.

616. Pehrson R, Stenman E, Andersson KE. Effects of tramadol on rat detrusor overactivity induced by experimental cerebral infarction. Eur Urol. 2003;44(4):495.

617. Pertwee RG, Howlett AC, Abood ME, et al. International Union of Basic and Clinical Pharmacology. LXXIX. Cannabinoid receptors and their ligands: beyond CB1 and CB2. Pharmacol Rev. 2010;62:588–631.

618. Peters SL, Schmidt M, Michel MC. Rho kinase: a target for treating urinary bladder dysfunction? Trends Pharmacol Sci. 2006;27(9):492.

619. Peters CA, Walsh PC. The effect of nafarelin acetate, a luteinizing-hormone-releasing hormone agonist, on benign prostatic hyperplasia. N Engl J Med. 1987;317:599.

620. Petkov GV. Role of potassium ion channels in detrusor smooth muscle function and dysfunction. Nat Rev Urol. 2011;9(1):30–40.

621. Pinto R, Lopes T, Frias B, et al. Trigonal injection of botulinum toxin A in patients with refractory bladder pain syndrome/interstitial cystitis. Eur Urol. 2010;58(3):360–5.

622. Planells-Cases R, Valente P, Ferrer-Montiel A, et al. Complex regulation of TRPV1 and related thermo-TRPs: implications for therapeutic intervention. Adv Exp Med Biol. 2011;704:491–515.

623. Porst H, Kim ED, Casabe AR, et al. Efficacy and safety of tadalafil once daily in the treatment of men with lower urinary tract symptoms suggestive of benign prostatic hyperplasia: results of an international randomized, double-blind, placebo-controlled trial. Eur Urol. 2011;60:1105–13.

624. Porst H, McVary KT, Montorsi F, et al. Effects of once-daily tadalafil on erectile function in men with erectile dysfunction and signs and symptoms of benign prostatic hyperplasia. Eur Urol. 2009;56:727–35.

625. Purkiss J, Welch M, Doward S, et al. Capsaicin-stimulated release of substance P from cultured dorsal root ganglion neurons: involvement of two distinct mechanisms. Biochem Pharmacol. 2000;59(11):1403.

626. Radley SC, Chapple CR, Bryan NP, et al. Effect of methoxamine on maximum urethral pressure in women with genuine stress incontinence: a placebo-controlled, double-blind crossover study. Neurourol Urodyn. 2001;20(1):43.

627. Rahnama'i MS, de Wachter SG, van Koeveringe GA, et al. The relationship between prostaglandin E receptor 1 and cyclooxygenase I expression in guinea pig bladder interstitial cells: proposition of a signal propagation system. J Urol. 2011;185(1):315–22.

628. Rahnama'i MS, van Koeveringe GA, Essers PB, et al. Prostaglandin receptor EP1 and EP2 site in guinea pig bladder urothelium and lamina propria. J Urol. 2010;183(3):1241–7.

629. Rapp DE, Turk KW, Bales GT, et al. Botulinum toxin type a inhibits calcitonin gene-related peptide release from isolated rat bladder. J Urol. 2006;175(3 Pt 1):1138.

630. Raz S, Zeigler M, Caine M. The effect of progesterone on the adrenergic receptors of the urethra. Br J Urol. 1973;45(2):131.

631. Razdan S, Leboeuf L, Meinbach DS, et al. Current practice patterns in the urologic surveillance and management of patients with spinal cord injury. Urology. 2003;61(5):893–6.

632. Rekik M, Rouget C, Palea S, et al. Effects of combining antimuscarinics and β3-adrenoceptor agonists on contractions induced by electrical field stimulation of rat isolated urinary bladder strips [AUA abstract]. J Urol. 2013;189(4 Suppl):e115–6.

633. Rembratt A, Riis A, Norgaard JP. Desmopressin treatment in nocturia; an analysis of risk factors for hyponatremia. Neurourol Urodyn. 2006;25(2):105.

634. Riedl CR, Stephen RL, Daha LK, et al. Electromotive administration of intravesical bethanechol and the clinical impact on acontractile detrusor management: introduction of a new test. J Urol. 2000;164(6):2108–11.

635. Rios LA, Panhoca R, Mattos Jr D, et al. Intravesical resiniferatoxin for the treatment of women with idiopathic detrusor overactivity and urgency incontinence: a single dose, 4 weeks, double-blind, randomized, placebo controlled trial. Neurourol Urodyn. 2007;26(6):773.

636. Rittig S, Jensen AR, Jensen KT, Pedersen EB. Effect of food intake on the pharmacokinetics and antidiuretic activity of oral desmopressin (DDAVP) in hydrated normal subjects. Clin Endocrinol (Oxf). 1998;48(2):235–41.

637. Robinson D, Cardozo L. The role of estrogens in female lower urinary tract dysfunction. Urology. 2003;62(4 Suppl 1):45.

638. Robinson D, Cardozo L. New drug treatments for urinary incontinence. Maturitas. 2010;65(4):340–7.

639. Robinson D, Cardozo L, Akeson M, et al. Antidiuresis: a new concept in managing female daytime urinary incontinence. BJU Int. 2004;93:996.

640. Robinson D, Cardozo L, Terpstra G, et al. A randomized double-blind placebo-controlled multicentre study to explore the efficacy and safety of tamsulosin and tolterodine in women with overactive bladder syndrome. BJU Int. 2007;100(4):840.

641. Robinson D, Rainer RO, Washburn SA, et al. Effects of estrogen and progestin replacement on the urogenital tract of the ovariectomized cynomolgus monkey. Neurourol Urodyn. 1996;15(3):215.

642. Robson WL, Leung AK, Norgaard JP. The comparative safety of oral versus intranasal desmopressin for the treatment of children with nocturnal enuresis. J Urol. 2007;178(1):24–30.

643. Roehrborn CG, Kaplan SA, Jones JS, et al. Tolterodine extended release with or without tamsulosin in men with lower urinary tract symptoms including overactive bladder symptoms: effects of prostate size. Eur Urol. 2009;55(2):472–9.

644. Roehrborn CG, Kaplan SA, Kraus SR, et al. Effects of serum PSA on efficacy of tolterodine extended release with or without tamsulosin in men with LUTS, including OAB. Urology. 2008;72(5):1061–7.

645. Roehrborn CG, McVary KT, Elion-Mboussa A, Viktrup L. Tadalafil administered once daily for lower urinary tract symptoms secondary to benign prostatic hyperplasia: a dose finding study. J Urol. 2008;180:1228–34.

646. Roehrborn CG, Siami P, Barkin J, et al., CombAT Study Group. The effects of combination therapy with dutasteride and tamsulosin on clinical outcomes in men with symptomatic benign prostatic hyperplasia: 4-year results from the CombAT study. Eur Urol. 2010;57(1):123-31.

647. Rogers R, Bachmann G, Jumadilova Z, et al. Efficacy of tolterodine on overactive bladder symptoms and sexual and emotional quality of life in sexually active women. Int Urogynecol J Pelvic Floor Dysfunct. 2008;19(11):1551.

648. Roosen A, Datta SN, Chowdhury RA, et al. Suburothelial myofibroblasts in the human overactive bladder and the effect of botulinum neurotoxin type A treatment. Eur Urol. 2009;55(6):1440–8.

649. Rosa GM, Bauckneht M, Scala C, Tafi E, Leone Roberti Maggiore U, Ferrero S, Brunelli C. Cardiovascular effects of antimuscarinic agents in overactive bladder. Expert Opin Drug Saf. 2013;12(6):815–27.

650. Rovner E, Kennelly M, Schulte-Baukloh H, et al. Urodynamic results and clinical outcomes with intradetrusor injections of onabotulinumtoxinA in a randomized, placebo-controlled dose-finding study in idiopathic overactive bladder. Neurourol Urodyn. 2011;30(4):556–62.

651. Rovner ES, Kreder K, Sussman DO, et al. Effect of tolterodine extended release with or without tamsulosin on measures of urgency and patient reported outcomes in men with lower urinary tract symptoms. J Urol. 2008;180(3):1034.

652. Rovner ES, Rackley R, Nitti VW, et al. Tolterodine extended release is efficacious in continent and incontinent subjects with overactive bladder. Urology. 2008;72(3):488.

653. Rudy D, Cline K, Harris R, et al. Multicenter phase III trial studying trospium chloride in patients with overactive bladder. Urology. 2006;67(2):275.

654. Ruffmann R. A review of flavoxate hydrochloride in the treatment of urge incontinence. J Int Med Res. 1988;16:317.

655. Rufford J, Hextall A, Cardozo L, et al. A double blind placebo controlled trial on the effects of 25 mg estradiol implants on the urge syndrome in post-menopausal women. Int Urogynecol J Pelvic Floor Dysfunct. 2003;14(2):78.

656. Ruggieri Sr MR. Cannabinoids: potential targets for bladder dysfunction. Handb Exp Pharmacol. 2011;202:425–51.

657. Ruggieri Sr MR, Braverman AS, Pontari MA. Combined use of alpha-adrenergic and muscarinic antagonists for the treatment of voiding dysfunction. J Urol. 2005;174(5):1743.

658. Sacco E, Bientinesi R. Mirabegron: a review of recent data and its prospects in the management of overactive bladder. Ther Adv Urol. 2012;4(6):315–24.

659. Safarinejad MR, Hosseini SY. Safety and efficacy of tramadol in the treatment of idiopathic detrusor overactivity: a double-blind, placebo-controlled, randomized study. Br J Clin Pharmacol. 2006;61(4):456.

660. Saffroy M, Torrens Y, Glowinski J, et al. Autoradiographic distribution of tachykinin NK2 binding sites in the rat brain: comparison with NK1 and NK3 binding sites. Neuroscience. 2003;116(3):761.

661. Sahai A, Dowson C, Khan MS, Dasgupta P. Improvement in quality of life after botulinum toxin-A injections for idiopathic detrusor overactivity: results from a randomized double-blind placebo-controlled trial. BJU Int. 2009;103(11):1509–15.

662. Sahai A, Khan MS, Dasgupta P. Efficacy of botulinum toxin-A for treating idiopathic detrusor overactivity: results from a single center, randomized, double-blind, placebo controlled trial. J Urol. 2007;177(6):2231.

663. Sahai A, Mallina R, Dowson C, et al. Evolution of transdermal oxybutynin in the treatment of overactive bladder. Int J Clin Pract. 2008;62(1):167.

664. Sairam K, Kulinskaya E, McNicholas TA, et al. Sildenafil influences lower urinary tract symptoms. BJU Int. 2002;90(9):836.

665. Saito H, Yamada T, et al. A comparative study of the efficacy and safety of tamsulosin hydrochloride alone and combination of propiverine hydrochloride and tamsulosin hydrochloride in the benign prostatic hypertrophy with pollakisuria and/or urinary incontinence. Jpn J Urol Surg. 1999;12:525–36.

666. Sakai H, Igawa T, Onita T, et al. Efficacy of naftopidil in patients with overactive bladder associated with benign prostatic hyperplasia: prospective randomized controlled study to compare differences in efficacy between morning and evening medication. Hinyokika Kiyo. 2011;57(1):7–13.

667. Sakakibara R, Ito T, Uchiyama T, et al. Effects of milnacipran and paroxetine on overactive bladder due to neurologic diseases: a urodynamic assessment. Urol Int. 2008;81:335–9.

668. Salvatore S, Serati M, Bolis P. Tolterodine for the treatment of overactive bladder. Expert Opin Pharmacother. 2008;9(7):1249.

669. Sand PK, Davila GW, Lucente VR, et al. Efficacy and safety of oxybutynin chloride topical gel for women with overactive bladder syndrome. Am J Obstet Gynecol. 2012;206(2):168.e1-6.

670. Sand PK, Heesakkers J, Kraus SR, et al. Long-term safety, tolerability and efficacy of fesoterodine in subjects with overactive bladder symptoms stratified

by age: pooled analysis of two open-label extension studies. Drugs Aging. 2012;29:119–31.

671. Sand PK, Johnson Ii TM, Rovner ES, et al. Trospium chloride once-daily extended release is efficacious and tolerated in elderly subjects (aged ≥75 years) with overactive bladder syndrome. BJU Int. 2011;107:612–20.

672. Sand PK, Rovner ES, Watanabe JH, Oefelein MG. Once-daily trospium chloride 60 mg extended release in subjects with overactive bladder syndrome who use multiple concomitant medications: Post hoc analysis of pooled data from two randomized, placebo-controlled trials. Drugs Aging. 2011;28(2): 151–60.

673. Santos-Silva A, Charrua A, Cruz CD, et al. Rat detrusor overactivity induced by chronic spinalization can be abolished by a transient receptor potential vanilloid 1 (TRPV1) antagonist. Auton Neurosci. 2012;166(1–2):35–8.

674. Schagen van Leeuwen JH, Lange RR, Jonasson AF, et al. Efficacy and safety of duloxetine in elderly women with stress urinary incontinence or stress-predominant mixed urinary incontinence. Maturitas. 2008;60(2):138.

675. Schneider T, Fetscher C, Krege S, Michel MC. Signal transduction underlying carbachol-induced contraction of human urinary bladder. J Pharmacol Exp Ther. 2004;309(3):1148–53.

676. Schneider T, Hein P, Michel MC. Signal transduction underlying carbachol-induced contraction of rat urinary bladder. I. Phospholipases and Ca2+ sources. J Pharmacol Exp Ther. 2004;308(1):47–53.

677. Schröder A, Colli E, Maggi M, et al. Effects of a vitamin D3 analogue in a rat model of bladder outflow obstruction. BJU Int. 2006;98:637.

678. Schroder A, Newgreen D, Andersson KE. Detrusor responses to prostaglandin E2 and bladder outlet obstruction in wild-type and Ep1 receptor knockout mice. J Urol. 2004;172:1166–70.

679. Schroeder FH, Westerhof M, Bosch RJLH, Kurth KH. Benign prostatic hyperplasia treated by castration or the LH-RH analogue buserelin: a report on 6 cases. Eur Urol. 1986;12:318.

680. Schulte-Baukloh H, Mürtz G, Henne T, et al. Urodynamic effects of propiverine hydrochloride in children with neurogenic detrusor overactivity: a prospective analysis. BJU Int. 2006;97(2):355.

681. Schulte-Baukloh H, Zurawski TH, Knispel HH, et al. Persistence of the synaptosomal-associated protein-25 cleavage product after intradetrusor botulinum toxin A injections in patients with myelomeningocele showing an inadequate response to treatment. BJU Int. 2007;100(5):1075.

682. Schwinn DA, Price DT, Narayan P. alpha1-Adrenoceptor subtype selectivity and lower urinary tract symptoms. Mayo Clin Proc. 2004;79(11):1423–34.

683. Schwinn DA, Roehrborn CG. Alpha1-adrenoceptor subtypes and lower urinary tract symptoms. Int J Urol. 2008;15(3):193–9.

684. Sears CL, Lewis C, Noel K, Albright TS, Fischer JR. Overactive bladder medication adherence when medication is free to patients. J Urol. 2010;183: 1077–81.

685. Seki S, Erickson KA, Seki M, et al. Elimination of rat spinal neurons expressing neurokinin 1 receptors reduces bladder overactivity and spinal c-fos expression induced by bladder irritation. Am J Physiol Renal Physiol. 2005;288(3):F466.

686. Serati M, Salvatore S, Uccella S, et al. Is there a synergistic effect of topical oestrogens when administered with antimuscarinics in the treatment of symptomatic detrusor overactivity? Eur Urol. 2009;55(3):713–9.

687. Serels SR, Toglia MR, Forero-Schwanhaeuser S, He W. Impact of solifenacin on diary-recorded and patient-reported urgency in patients with severe overactive bladder (OAB) symptoms. Curr Med Res Opin. 2010;26(10):2277–85.

688. Serra DB, Affrime MB, Bedigian MP, et al. QT and QTc interval with standard and supratherapeutic doses of darifenacin, a muscarinic M3 selective receptor antagonist for the treatment of overactive bladder. J Clin Pharmacol. 2005;45(9):1038.

689. Shaban A, Drake M, Hashim H. The medical management of urinary incontinence. Auton Neurosci. 2010;152(1–2):4–10.

690. Sharma A, Goldberg MJ, Cerimele BJ. Pharmacokinetics and safety of duloxetine, a dual-serotonin and norepinephrine reuptake inhibitor. J Clin Pharmacol. 2000;40(2):161.

691. Sheldon JH, Norton NW, Argentieri TM. Inhibition of guinea pig detrusor contraction by NS-1619 is associated with activation of BKCa and inhibition of calcium currents. J Pharmacol Exp Ther. 1997;283: 1193.

692. Sheu MT, Yeh GC, Ke WT, et al. Development of a high-performance liquid chromatographic method for bioequivalence study of flavoxate tablets. J Chromatogr B Biomed Sci Appl. 2001;751(1):79.

693. Shieh C-C, Brune ME, Buckner SA, et al. Characterization of a novel ATP-sensitive K+ channel opener, A-251179, on urinary bladder relaxation and cystometric parameters. Br J Pharmacol. 2007;151:467.

694. Shore N. NX-1207: a novel investigational drug for the treatment of benign prostatic hyperplasia. Expert Opin Investig Drugs. 2010;19(2):305–10.

695. Siddiqui MA, Perry CM, Scott LJ. Oxybutynin extended-release: a review of its use in the management of overactive bladder. Drugs. 2004; 64(8):885.

696. Silva C, Ribeiro MJ, Cruz F. The effect of intravesical resiniferatoxin in patients with idiopathic detrusor instability suggests that involuntary detrusor contractions are triggered by C-fiber input. J Urol. 2002;168(2):575.

697. Silva C, Rio ME, Cruz F. Desensitization of bladder sensory fibers by intravesical resiniferatoxin, a

capsaicin analog: long-term results for the treatment of detrusor hyperreflexia. Eur Urol. 2000;38(4):444.

698. Silva C, Silva J, Castro H, et al. Bladder sensory desensitization decreases urinary urgency. BMC Urol. 2007;11(7):9.

699. Silva C, Silva J, Ribeiro MJ, et al. Urodynamic effect of intravesical resiniferatoxin in patients with neurogenic detrusor overactivity of spinal origin: results of a double-blind randomized placebo-controlled trial. Eur Urol. 2005;48(4):650.

700. Silver N, Sandage B, Sabounjian L, et al. Pharmacokinetics of once-daily trospium chloride 60 mg extended release and twice-daily trospium chloride 20 mg in healthy adults. J Clin Pharmacol. 2010;50(2):143–50.

701. Singh SK, Agarwal MM, Batra YK, et al. Effect of lumbar-epidural administration of tramadol on lower urinary tract function. Neurourol Urodyn. 2008;27(1):65.

702. Singh R, Browning JL, Abi-Habib R, et al. Recombinant prostate-specific antigen proaerolysin shows selective protease sensitivity and cell cytotoxicity. Anticancer Drugs. 2007;18(7):809–16.

703. Sjögren C, Andersson K-E, Husted S, et al. Atropine resistance of the transmurally stimulated isolated human bladder. J Urol. 1982;128:1368.

704. Skerjanec A. The clinical pharmacokinetics of darifenacin. Clin Pharmacokinet. 2006;45(4):325.

705. Smet PJ, Moore KH, Jonavicius J. Distribution and colocalization of calcitonin gene-related peptide, tachykinins, and vasoactive intestinal peptide in normal and idiopathic unstable human urinary bladder. Lab Invest. 1997;77(1):37.

706. Smith PH, Cook JB, Prasad EW. The effect of ubretid on bladder function after recent complete spinal cord injury. Br J Urol. 1974;46(2):187.

707. Smith CP, Gangitano DA, Munoz A, et al. Botulinum toxin type A normalizes alterations in urothelial ATP and NO release induced by chronic spinal cord injury. Neurochem Int. 2008;52(6):1068.

708. Smith N, Grimes I, Ridge S, et al. YM905 is effective and safe as treatment of overactive bladder in women and men: results from phase II study. ICS Proceedings, Heidelberg, Germany; 2002. p. 138 (abstract 222).

709. Smith P, Heimer G, Norgren A, et al. Steroid hormone receptors in pelvic muscles and ligaments in women. Gynecol Obstet Investig. 1990;30(1):27.

710. Smulders RA, Krauwinkel WJ, Swart PJ, et al. Pharmacokinetics and safety of solifenacin succinate in healthy young men. J Clin Pharmacol. 2004;44(9):1023.

711. Smulders R, Tan H, Krauwinkel W, et al. A placebo-controlled, dose–rising study in healthy male volunteers to evaluate safety, tolerability, pharmacokinetics and pharmacodynamics of single oral doses of YM905. Presented at the 32nd International Continence Society Annual Meeting, Heidelberg, Germany, August 2002.

712. Song C, Park JT, Heo KO, et al. Effects of bladder training and/or tolterodine in female patients with overactive bladder syndrome: a prospective, randomized study. J Korean Med Sci. 2006;21(6):1060.

713. Stahl MM, Ekstrom B, Sparf B, et al. Urodynamic and other effects of tolterodine: a novel antimuscarinic drug for the treatment of detrusor overactivity. Neurourol Urodyn. 1995;14(6):647.

714. Stanton SL. A comparison of emepronium bromide and flavoxate hydrochloride in the treatment of urinary incontinence. J Urol. 1973;110:529.

715. Staskin DR, Dmochowski RR, Sand PK, et al. Efficacy and safety of oxybutynin chloride topical gel for overactive bladder: a randomized, double-blind, placebo controlled, multicenter study. J Urol. 2009;181(4):1764–72.

716. Staskin D, Kay G, Tannenbaum C, et al. Trospium chloride has no effect on memory testing and is assay undetectable in the central nervous system of older patients with overactive bladder. Int J Clin Pract. 2010;64(9):1294–300.

717. Staskin DR, Robinson D. Oxybutynin chloride topical gel: a new formulation of an established antimuscarinic therapy for overactive bladder. Expert Opin Pharmacother. 2009;10(18):3103–11.

718. Staskin DR, Salvatore S. Oxybutynin topical and transdermal formulations: an update. Drugs Today (Barc). 2010;46(6):417–25.

719. Staskin D, Sand P, Zinner N, et al., Trospium Study Group. Once daily trospium chloride is effective and well tolerated for the treatment of overactive bladder: results from a multicenter phase III trial. J Urol. 2007;178(3 Pt 1):978.

720. Staskin DR, Te AE. Short- and long-term efficacy of solifenacin treatment in patients with symptoms of mixed urinary incontinence. BJU Int. 2006;97(6):1256.

721. Steers W, Corcos J, Foote J, et al. An investigation of dose titration with darifenacin, an M3-selective receptor antagonist. BJU Int. 2005;95(4):580.

722. Steers WD, Herschorn S, Kreder KJ, et al. Duloxetine compared with placebo for treating women with symptoms of overactive bladder. BJU Int. 2007;100(2):337.

723. Stewart DA, Taylor J, Ghosh S, et al. Terodiline causes polymorphic ventricular tachycardia due to reduced heart rate and prolongation of QT interval. Eur J Clin Pharmacol. 1992;42(6):577.

724. Stief CG, Porst H, Neuser D, et al. A randomised, placebo-controlled study to assess the efficacy of twice-daily vardenafil in the treatment of lower urinary tract symptoms secondary to benign prostatic hyperplasia. Eur Urol. 2008;53(6):1236.

725. Stöhrer M, Bauer P, Giannetti BM, et al. Effect of trospium chloride on urodynamic parameters in patients with detrusor hyperreflexia due to spinal cord injuries: a multicentre placebo controlled double-blind trial. Urol Int. 1991;47:138.

726. Stöhrer M, Madersbacher H, Richter R, et al. Efficacy and safety of propiverine in SCI-patients suffering from detrusor hyperreflexia—a double-blind, placebo-controlled clinical trial. Spinal Cord. 1999;37:196.

727. Stöhrer M, Mürtz G, Kramer G, et al. Propiverine compared to oxybutynin in neurogenic detrusor overactivity–results of a randomized, double-blind, multicenter clinical study. Eur Urol. 2007;51(1):235.

728. Streng T, Andersson KE, Hedlund P, et al. Effects on bladder function of combining elocalcitol and tolterodine in rats with outflow obstruction. BJU Int. 2012;110(2 Pt 2):E125–31.

729. Streng T, Christoph T, Andersson K-E. Urodynamic effects of the K+ channel (KCNQ) opener retigabine in freely moving, conscious rats. J Urol. 2004;172:2054.

730. Striano P, Striano S. Gabapentin: a Ca2+ channel alpha 2-delta ligand far beyond epilepsy therapy. Drugs Today (Barc). 2008;44(5):353.

731. Strittmatter F, Gandaglia G, Benigni F, et al. Expression of fatty acid amide hydrolase (FAAH) in human, mouse, and rat urinary bladder and effects by FAAH inhibition on bladder function in awake rats. Eur Urol. 2012;61:98–106.

732. Suckling J, Lethaby A, Kennedy R. Local oestrogen for vaginal atrophy in postmenopausal women. Cochrane Database Syst Rev. 2003;(4):CD001500.

733. Sugiyama Y, Yoshida M, Masunaga K, et al. Pharmacological effects of propiverine and its active metabolite, M-1, on isolated human urinary bladder smooth muscle, and on bladder contraction in rats. Int J Urol. 2008;15(1):76.

734. Sultana CJ, Walters MD. Estrogen and urinary incontinence in women. Maturitas. 1990;20:129.

735. Sundin T, Dahlström A, Norlén L, Svedmyr N. The sympathetic innervation and adrenoreceptor function of the human lower urinary tract in the normal state and after parasympathetic denervation. Invest Urol. 1977;14(4):322–8.

736. Sussman D, Garely A. Treatment of overactive bladder with once-daily extended-release tolterodine or oxybutynin: the antimuscarinic clinical effectiveness trial (ACET). Curr Med Res Opin. 2002;18(4):177.

737. Swart PJ, Krauwinkel WJ, Smulders RA, et al. Pharmacokinetic effect of ketoconazole on solifenacin in healthy volunteers. Basic Clin Pharmacol Toxicol. 2006;99(1):33.

738. Swierzewski III SJ, Gormley EA, Belville WD, Sweetser PM, Wan J, McGuire EJ. The effect of terazosin on bladder function in the spinal cord injured patient. J Urol. 1994;151(4):951–4.

739. Swithinbank LV, Vestey S, Abrams P. Nocturnal polyuria in community-dwelling women. BJU Int. 2004;93(4):523–7.

740. Szollar SM, Lee SM. Intravesical oxybutynin for spinal cord injury patients. Spinal Cord. 1996;34:284.

741. Szonyi G, Collas DM, Ding YY, et al. Oxybutynin with bladder retraining for detrusor instability in elderly people: a randomized controlled trial. Age Aging. 1995;24:287.

742. Takao T, Tsujimura A, Yamamoto K, et al. Solifenacin may improve sleep quality in patients with overactive bladder and sleep disturbance. Urology. 2011;78(3):648–52.

743. Takasu T, Ukai M, Sato S, et al. Effect of (R)-2-(2-aminothiazol-4-yl)-4′-{2-[(2-hydroxy-2-phenylethyl)amino]ethyl} acetanilide (YM178), a novel selective beta3-adrenoceptor agonist, on bladder function. J Pharmacol Exp Ther. 2007;321(2):642.

744. Take H, Shibata K, Awaji T, et al. Vascular alpha1-adrenoceptor subtype selectivity and alpha1-blocker-induced orthostatic hypotension. Jpn J Pharmacol. 1998;77(1):61–70.

745. Takeda M, Obara K, Mizusawa T, et al. Evidence for beta3-adrenoceptor subtypes in relaxation of the human urinary bladder detrusor: analysis by molecular biological and pharmacological methods. J Pharmacol Exp Ther. 1999;288(3):1367.

746. Takeda H, Yamazaki Y, Igawa Y, et al. Effects of beta(3)-adrenoceptor stimulation on prostaglandin E(2)-induced bladder hyperactivity and on the cardiovascular system in conscious rats. Neurourol Urodyn. 2002;21(6):558.

747. Takusagawa S, Miyashita A, Iwatsubo T, et al. In vitro inhibition and induction of human cytochrome P450 enzymes by mirabegron, a potent and selective β3-adrenoceptor agonist. Xenobiotica. 2012;42(12):1187–96.

748. Takusagawa S, van Lier JJ, Suzuki K, Nagata M. Absorption, metabolism and excretion of [14C] mirabegron (YM178), a potent and selective β3-adrenoceptor agonist, after oral administration to healthy male volunteers. Drug Metab Dispos. 2012;40(4):815–24.

749. Takusagawa S, Yajima K, Miyashita A, et al. Identification of human cytochrome P450 isoforms and esterases involved in the metabolism of mirabegron, a potent and selective β3-adrenoceptor agonist. Xenobiotica. 2012;42(10):957–67.

750. Tamimi NA, Mincik I, Haughie S, et al. A placebo-controlled study investigating the efficacy and safety of the phosphodiesterase type 5 inhibitor UK-369,003 for the treatment of men with lower urinary tract symptoms associated with clinical benign prostatic hyperplasia. BJU Int. 2010;106:674–80.

751. Tanaka Y, Masumori N, Tsukamoto T. Urodynamic effects of solifenacin in untreated female patients with symptomatic overactive bladder. Int J Urol. 2010;17(9):796–800.

752. Tanaka M, Sasaki Y, Kimura Y, et al. A novel pyrrole derivative, NS-8, suppresses the rat micturition reflex by inhibiting afferent pelvic nerve activity. BJU Int. 2003;92:1031.

753. Tatemichi S, Akiyama K, Kobayashi M, et al. A selective alpha1A-adrenoceptor antagonist inhibits detrusor overactivity in a rat model of benign prostatic hyperplasia. J Urol. 2006;176(3):1236–41.

754. Tatemichi S, Tomiyama Y, Maruyama I, et al. Uroselectivity in male dogs of silodosin (KMD-3213), a novel drug for the obstructive component of

benign prostatic hyperplasia. Neurourol Urodyn. 2006;25(7):792–9.

755. Taylor MC, Bates CP. A double-blind crossover trial of baclofen—a new treatment for the unstable bladder syndrome. Br J Urol. 1979;51(6):504.

756. Thor KB, de Groat WC. Neural control of the female urethral and rhabdosphincteris and pelvic floor muscles. Am J Physiol Regul Integr Comp Physiol. 2010;299(2):R416–38.

757. Thor K, Katofiasc MA. Effects of duloxetine, a combined serotonin and norepinephrine reuptake inhibitor, on central neural control of lower urinary tract function in the chloralose-anesthetized female cat. J Pharmacol Exp Ther. 1995;274(2):1014.

758. Thor K, Kirby M, Viktrup L. Serotonin and noradrenaline involvement in urinary incontinence, depression and pain: scientific basis for overlapping clinical efficacy from a single drug. Int J Clin Pract. 2007;61(8):1349–55.

759. Thumfart J, Roehr CC, Kapelari K, et al. Desmopressin associated symptomatic hyponatremic hypervolemia in children. Are there predictive factors? J Urol. 2005;174(1):294–8.

760. Thüroff JW, Bunke B, Ebner A, et al. Randomized, double-blind, multicenter trial on treatment of frequency, urgency and incontinence related to detrusor hyperactivity: oxybutynin versus propantheline versus placebo. J Urol. 1991;145:813.

761. Thüroff JW, Chartier-Kastler E, Corcus J, et al. Medical treatment and medical side effects in urinary incontinence in the elderly. World J Urol. 1998;16 Suppl 1:S48–61.

762. Tincello DG, Kenyon S, Abrams KR, et al. Botulinum toxin a versus placebo for refractory detrusor overactivity in women: a randomised blinded placebo-controlled trial of 240 women (the RELAX study). Eur Urol. 2012;62(3):507–14.

763. Tiwari A. Elocalcitol, a vitamin D3 analog for the potential treatment of benign prostatic hyperplasia, overactive bladder and male infertility. IDrugs. 2009;12(6):381–93.

764. Todorova A, Vonderheid-Guth B, Dimpfel W. Effects of tolterodine, trospium chloride, and oxybutynin on the central nervous system. J Clin Pharmacol. 2001;41(6):636.

765. Toglia MR, Serels SR, Laramée C, et al. Solifenacin for overactive bladder: patient-reported outcomes from a large placebo-controlled trial. Postgrad Med. 2009;121(5):151–8.

766. Tokuno H, Chowdhury JU, Tomita T. Inhibitory effects of propiverine on rat and guinea-pig urinary bladder muscle. Naunyn Schmiedebergs Arch Pharmacol. 1993;348:659.

767. Tominaga M, Caterina MJ, Malmberg AB, et al. The cloned capsaicin receptor integrates multiple pain-producing stimuli. Neuron. 1998;21(3):531–43.

768. Truss MC, Stief CG, Uckert S, et al. Initial clinical experience with the selective phosphodiesterase-I isoenzyme inhibitor vinpocetine in the treatment of urge incontinence and low compliance bladder. World J Urol. 2000;18:439.

769. Truss MC, Stief CG, Uckert S, et al. Phosphodiesterase 1 inhibition in the treatment of lower urinary tract dysfunction: from bench to bedside. World J Urol. 2001;19:344.

770. Tsakiris P, de la Rosette JJ, Michel M, et al. Pharmacologic treatment of male stress urinary incontinence: systemic review of the literature and levels of evidence. Eur Urol. 2008;53:53–9.

771. Tseng LH, Wang AC, Chang YL, et al. Randomised comparison of tolterodine with vaginal oestrogen cream versus tolterodine alone for the treatment of postmenopausal women with overactive bladder syndrome. Neurourol Urodyn. 2009;28(1):47–51.

772. Tuncel A, Nalcacioglu V, Ener K, et al. Sildenafil citrate and tamsulosin combination is not superior to monotherapy in treating lower urinary tract symptoms and erectile dysfunction. World J Urol. 2010;28:17–22.

773. Tyagi V, Philips BJ, Su R, et al. Differential expression of functional cannabinoid receptors in human bladder detrusor and urothelium. J Urol. 2009;181:1932–8.

774. Uchida H, Shishido K, Nomiya M, et al. Involvement of cyclic AMP-dependent and -independent mechanisms in the relaxation of rat detrusor muscle via beta-adrenoceptors. Eur J Pharmacol. 2005;518(2–3):195.

775. Uckert S, Hedlund P, Andersson KE, et al. Update on phosphodiesterase (PDE) isoenzymes as pharmacologic targets in urology: present and future. Eur Urol. 2006;50(6):1194–207.

776. Uckert S, Stief CG, Odenthal KP, et al. Responses of isolated normal human detrusor muscle to various spasmolytic drugs commonly used in the treatment of the overactive bladder. Arzneimittelforschung. 2000;50(5):456.

777. Valiquette G, Herbert J, Maede-D'Alisera P. Desmopressin in the management of nocturia in patients with multiple sclerosis. A double-blind, crossover trial. Arch Neurol. 1996;53:1270.

778. Van de Walle J, Van Herzeele C, Raes A. Is there still a role for desmopressin in children with primary monosymptomatic nocturnal enuresis?: a focus on safety issues. Drug Saf. 2010;33(4):261–71.

779. van Gelderen EM, Li Q, Meijer J, et al. An exploratory comparison of the single dose pharmacokinetics of the beta3-adrenoceptor agonist mirabegron in healthy CYP2D6 poor and extensive metabolizers. Clin Pharmacol Ther. 2009;85:S88.

780. Van Kerrebroeck P, Abrams P, Lange R, et al. Duloxetine vs. placebo in the treatment of European and Canadian women with stress urinary incontinence. Br J Obstet Gynaecol. 2004;111:249.

781. Van Kerrebroeck P, Kreder K, Jonas U, et al. Tolterodine once-daily: superior efficacy and tolerability in the treatment of the overactive bladder. Urology. 2001;57(3):414.

782. van Kerrebroeck P, Rezapour M, Cortesse A, et al. Desmopressin in the treatment of nocturia: a double-blind, placebo-controlled study. Eur Urol. 2007;52:221.

783. van Rey F, Heesakkers J. Solifenacin in multiple sclerosis patients with overactive bladder: a prospective study. Adv Urol. 2011;2011:834753.

784. Vande Walle JGJ, Bogaert GA, Mattsson S, et al. A new fast-melting oral formulation of desmopressin: a pharmacodynamic study in children with primary nocturnal enuresis. BJU Int. 2006;97:603.

785. Vardy MD, Mitcheson HD, Samuels TA, et al. Effects of solifenacin on overactive bladder symptoms, symptom bother and other patient-reported outcomes: results from VIBRANT—a double-blind, placebo-controlled trial. Int J Clin Pract. 2009;63(12):1702–14.

786. Vaughan CP, Johnson II TM, Ala-Lipasti MA, et al. The prevalence of clinically meaningful overactive bladder: bother and quality of life results from the population-based FINNO study. Eur Urol. 2011;59(4):629–36.

787. Vella M, Duckett J, Basu M. Duloxetine 1 year on: the long-term outcome of a cohort of women prescribed duloxetine. Int Urogynecol J Pelvic Floor Dysfunct. 2008;19(7):961–4.

788. Vemulakonda VM, Somogyi GT, Kiss S, et al. Inhibitory effect of intravesically applied botulinum toxin A in chronic bladder inflammation. J Urol. 2005;173(2):621–4.

789. Versi E, Appell R, Mobley D, et al. Dry mouth with conventional and controlled-release oxybutynin in urinary incontinence. The Ditropan XL Study Group. Obstet Gynecol. 2000;95(5):718–21.

790. Versi E, Cardozo LD. Urethral instability: diagnosis based on variations in the maximum urethral pressure in normal climacteric women. Neurourol Urodyn. 1986;5(6):535.

791. Vijaya G, Digesu GA, Derpapas A, et al. Antimuscarinic effects on current perception threshold: a prospective placebo control study. Neurourol Urodyn. 2012;31(1):75–9.

792. Visco AG, Brubaker L, Richter HE, et al., Pelvic Floor Disorders Network. Anticholinergic versus botulinum toxin A comparison trial for the treatment of bothersome urge urinary incontinence: ABC trial. Contemp Clin Trials. 2012;33(1):184–96.

793. Wada N, Watanabe M, Kita M, et al. Efficacy and safety of propiverine and solifenacin for the treatment of female patients with overactive bladder: a crossover study. Low Urin Tract Symptoms. 2011;3:36–42.

794. Waetjen LE, Brown JS, Modelska K, et al. Effect of raloxifene on urinary incontinence: a randomized controlled trial. Obstet Gynaecol. 2004;103(2):261.

795. Wagg A, Compion G, Fahey A, Siddiqui E. Persistence with prescribed antimuscarinic therapy for overactive bladder: a UK experience. BJU Int. 2012;110(11):1767–74. doi:10.1111/j.1464-410X.2012.11023.x.

796. Wagg A, Verdejo C, Molander U. Review of cognitive impairment with antimuscarinic agents in elderly patients with overactive bladder. Int J Clin Pract. 2010;64:1279–86.

797. Wagg A, Wyndaele JJ, Sieber P. Efficacy and tolerability of solifenacin in elderly subjects with overactive bladder syndrome: a pooled analysis. Am J Geriatr Pharmacother. 2006;4(1):14.

798. Walczak JS, Cervero F. Local activation of cannabinoid CB1 receptors in the urinary bladder reduces the inflammation-induced sensitization of bladder afferents. Mol Pain. 2011;7:31–42.

799. Waldeck K, Larsson B, Andersson K-E. Comparison of oxybutynin and its active metabolite, N-desethyl-oxybutynin, in the human detrusor and parotid gland. J Urol. 1997;157:1093.

800. Walter P, Grosse J, Bihr AM, et al. Bioavailability of trospium chloride after intravesical instillation in patients with neurogenic lower urinary tract dysfunction: a pilot study. Neurourol Urodyn. 1999;18(5):447–53.

801. Walter R, Ullmann C, Thummler D, et al. Influence of propiverine on hepatic microsomal cytochrome p450 enzymes in male rats. Drug Metab Dispos. 2003;31(6):714.

802. Wammack R, Weihe E, Dienes H-P, Hohenfellner R. Die Neurogene Blase in vitro. Akt Urol. 1995;26:16.

803. Wang CJ, Lin YN, Huang SW, Chang CH. Low dose oral desmopressin for nocturnal polyuria in patients with benign prostatic hyperplasia: a double-blind, placebo controlled, randomized study. J Urol. 2011;185(1):219–23.

804. Wang X, Momota Y, Yanase H, Narumiya S, Maruyama T, Kawatani M. Urothelium EP1 receptor facilitates the micturition reflex in mice. Biomed Res. 2008;29:105–11.

805. Weatherall M. The risk of hyponatremia in older adults using desmopressin for nocturia: a systematic review and meta-analysis. Neurourol Urodyn. 2004;23(4):302.

806. Wegener JW, Schulla V, Lee T-S, et al. An essential role of CaV1.2L-type calcium channel for urinary bladder function. FASEB J. 2004;18:1159.

807. Wehnert J, Sage S. Comparative investigations to the action of Mictonorm (propiverin hydrochloride) and Spasuret (flavoxat hydrochloride) on detrusor vesicae. Z Urol Nephrol. 1989;82:259.

808. Wehnert J, Sage S. Therapie der Blaseninstabilität und Urge-Inkontinenz mit Propiverin hydrochlorid (Mictonorm®) und Oxybutynin chlorid (Dridase®)—eine randomisierte Crossover-Vergleichsstudie. Akt Urol. 1992;23:7.

809. Weil EH, Eerdmans PH, Dijkman GA, et al. Randomized double-blind placebo controlled multicenter evaluation of efficacy and dose finding of midodrine hydrochloride in women with mild to moderate stress urinary incontinence: a phase II study. Int Urogynecol J Pelvic Floor Dysfunct. 1998;9(3):145.

810. Wein AJ. Pathophysiology and classification of lower urinary tract dysfunction. In: Wein AJ, Kavoussi LR, Novick AC, Partin AW, Peters CA, editors. Campbell-Walsh urology, vol. 3. 10th ed. Philadelphia, PA: Elsevier Saunders; 2012. p. 1834–46.

811. Wein AJ, Dmochoski RR. Neuromuscular dysfunction of the lower urinary tract. In: Wein AJ, Kavoussi LR, Novick AC, Partin AW, Peters CA, editors. Campbell-Walsh urology, vol. 3. 10th ed. Philadelphia, PA: Elsevier Saunders; 2012. p. 1909–46.

812. Weiss JP, Blaivas J, Bliwise D, et al. The evaluation and treatment of nocturia: a consensus statement. BJU Int. 2011;108(1):6–21.

813. Weiss JP, van Kerrebroeck PE, Klein BM, Nørgaard JP. Excessive nocturnal urine production is a major contributing factor to the etiology of nocturia. J Urol. 2011;186(4):1358–63.

814. Werkström V, Svensson A, Andersson KE, et al. Phosphodiesterase 5 in the female pig and human urethra: morphological and functional aspects. BJU Int. 2006;98(2):414.

815. Wesnes KA, Edgar C, Tretter RN, Bolodeoku J. Exploratory pilot study assessing the risk of cognitive impairment or sedation in the elderly following single doses of solifenacin 10 mg. Expert Opin Drug Saf. 2009;8(6):615–26.

816. Wiedemann A, Füsgen I, Hauri D. New aspects of therapy with trospium chloride for urge incontinence. Eur J Geriatr. 2002;3:41.

817. Wiseman OJ, Fowler CJ, Landon DN. The role of the human bladder lamina propria myofibroblast. BJU Int. 2003;91(1):89–93.

818. Woods M, Carson N, Norton NW, et al. Efficacy of the beta3-adrenergic receptor agonist CL-316243 on experimental bladder hyperreflexia and detrusor instability in the rat. J Urol. 2001;166(3):1142.

819. Wuest M, Hiller N, Braeter M, et al. Contribution of Ca2+ influx to carbachol-induced detrusor contraction is different in human urinary bladder compared to pig and mouse. Eur J Pharmacol. 2007;565:180.

820. Wuest M, Weiss A, Waelbroeck M, et al. Propiverine and metabolites: differences in binding to muscarinic receptors and in functional models of detrusor contraction. Naunyn Schmiedebergs Arch Pharmacol. 2006;374(2):87.

821. Wyndaele JJ, Goldfischer ER, Morrow JD, et al. Effects of flexible-dose fesoterodine on overactive bladder symptoms and treatment satisfaction: an open-label study. Int J Clin Pract. 2009;63(4):560–7.

822. Wyndaele JJ, Van Dromme SA. Muscular weakness as side effect of botulinum toxin injection for neurogenic detrusor overactivity. Spinal Cord. 2002;40(11):599.

823. Yamada S, Seki M, Ogoda M, et al. Selective binding of bladder muscarinic receptors in relation to the pharmacokinetics of a novel antimuscarinic agent, imidafenacin, to treat overactive bladder. J Pharmacol Exp Ther. 2011;336(2):365–71.

824. Yamaguchi O, Marui E, Kakizaki H, et al. Randomized, double-blind, placebo- and propiverine-controlled trial of the once-daily antimuscarinic agent solifenacin in Japanese patients with overactive bladder. BJU Int. 2007;100(3):579.

825. Yamanishi T, Mizuno T, Tatsumiya K, et al. Urodynamic effects of silodosin, a new alpha 1A-adrenoceptor selective antagonist, for the treatment of benign prostatic hyperplasia. Neurourol Urodyn. 2009;29:558–62.

826. Yaminishi T, Yasuda K, Tojo M, et al. Effects of beta-2 stimulants on contractility and fatigue of canine urethral sphincter. J Urol. 1994;151:1073.

827. Yarker YE, Goa KL, Fitton A. Oxybutynin—a review of its pharmacodynamic and pharmacokinetic properties, and its therapeutic use in detrusor instability. Drugs Aging. 1995;6:243.

828. Yashiro K, Thor K, Burgard E. Properties of urethral rhabdosphincter motoneurons and their regulation by noradrenaline. J Physiol. 2010;588(Pt 24):4951–67.

829. Yasuda K, Kawabe K, Takimoto Y, et al. A double blind clinical trial of a beta-2 adrenergic agonist in stress incontinence. Int Urogynecol J. 1993;4:146.

830. Yokoyama T, Uematsu K, Watanabe T, et al. Naftopidil and propiverine hydrochloride for treatment of male lower urinary tract symptoms suggestive of benign prostatic hyperplasia and concomitant overactive bladder: a prospective randomized controlled study. Scand J Urol Nephrol. 2009;43:307–14.

831. Yokoyama O, Yamaguchi O, Kakizaki H, et al. Efficacy of solifenacin on nocturia in Japanese patients with overactive bladder: impact on sleep evaluated by bladder diary. J Urol. 2011;186(1):170–4.

832. Yoo DS, Han JY, Lee KS, Choo MS. Prescription pattern of oxybutynin ER in patients with overactive bladder in real life practice: a multicentre, open-label, prospective observational study. Int J Clin Pract. 2012;66(2):132–8.

833. Yoong HF, Sundaram MB, Aida Z. Prevalence of nocturnal polyuria in patients with benign prostatic hyperplasia. Med J Malaysia. 2005;60(3):294–6.

834. Yoshida M, Homma Y, Inadome A, et al. Age-related changes in cholinergic and purinergic neurotransmission in human isolated bladder smooth muscles. Exp Gerontol. 2001;36(1):99.

835. Yoshida M, Homma Y, Kawabe K. Silodosin, a novel selective alpha 1A-adrenoceptor selective antagonist for the treatment of benign prostatic hyperplasia. Expert Opin Investig Drugs. 2007;16(12):1955–65.

836. Yoshida M, Inadome A, Maeda Y, et al. Non-neuronal cholinergic system in human bladder urothelium. Urology. 2006;67(2):425.

837. Yoshida M, Kudoh J, Homma Y, Kawabe K. Safety and efficacy of silodosin for the treatment of benign prostatic hyperplasia. Clin Interv Aging. 2011;6:161–72.

838. Yoshida M, Masunaga K, Satoji Y, et al. Basic and clinical aspects of non-neuronal acetylcholine: expression of non-neuronal acetylcholine in urothelium and its clinical significance. J Pharmacol Sci. 2008;106(2):193.

839. Yoshida M, Miyamae K, Iwashita H, et al. Management of detrusor dysfunction in the elderly: changes in acetylcholine and adenosine triphosphate release during aging. Urology. 2004;63(3 Suppl 1):17.

840. Yossepowitch O, Gillon G, Baniel J, et al. The effect of cholinergic enhancement during filling cystometry: can edrophonium chloride be used as a provocative test for overactive bladder? J Urol. 2001;165(5):1441.

841. Zahariou A, Karagiannis G, Papaionnou P, et al. The use of desmopressin in the management of nocturnal enuresis in patients with spinal cord injury. Eura Medicophys. 2007;43:333.

842. Zaitsu M, Mikami K, Ishida N, Takeuchi T. Comparative evaluation of the safety and efficacy of long-term use of imidafenacin and solifenacin in patients with overactive bladder: a prospective, open, randomized, parallel-group trial (the LIST Study). Adv Urol. 2011;2011:854697.

843. Zhu HL, Brain KL, Aishima M, et al. Actions of two main metabolites of propiverine (M-1 and M-2) on voltage-dependent L-type Ca2+ currents and Ca2+ transients in murine urinary bladder myocytes. J Pharmacol Exp Ther. 2008;324(1):118.

844. Zinner N. Darifenacin: a muscarinic M3-selective receptor antagonist for the treatment of overactive bladder. Expert Opin Pharmacother. 2007 Mar;8(4):511–23.

845. Zinner NR, Dmochowski RR, Staskin DR, et al. Once-daily trospium chloride 60 mg extended-release provides effective, long-term relief of overactive bladder syndrome symptoms. Neurourol Urodyn. 2011;30(7):1214–9.

846. Zinner N, Gittelman M, Harris R, et al. Trospium Study Group. Trospium chloride improves overactive bladder symptoms: a multicenter phase III trial. J Urol. 2004;171(6 Pt 1):2311.

847. Zinner NR, Mattiasson A, Stanton SL. Efficacy, safety, and tolerability of extended-release once-daily tolterodine treatment for overactive bladder in older versus younger patients. J Am Geriatr Soc. 2002;50(5):799.

848. Zinner N, Susset J, Gittelman M, et al. Efficacy, tolerability and safety of darifenacin, an M(3) selective receptor antagonist: an investigation of warning time in patients with OAB. Int J Clin Pract. 2006;60(1):119.

849. Zinner N, Tuttle J, Marks L. Efficacy and tolerability of darifenacin, a muscarinic M3 selective receptor antagonist (M3 SRA), compared with oxybutynin in the treatment of patients with overactive bladder. World J Urol. 2005;23(4):248–52.

Electrical Stimulation and Neuromodulation

Alex Gomelsky and Roger R. Dmochowski

Electrical Stimulation and Neuromodulation

Electrical stimulation of the urinary tract is a concept that dates back to the 1800s, when Saxtorph stimulated the detrusor of a patient with urinary retention intravesically with a metal electrode [1]. In the last 50 years, this technique has been altered and refined for different end-organs in the lower urinary tract [2, 3]. While the results of electrical stimulation have often been encouraging, very little has been published about this therapeutic modality in the last decade. On the other hand, the modes and potential uses for neuromodulation only continue to increase. The following is a brief review of neurostimulation and neuromodulation.

Pathophysiology of Urinary Storage and Emptying

Prior to a discussion of neurostimulation and neuromodulation, it is important to review the normal physiologic adaptations of the urinary tract

A. Gomelsky, M.D.
Department of Urology, LSU Health Shreveport, Shreveport, LA, USA

R.R. Dmochowski, M.D., M.M.H.C. (✉)
Department of Urologic Surgery, Vanderbilt University Medical Center, A1302 Medical Center North, Nashville, TN 37232-2765, USA
e-mail: roger.dmochowski@vanderbilt.edu

during urine storage and emptying. The ultimate result of all bladder functions is low-pressure urinary storage, complete urinary continence, and low-pressure emptying when a threshold bladder capacity is reached [4]. The normal adaptations during urinary storage and emptying are facilitated by cooperation between the bladder body and outlet, where both are innervated by peripheral nerves from the sympathetic, parasympathetic, and somatic nervous systems [5]. Efferent axons in the sympathetic nerves inhibit bladder contraction and stimulate the urethra to promote urinary storage, while parasympathetic nerves stimulate bladder contraction and relax the bladder outlet to promote urinary emptying. The somatic nervous system controls the external urethral sphincter and pelvic floor musculature.

Urinary storage is achieved by CNS reflex pathways coordinated through the Periaqueductal Grey (PAG) in the midbrain, which regulates activity in the brainstem pontine micturition center (PMC) and putative pontine storage center. Increasing wall tension during bladder filling activates afferent nerves, which reflexively activate sympathetic outflow to the lower urinary tract from the lumbosacral spinal cord [6, 7]. As a result, there is internal sphincter contraction and ganglionic inhibition via the hypogastric nerve, as well as contraction of the external sphincter and pelvic floor striated musculature via the pudendal nerve. The sacral parasympathetic outflow is typically inactive during the storage phase. The outcome of detrusor inhibition and outlet excitation is low-pressure urinary storage and continence.

A.J. Wein et al. (eds.), *Bladder Dysfunction in the Adult: The Basis for Clinical Management*, Current Clinical Urology, DOI 10.1007/978-1-4939-0853-0_14, © Springer Science+Business Media New York 2014

The storage phase of the bladder can be switched to the voiding phase either reflexively or voluntarily [8, 9]. When the volume of urine exceeds micturition threshold, the PMC is activated, reversing the efferent outflow and inhibiting the spinal guarding reflexes (sympathetic outflow to the detrusor and somatic outflow to the external sphincter). The PMC also stimulates parasympathetic outflow which is excitatory to the detrusor (bladder contraction mainly via muscarinic M3 receptors) and inhibitory to the internal urethral sphincter smooth muscle. The expulsion phase consists of an initial relaxation of the urethral sphincter, followed in a few seconds by a phasic, sustained detrusor contraction, an increase in bladder pressure, and the flow of urine. There is quiescence of striated muscle activity on electromyography due to inhibition of Onuf's nucleus.

Any disruption in the routine communication between the brain, central nervous system, peripheral nervous system, the bladder, outlet, and pelvic floor musculature can result in lower urinary tract dysfunction. These dysfunctions can be grouped as failure to store urine, manifesting in urinary urgency, frequency, and urinary incontinence, and failure to empty urine or urinary retention [4]. Treatment options may include behavioral intervention, intermittent or indwelling catheterization, pelvic floor muscle training with biofeedback, pharmaceutical intervention, and invasive surgical therapy. All of these options are associated with varying degrees of success and adverse event profiles.

Electrical Stimulation for Disorders of Urinary Storage

During electrical neurostimulation, nerves or muscles are directly stimulated by an electrical current to achieve an immediate response. Several mechanisms have been proposed for the efficacy of neurostimulation in treating urinary storage disorders such as stress or urgency urinary incontinence (SUI; UUI), overactive bladder (OAB), and interstitial cystitis (IC). First, direct electrical stimulation of local nerves may lead to contraction

of the pelvic floor musculature and/or the external urinary sphincter. This mechanism may be applicable to treatment of urinary incontinence resulting from external sphincter or pelvic floor dysfunction. The second mechanism involves local stimulation of afferents in the micturition reflex arc, resulting in detrusor inhibition and improvement of idiopathic or neurogenic detrusor overactivity (IDO; NDO) in conditions such as spinal cord injury (SCI) and multiple sclerosis (MS) [10, 11]. Additionally, electrically mediated external sphincter contraction has been shown to cause reflex detrusor inhibition [11].

In most commercially available electrical stimulation units, the voltage is fixed at 9–12 V to minimize the potential for thermal injury [11]. The ratio of stimulation time to rest time is usually 1:2 and the frequency is chosen based on the patient's diagnosis and symptoms. Frequencies of 5–10 Hz typically inhibit reflex detrusor contractions in DO, while frequencies of 20–50 Hz lead to pelvic floor and external sphincter contraction in patients with SUI [11–13]. Stimulation can be performed in several locations and via several approaches (suprapubic, vaginal, perineal, and rectal). The best responses have been reported when the stimulating probe was in close proximity to the nerve [11].

Transcutaneous electrical nerve stimulation (TENS) has been employed for urinary storage dysfunction due to IDO, NDO, and IC [14, 15]. The mechanism of efficacy of this approach is based on stimulating the cutaneous distribution of the common peroneal or posterior tibial nerves that have common and overlapping afferent central pathways with the pudendal nerve [11]. Two electrodes are positioned suprapubically 10–15 cm apart and stimulation is given at maximum tolerable intensity up to 2 h twice daily [1]. Frequencies may vary from 2 Hz, at which pudendal nerve afferents are stimulated, to 50 Hz, at which the striated paraurethral musculature is stimulated [16, 17]. In placebo-controlled studies, urodynamic outcomes are conflicting. Hasan et al. reported no significant changes in urodynamic variables after TENS [18], while Bower et al. reported significant changes in the first desire to void, maximum cystometric capacity, and threshold volume in the suprapubic TENS group [19]. Additionally, transurethral electrical bladder stimulation (TEBS) has been used in pediatric myelomeningocele patients with the intent of increasing bladder capacity at low pressures [20, 21].

The evidence to support the use of electrical stimulation for treatment of urinary storage disorders has been inconsistent. Patients using chronic daily electrical stimulation via a vaginal or anal probe have reported 6–30 % cure rates, with most studies reporting less than 1 year of follow-up [11]. In one multicenter RCT, Sand et al. demonstrated significant subjective and objective improvement in women with SUI undergoing vaginal stimulation versus sham treatment [22]. However, only 48 % of the women in the active treatment arm were considered improved and the follow-up period was just 15 weeks. In another multicenter, placebo-controlled (non-randomized) trial, Richardson et al. reported that 68 % of women in the active treatment arm were improved at 1 year of follow-up [23]. While the technique can be performed by patients at home, treatment must be typically given for a long period of time. Additionally, the transvaginal mode of treatment may not be well accepted by many patients due to high intensity of stimulation and pain during treatment may be reported by up to half of the patients [22, 24].

Electrical Stimulation to Enhance Bladder Emptying

SCI may lead to failure to empty urine due to an absence of a sustained detrusor contraction. Direct stimulation of the detrusor has been attempted by several groups since the 1960s and the practice has often met with limited success [11, 25]. Low post-void residuals and sterile urine were only reported in 50–60 % of patients with hypotonic and areflexic bladders and secondary failure due to bladder fibrosis and device malfunction was common [26]. Furthermore, the spread of current to other pelvic structures resulted in pain and lower extremity spasms, as well as defecatory, erectile, and ejaculatory dysfunction [26, 27].

Techniques of electrical stimulation of the anterior sacral nerve roots for treatment of emptying dysfunction were introduced and modified by groups led by Brindley and Tanagho over 30 years ago and continue to be used to this day [28–30]. The Brindley device is the most common sacral anterior root stimulator (SARS) used and consists of an implantable receiver with stimulation wires and an external transmitter. The electrodes of the SARS can be placed either extradurally or intradurally via a dorsal lumbosacral laminectomy [30, 31]. Anterior sacral nerve stimulation is typically combined with a dorsal or posterior rhizotomy which eliminates striated sphincter stimulation and reflex incontinence, and may also increase bladder compliance [30, 32, 33]. In brief, after laminectomy from L3-4 to S2, the sacral roots are identified intradurally and separated into their anterior and posterior components with a hook electrode [1]. After transection of the S2–S4 posterior roots, the remaining anterior roots are placed in the electrodes, the dura is closed, and the receiver is placed in a subcutaneous pocket. The procedure can also be performed extradurally and it may have beneficial effects on erectile function and defecation [34]. As stimulation induces simultaneous contractions of the detrusor and external sphincter, micturition occurs by post-stimulus voiding since the relaxation time of the sphincter is shorter than that of detrusor smooth muscle [1]. Therefore, bursts of impulses are given to aid in bladder emptying. The only two prerequisites for the placement of a SARS are (1) a detrusor that is capable of contracting following stimulation and, (2) an intact sacral motor neuron [35]. The results in patients with neurogenic bladder due to SCI vary [11]. When reported, postoperative bladder capacity may approach 500 mL and successful implant-driven micturition may be achieved in 73–100 %. Continence is maintained in 69–100 % of patients. The main complications appear to be related to mechanical malfunction of the device and the need for readjustment and replacement [32]. Although it is not performed at many centers worldwide, SARS after dorsal rhizotomy remains a well-accepted treatment option in patients with a complete suprasacral SCI who suffer from complications such as significant urinary incontinence, recurrent urinary tract infections, or upper urinary tract compromise.

Neuromodulation of Bladder Storage and Emptying

Neuromodulation is the electrical or chemical modulation of a nerve to influence the physiologic behavior of an organ [36]. While electrical stimulation has a direct effect on efferent nerves and has been around since the late nineteenth century, neuromodulation was pioneered a century later through the work of Tanagho et al. [30] The authors implanted an electrode in S3–S4 via an extensive dorsal rhizotomy and observed a complete or partial response in 18 of 19 patients available for long-term follow-up. Thus, neuromodulation produces an indirect effect via a central afferent mechanism by targeting reflex centers in the spinal cord and pons to influence reflexes between the bladder, urethral sphincter, and pelvic floor. Since that experience, the use of neuromodulation in urology has expanded to include several approaches and has become an integral part of the treatment algorithm for idiopathic or neurogenic detrusor overactivity (IDO; NDO) and nonobstructive urinary retention (NOUR).

Sacral Neuromodulation

Sacral neuromodulation (SNM) is internationally marketed as InterStim® (Medtronic, Inc., Minneapolis, MN) and was approved by the U.S. Food and Drug Administration in 1997 for the treatment of refractory UUI. FDA approval was obtained for treatment of urinary frequency and NOUR in 1999 and for OAB in 2002. While the mechanism of action of SNM is not completely understood, it is postulated that symptoms of incontinence and voiding dysfunction may represent an alteration of the pelvic neuromuscular environment by changes in the inhibitory and excitatory signals of the voiding reflex [37]. It is thought that electrical stimulation of the sacral nerve roots modulates the afferent neural reflex pathways between the spinal cord/pons and pelvic floor, bladder, and outlet [38]. As the ascending sensory pathway inputs and guarding reflex pathway are modulated, storage and emptying may be facilitated [39]. This is considered as a nonselective neuromodulation procedure, as opposed to more selective modulation of branches of the pudendal nerve.

Therapy is typically performed in two stages. The first stage consists of either a percutaneous nerve evaluation (PNE), where a temporary lead is placed bilaterally for up to a week of testing, or an implant of a potentially permanent tined lead that is attached to a temporary generator (Stage 1) which may be tested for up to 4 weeks. If patients experience >50 % improvement in their symptoms during a testing period, they may opt to proceed to the second stage of implantation. For patients who responded to a PNE, a permanent lead and implantable pulse generator (IPG) are implanted, while patients who already underwent permanent lead implant undergo only IPG placement (Stage 2). Evidence exists that significantly more patients who undergo a Stage 1 lead implant (88 %) go on to device implantation as compared to those undergoing PNE as their test procedure (46 %), with failures attributed to lead migration and inadequate length of testing [40].

Long-term outcomes of SNM have been recently reported by several groups. In an international, multi-institutional, prospective study at 17 centers, van Kerrebroeck et al. reported a significant reduction in the number of mean daily incontinence episodes and mean number of daily voids compared to baseline in 163 patients at 5 years of follow-up [41]. Mean voided volume (MVV) also increased significantly. For patients with NOUR, the mean volume per catheterization decreased significantly and the mean number of daily catheterizations also decreased. Likewise, at a mean follow-up of 53 months, Marcelissen et al. reported that 64 % of their 59 living patients achieved greater than 50 % improvement in daily incontinence episodes, daily pad use, number of daily voids, or an increase in MVV [42]. One patient underwent a lead revision due to suspected lead migration and 33 % underwent surgical revision due to an adverse event (AE). Additionally, a systematic review of the literature of SNM outcomes included 26 independent studies encompassing 357 patients [43]. The evidence level ranged from 2b to 4. The pooled success rate was 68 % for the test phase and 92 % for permanent SNM at a mean follow-up of 26 months. The pooled AE rate was 0 % for the test phase and 24 % for permanent SNM. Finally, a Cochrane Review identified eight randomized studies that evaluated implants which provided continuous stimulation [44]. Although it was unclear whether some reports included patients who also appeared in other reports, and no data were pooled, the authors concluded that continuous stimulation offered benefits for carefully selected patients with OAB syndrome and for those with NOUR. The contemporary revision rates (other than for battery replacement) after SNM implant range from 7 to 18 %, with loss of efficacy over time representing the most common reason for reoperation [45]. Overall long-term satisfaction with SNM obtained via a postal questionnaire approaches 90 %, and, while AEs were reported by 56 % of patients, 89 % of these patients did not seek further therapy [46].

SNM has also been used for alleviation of symptoms associated with other conditions impacting the lower urinary tract. At a mean follow-up of 14 months, Comiter reported an improvement in mean diurnal frequency episodes, MVV, pain scores, and IC Symptom and Problem Index scores after permanent SNM implantation in 17 patients with IC refractory to conservative therapy [47]. At a median follow-up of 86 months, Marinkovic et al. reported a significant improvement in pelvic pain and urgency/frequency scores and mean visual analog pain scores in 34 women with refractory IC [48]. Sievert et al. implanted ten patients with neurologically confirmed complete SCI with bilateral SNM electrodes during the detrusor atony phase [49]. At a mean follow-up of 26 months, urinary continence was achieved and a significant reduction in urinary tract infections was observed. Marinkovic and Gillen cited a significant increase in urinary flow rate and decrease in post-void

residual in a cohort of women with MS and NOUR at a mean follow-up of 4.3 years [50].

Percutaneous Tibial Nerve Stimulation

The posterior tibial nerve is a mixed sensory-motor nerve that originates from spinal roots L4 through S3, which also contribute directly to sensory and motor control of the bladder and pelvic floor musculature [36]. Percutaneous tibial nerve stimulation (PTNS) was developed as a method to stimulate sacral nerve roots through peripheral pathways and was approved by the Food and Drug Administration in 2000. This therapy consists of temporarily implanting a 34 gauge disposable needle cephalad to the medial malleolus of the ankle while a grounding pad is placed on the arch of the ipsilateral foot [51]. Electrical stimulation is applied unilaterally from the medial malleolus and posterior to the edge of the tibia by using charge-compensated 200 µs pulses and a pulse rate of 20 Hz. The stimulator is programmed with amplitude of 1–10 mA and the amplitude of the stimulation is gradually increased until a motor response (toe flexion and/or fanning) and a sensory response (radiating sensation in the sole of the foot) are generated. Stimulation of the underlying nerve is performed in weekly 30-min sessions over a 3-month period, but sessions may be performed biweekly. Where symptom improvement is seen it is usually manifested after 6–8 sessions. In successful cases, treatment may be continued as the patient requires (e.g., once every 2–3 weeks). PTNS is currently marketed as the Urgent® PC (Uroplasty, Inc., Minnetonka, MN). It has been suggested that 20–30 PTNS sessions may be required annually to maintain efficacy [52].

Several recent studies have focused on the efficacy of PTNS in treating patients with refractory OAB. Peters et al. performed a randomized, multicenter, controlled study comparing PTNS to tolterodine ER and found a similar reduction in urinary frequency, number of UUI episodes, urge severity, voided volume (VV), and number of nighttime voids [53]. Although objective outcomes were similar between the two groups, subjectively, there was a clear preference for PTNS over tolterodine. A placebo effect for PTNS could not be excluded as there was no sham arm in this study. A follow-up study by MacDiarmid et al. concluded that the outcomes of PTNS are durable, as patients completing 12 weekly treatments maintained benefits at 12 months of follow-up [52]. Two recent studies have compared PTNS with sham treatment. Peters et al. found that 54.5 % of patients reported moderate or marked improvement in their symptoms after PTNS, compared with 20.9 % after sham therapy [54]. Finazzi-Agro et al. likewise found a 71 % responder rate in patients completing 12 PTNS sessions, with ≥50 % reduction in UUI episodes denoting a positive response [55].

The effects of PTNS have been evaluated for NDO and pelvic pain. Kabay et al. showed that PTNS treatment in patients with Parkinson's disease and MS resulted in a statistically significant increase in mean volume at first detrusor contraction and MCC [56, 57]. After 12 weeks, the improvements in both urodynamic indices remained statistically significant [58]. PTNS has also been tested in patients with pelvic pain. Kabay et al. randomized 89 patients with therapy-resistant, category IIIB chronic, non-bacterial prostatitis/chronic pelvic pain syndrome to undergo PTNS or sham treatment [59]. An objective response was observed with the pain and symptom scores after 12 weeks of PTNS in 40 % and 67 % of the patients and a partial response was observed in 60 % and 33 % of the patients, respectively. Mean symptom scores and visual analog scores for pain and urgency improved significantly after PTNS treatment, while scores for symptoms, urgency, and pain remained unchanged after sham treatment. Finally, De Gennaro et al. performed PTNS in 23 children (ages 4–17 years) with refractory lower urinary symptoms [36, 60]. Ten patients had idiopathic OAB, seven had non-neurogenic urinary retention, and six had neuropathic bladder. Symptoms improved in the majority of children with idiopathic OAB and non-neurogenic urinary retention, while symptoms and urodynamics did not significantly change in the neuropathic bladder

group. PTNS therapy was well tolerated in the pediatric age group.

Pudendal Nerve Stimulation

The pudendal nerve is a peripheral nerve that is mainly composed of afferent sensory fibers from sacral nerve roots S1–S3, thus contributing significantly to the afferent regulation of bladder function [36]. In 2005, Spinelli et al. described a staged procedure similar to SNM to place a tined lead near the pudendal nerve through a perineal or posterior approach using neurophysiological guidance [61]. Fifteen patients with NDO had a significant reduction in daily incontinence episodes, while eight became continent, two improved by more than 88 %, and two patients reduced the number of incontinence episodes by 50 %. In 12 patients who underwent IPG implantation, 6-month urodynamic evaluation revealed a significant objective improvement in MCC and the maximum pressure decreased. The Bion® device (Boston Scientific, Natick, MA) is an implantable stimulator used with an electrode placed near the pudendal nerve as it exits Alcock's canal, and a pilot study with this device has reported improvements in daily incontinence episodes, pad use, and leakage severity [62]. Peters et al. recently reported outcomes of 55 of 84 patients who continued on chronic pudendal nerve stimulation (PNS) at a median of 24 months [63]. Over the follow-up period, significant improvement was observed in VV, urinary frequency, urgency, and incontinence episodes. Peters et al. also compared SNM to PNS in 30 patients with voiding dysfunction [64]. At the time of SNM implantation, the patients consented to having an additional tined lead placed at the pudendal nerve via a posterior approach and, in a blinded, randomized fashion, each lead was tested for 7 days. Eighty percent of the patients responded, with PNS chosen as a superior lead in 79.2 % and SNM in 20.8 %. The overall reduction in symptoms was significantly higher for PNS (63 %) versus SNM (46 %), and the pudendal lead was superior to the sacral lead for scores relating to pelvic pain, urgency, frequency, and bowel function.

Dorsal Genital Nerve Stimulation

The dorsal nerve of the penis in men and the clitoral nerve in women are the most superficial and terminal branches of the pudendal nerve and are located at the level of the pubic symphysis [65]. As the DGN is a sensory afferent branch of the pudendal nerve, stimulation of this nerve may affect bladder activity. Goldman et al. performed a prospective, multicenter trial of percutaneous dorsal genital nerve stimulation (DGNS) under local anesthesia in 21 women with UUI [66]. Test stimulation was applied to confirm electrode placement and CMG was recorded with and without application of electrical stimulation. A 7-day testing period with the electrode connected to an external pulse generator was performed and was followed by a 3-day posttreatment test period. Percutaneous electrode placement required under 10 min and was well tolerated. Pad weight was reduced by ≥50 % in 76 % of patients and 47 % of subjects reported ≥50 % reduction in daily incontinence episodes. Of the patients with severe urgency at baseline, 81 % experienced ≥50 % improvement. Seven patients experienced nine adverse events ranging from skin irritation to pain and bruising around the electrode exit site. Successful percutaneous DGN electrode implantation using genital-anal reflex guidance has also been described in patients with SCI [67].

Conclusions

Although electrical neurostimulation and neuromodulation to treat symptoms of lower urinary tract dysfunction have been extensively studied, there is a dearth of well-designed, randomized, placebo-controlled studies. Studies are also challenging to compare due to variations in treatment parameters and schedules, definitions of success, and lack of consistent long-term follow-up. Despite these obvious shortcomings in the available data, both neurostimulation and neuromodulation result in 30–50 % clinical success on an intent to treat basis [1]. Neuromodulation, especially, continues to emerge rapidly as a mainstream option in the treatment algorithm for lower urinary tract dysfunction. This therapy may be useful for both refractory OAB symptoms and NOUR, and may have a role in the treatment of NDO, pelvic pain, and in the pediatric population. The adverse event profile is quite favorable. In conclusion, the base of knowledge regarding neurostimulation and neuromodulation continues to grow exponentially, which should only improve our ability as physicians to deliver more therapeutic options to our patients with urinary and pelvic dysfunction.

References

1. van Balken MR, Vergunst H, Bemelmans BL. Electrical stimulation of the bladder. J Urol. 2004; 172:846–51.
2. Caldwell KP. The electrical control of sphincter incompetence. Lancet. 1963;2:174–5.
3. Katona F, Berenyi M. Intravesical transurethral electrotherapy of bladder paralysis. Orv Hetil. 1975;116: 854–6.
4. Wein AJ. Pathophysiology and classification of voiding dysfunction. In: Wein AJ, Kavoussi LR, Novick AC, Partin AW, Peters CA, editors. Campbell-Walsh Urology. 9th ed. Philadelphia: Saunders Elsevier; 2007. p. 1973–85.
5. Morrison J, Birder L, Craggs M, et al. Neural control. In: Abrams P, Cardozo L, Khoury S, Wein AJ, editors. Incontinence. Jersey: Health Publications, Ltd; 2005. p. 363–422.
6. de Groat WC, Theobald RJ. Reflex activation of sympathetic pathways to vesical smooth muscle and parasympathetic ganglia by electrical stimulation of vesical afferents. J Physiol. 1976;259:223–37.
7. de Groat WC. Integrative control of the lower urinary tract: preclinical perspective. Br J Pharmacol. 2006; 147 Suppl 2:S25–40.
8. Andersson KE. Antimuscarinics for treatment of overactive bladder. Lancet Neurol. 2004;3:46–53.
9. Yoshimura N, Chancellor MB. Physiology and pharmacology of the bladder and urethra. In: Wein AJ, Kavoussi LR, Novick AC, Partin AW, Peters CA, editors. Campbell-Walsh Urology. 9th ed. Philadelphia: Saunders Elsevier; 2007. p. 1922–72.
10. Teague CT, Merrill DC. Electric pelvic floor stimulation—mechanism of action. Investig Urol. 1977;15: 65–9.

11. Kohn IJ, Te AE, Kaplan SA. Electrical stimulation and neuromodulation in the treatment of lower urinary tract dysfunction. AUA Update Series 2003, Volume XXII, Lesson 9.

12. Erlandson BE, Magnus F, Sundin J. Intravaginal electrical stimulation. Clinical experiments urethral closure. Scand J Urol Nephrol. 1977;44(Suppl):31–9.

13. Fall M, Erlandson BE, Sundin T, Waagstein F. Intravaginal electrical stimulation. Clinical experiments on bladder inhibition. Scand J Urol Nephrol Suppl. 1977;44:41–7.

14. McGuire EJ, Zhang SC, Horwinski ER, Lytton B. Treatment of motor and sensory detrusor instability by electrical stimulation. J Urol. 1983;129:78–9.

15. Fall M, Lindstrom S. Transcutaneous electrical nerve stimulation in classic and nonulcer interstitial cystitis. Urol Clin North Am. 1994;21:131–9.

16. Lindstrom S, Fall M, Carlsson CA, Erlandson BE. The neurophysiological basis of bladder inhibition in response to intravaginal electrical stimulation. J Urol. 1983;129:405–10.

17. Fall M, Lindstrom S. Electrical stimulation. A physiologic approach to the treatment of urinary incontinence. Urol Clin North Am. 1991;18:393–407.

18. Hasan ST, Robson WA, Pridie AK, Neal DE. Transcutaneous electrical nerve stimulation and temporary S3 neuromodulation in idiopathic detrusor instability. J Urol. 1996;155:2005–11.

19. Bower WF, Moore KH, Adams RD, Shepherd R. A urodynamic study of surface neuromodulation versus sham in detrusor instability and sensory urgency. J Urol. 1998;160:2133–6.

20. Kaplan WE, Richards TW, Richards I. Intravesical transurethral bladder stimulation to increase bladder capacity. J Urol. 1989;142(Pt 2):600–2.

21. Decter RM, Snyder P, Laudermilch C. Transurethral electrical bladder stimulation: a follow-up report. J Urol. 1994;152:812–7.

22. Sand PK, Richardson DA, Staskin DR, et al. Pelvic floor electrical stimulation in the treatment of genuine stress incontinence: a multicenter, placebo-controlled trial. Am J Obstet Gynecol. 1995;173:72–9.

23. Richardson DA, Miller KL, Siegel SW, Karram MM, Blackwood NB, Staskin DR. Pelvic floor electrical stimulation: a comparison of daily and every-other-day therapy for genuine stress incontinence. Urology. 1996;48:110–8.

24. Bent AE, Sand PK, Ostergard DR. Transvaginal electrical stimulation in the treatment of genuine stress incontinence and detrusor instability. Neurourol Urodyn. 1989;8:363–4.

25. Wein AJ, Barrett DM. Voiding function and dysfunction—a logical and practical approach. Chicago: Year Book; 1988.

26. Vasavada SP, Rackley RR. Electrical stimulation for storage and emptying disorders. In: Wein AJ, Kavoussi LR, Novick AC, Partin AW, Peters CA, editors. Campbell-Walsh Urology. 9th ed. Philadelphia: Saunders Elsevier; 2007. p. 2147–67.

27. Hald T, Meier W, Khalili A, Agrawal G, Benton JG, Kantrowitz A. Clinical experience with a radio-linked bladder stimulator. J Urol. 1967;97:73–8.

28. Brindley GS. Physiological considerations in the use of sacral anterior root stimulators. Neurourol Urodyn. 1993;12:485–6.

29. Tanagho EA, Schmidt RA. Electrical stimulation in the clinical management of the neurogenic bladder. J Urol. 1988;140:1331–9.

30. Tanagho EA, Schmidt RA, Orvis BR. Neural stimulation for control of voiding dysfunction: a preliminary report in 22 patients with serious neuropathic voiding disorders. J Urol. 1989;142:340–5.

31. Van Kerrebroeck E, Koldewijn E, Wijkstra H, Debruyne FM. Intradural sacral rhizotomies and implantation of an anterior sacral nerve root stimulator in the treatment of neurogenic bladder dysfunction after spinal cord injury: surgical technique and complications. World J Urol. 1991;9:126–32.

32. Brindley GS. The first 500 patients with sacral anterior root stimulator implants: general description. Paraplegia. 1994;32:795–805.

33. Sauerwein D. Surgical treatment of spastic bladder paralysis in paraplegic patients. Sacral deafferentation with implantation of a sacral anterior root stimulator. Urologe A. 1990;29:196–203.

34. Brindley GS, Polkey CE, Rushton DN, Cardozo L. Sacral anterior root stimulators for bladder control in paraplegia: the first 50 cases. J Neurol Neurosurg Psychiatry. 1986;49:1104–14.

35. Fischer J, Madersbacher H, Zechberger J, Russegger L, Huber A. Sacral anterior root stimulation to promote micturition in transverse spinal cord lesions. Zentralbl Neurochir. 1993;54:77–9.

36. Peters KM. Alternative approaches to sacral nerve stimulation. Int Urogynecol J Pelvic Floor Dysfunct. 2010;21:1559–63.

37. Thompson JH, Sutherland SE, Siegel SW. Sacral neuromodulation: therapy evolution. Indian J Urol. 2010;26:379–84.

38. Starkman JS, Smith CP, Staskin DR. Surgical options for drug-refractory overactive bladder patients. Rev Urol. 2010;12:e97–110.

39. Leng WW, Chancellor MB. How sacral nerve stimulation neuromodulation works. Urol Clin North Am. 2005;32:11–8.

40. Borawski KM, Foster RT, Webster GD, Amundsen CL. Predicting implantation with a neuromodulator using two different test stimulation techniques: a prospective randomized study in urge incontinent women. Neurourol Urodyn. 2007;26:14–8.

41. Van Kerrebroeck PE, van Voskuilen AC, Heesakkers JP, et al. Results of sacral neuromodulation therapy for urinary voiding dysfunction: outcomes of a prospective, worldwide clinical study. J Urol. 2007;178:2029–34.

42. Marcelissen TA, Leong RK, de Bie RA, van Kerrebroeck PE, de Wachter SG. Long-term results of sacral neuromodulation with the tined lead procedure. J Urol. 2010;184:1997–2000.

43. Kessler TM, La Framboise D, Trelle S, et al. Sacral neuromodulation for neurogenic lower urinary tract dysfunction: systematic review and meta-analysis. Eur Urol. 2010;58:865–74.
44. Herbison GP, Arnold EP. Sacral neuromodulation with implanted devices for urinary storage and voiding dysfunction in adults. Cochrane Database Syst Rev. 2009;2:CD004202.
45. Pettit P. Current opinion: complications and troubleshooting of sacral neuromodulation. Int Urogynecol J Pelvic Floor Dysfunct. 2010;21:S491–6.
46. Leong RK, Marcelissen TA, Nieman FH, De Bie RA, Van Kerrebroeck PE, De Wachter SG. Satisfaction and patient experience with sacral neuromodulation: results of a single center sample survey. J Urol. 2011;185:588–92.
47. Comiter CV. Sacral neuromodulation for the symptomatic treatment of refractory interstitial cystitis: a prospective study. J Urol. 2003;169:1369–73.
48. Marinkovic SP, Gillen LM, Marinkovic CM. Minimum 6-year outcomes for interstitial cystitis treated with sacral neuromodulation. Int Urogynecol J Pelvic Floor Dysfunct. 2011;22:407–12.
49. Sievert KD, Amend B, Gakis G, et al. Early sacral neuromodulation prevents urinary incontinence after complete spinal cord injury. Ann Neurol. 2010;67:74–84.
50. Marinkovic SP, Gillen LM. Sacral neuromodulation for multiple sclerosis patients with urinary retention and clean intermittent catheterization. Int Urogynecol J Pelvic Floor Dysfunct. 2010;21:223–8.
51. Govier FE, Litwiller S, Nitti V, Kreder KJ, Rosenblatt P. Percutaneous afferent neuromodulation for the refractory overactive bladder: results of a multicenter study. J Urol. 2001;165:1193–8.
52. MacDiarmid SA, Peters KM, Shobeiri SA, et al. Long-term durability of percutaneous tibial nerve stimulation for the treatment of overactive bladder. J Urol. 2010;183:234–40.
53. Peters KM, MacDiarmid SA, Wooldridge LS, et al. Randomized trial of percutaneous tibial nerve stimulation versus extended-release tolterodine: results from the Overactive Bladder Innovative Therapy trial. J Urol. 2009;182:1055–61.
54. Peters KM, Carrico DJ, Perez-Marrero RA, et al. Randomized trial of percutaneous tibial nerve stimulation versus sham efficacy in the treatment of overactive bladder syndrome: results from the SUmiT trial. J Urol. 2010;183:1438–43.
55. Finazzi-Agro E, Petta F, Sciobica F, Pasqualetti P, Musco S, Bove P. Percutaneous tibial nerve stimulation effects on detrusor overactivity incontinence are not due to a placebo effect: a randomized, double-blind, placebo controlled trial. J Urol. 2010;184:2001–6.
56. Kabay SC, Kabay S, Yucel M, Ozden H. Acute urodynamic effects of percutaneous posterior tibial nerve stimulation on neurogenic detrusor overactivity in patients with Parkinson's disease. Neurourol Urodyn. 2009;28:62–7.
57. Kabay SC, Yucel M, Kabay S. Acute effect of posterior tibial nerve stimulation on neurogenic detrusor overactivity in patients with multiple sclerosis: urodynamic study. Urology. 2008;71:641–5.
58. Kabay S, Kabay SC, Yucel M, et al. The clinical and urodynamic results of a 3-month percutaneous posterior tibial nerve stimulation treatment in patients with multiple sclerosis-related neurogenic bladder dysfunction. Neurourol Urodyn. 2009;28:964–8.
59. Kabay S, Kabay SC, Yucel M, Ozden H. Efficiency of posterior tibial nerve stimulation in category IIIB chronic prostatitis/chronic pelvic pain: a sham-controlled comparative study. Urol Int. 2009;83:33–8.
60. De Gennaro M, Capitanucci ML, Mastracci P, Silveri M, Gatti C, Mosiello G. Percutaneous tibial nerve neuromodulation is well tolerated in children and effective in treating refractory vesical dysfunction. J Urol. 2004;171:1911–3.
61. Spinelli M, Malaguti S, Giardiello G, Lazzeri M, Tarantola J, Van Den Hombergh U. A new minimally invasive procedure for pudendal nerve stimulation to treat neurogenic bladder: description of the method and preliminary data. Neurourol Urodyn. 2005;24:305–9.
62. Groen J, Amiel C, Ruud Bosch JL. Chronic pudendal nerve neuromodulation in women with idiopathic refractory detrusor overactivity incontinence: results of a pilot study with a novel minimally invasive implantable mini-stimulator. Neurourol Urodyn. 2005;24:226–30.
63. Peters KM, Killinger KA, Boguslawski BM, Boura JA. Chronic pudendal neuromodulation: expanding available treatment options for refractory urologic symptoms. Neurourol Urodyn. 2010;29:1267–71.
64. Peters KM, Feber KM, Bennett RC. Sacral versus pudendal nerve stimulation for voiding dysfunction: a prospective, single-blinded, randomized, crossover trial. Neurourol Urodyn. 2005;24:643–7.
65. Vasavada SP, Goldman HB, Rackley RR. Neuromodulation techniques: a comparison of available new therapies. Curr Urol Rep. 2007;8:455–60.
66. Goldman HB, Amundsen CL, Mangel J, et al. Dorsal genital nerve stimulation for the treatment of overactive bladder symptoms. Neurourol Urodyn. 2008;27:499–503.
67. Martens FM, Heesakkers JP, Rijkhoff NJ. Minimal invasive electrode implantation for conditional stimulation of the dorsal genital nerve in neurogenic detrusor overactivity. Spinal Cord. 2011;49:566–72.

Surgery for Bladder Outlet Obstruction in the Male

15

Alex Gomelsky and Roger R. Dmochowski

The term benign prostatic hypertrophy (BPH) refers to a histological condition that involves the presence of stromal–glandular hyperplasia within the prostate gland [1]. BPH is clinically significant when it is associated with lower urinary tract symptoms (LUTS), which in turn may be related to urinary storage or emptying. The relationship between BPH and LUTS is incompletely understood, as not all men with BPH develop bothersome LUTS and men with significant LUTS may not have histological BPH. The relationship of benign prostatic enlargement (BPE) to BPH and LUTS is likewise incompletely understood [1]. Finally, bladder outlet obstruction (BOO) refers to the pressure gradient that develops between the bladder neck/prostatic urethra and the bladder, resulting in urethral compression, compromised urinary outflow, and potential compromise of the upper urinary tracts [1]. While BOO has most commonly been associated with BPH/BPE, primary bladder neck obstruction is another condition potentially responsible for BOO. The objective is to review the surgical treatment options for BOO in the male. Contracture of the

bladder neck after radical prostatectomy, urethral stricture disease, and external sphincter dyssynergia are additional factors potentially responsible for BOO, but will not be discussed further.

Evaluation of LUTS/BPH/BPE

Several longitudinal studies have demonstrated that symptom progression associated with BPH increases with advancing age. The Olmstead County Study cited an annual increase in the AUA Symptom Score (AUASS) of 0.34 points in men followed over 7 years [2], while the Medical Therapy of Prostatic Symptoms (MTOPS) study found a 17.4 % rate of clinical symptom progression in men followed for 4 years [3]. Symptom progression in the study was defined as an increase in AUASS ≥ 4 points, acute urinary retention (AUR), urinary incontinence, recurrent urinary tract infection (UTI), or renal insufficiency. In light of the significant potential for symptom progression, multiple diagnostic and therapeutic options are available for the male with BPH/LUTS.

The AUA Guideline Panel on the Management of BPH is one group that has made recommendations regarding the initial evaluation of male LUTS [4]. All men presenting with LUTS suggestive of BPH should undergo a medical history focusing on the urinary tract, previous surgical procedures, and medical conditions and symptoms that lead to bladder dysfunction or polyuria.

A. Gomelsky, M.D.
Department of Urology, LSU Health—Shreveport, Shreveport, LA, USA

R.R. Dmochowski, M.D., M.M.H.C. (✉)
Department of Urologic Surgery, Vanderbilt University Medical Center, A1302 Medical Center North, Nashville, TN 37232-2765, USA
e-mail: roger.dmochowski@vanderbilt.edu

A.J. Wein et al. (eds.), *Bladder Dysfunction in the Adult: The Basis for Clinical Management*, Current Clinical Urology, DOI 10.1007/978-1-4939-0853-0_15, © Springer Science+Business Media New York 2014

A family history of BPH and prostate cancer should be elicited, and fitness for a possible surgical procedure should be assessed. Digital rectal examination (DRE) should evaluate for the presence of locally advanced prostate cancer and a focused neurologic examination should assess the patient's general mental status, ambulatory status, lower extremity neuromuscular function, and anal sphincter tone. A dipstick urinalysis ± microscopic examination should screen for hematuria and UTI. Finally, AUASS should be administered, as this scale has been found to be superior to an unstructured interview in quantifying symptom frequency and severity [5]. Optional tests following the initial evaluation include urinary flow rate recording and measurement of post-void residual urine (PVR). These tests were felt to be helpful in patients with a complex medical history (e.g., neurologic or other diseases known to affect bladder function or prior failure of BPH therapy) and in those desiring invasive therapy.

The 6th International Consultation on New Developments in Prostate Cancer and Prostate Disease also recently published its recommendations regarding the initial evaluation of LUTS in men [6]. The recommended tests (history, physical examination, assessment of symptom bother, and urinalysis) were the same as those recommended by the AUA BPH Guidelines Panel. The International Panel also recommended a serum prostate-specific antigen (PSA) in those men with a life expectancy exceeding 10 years or when a diagnosis of prostate cancer can modify the management, as well as a frequency–volume chart in those men with nocturia as a predominant symptom. Additionally, the International Panel recommended validated questionnaires, frequency–volume charting, urinary flow rate recording, and PVR for those men with persistent bothersome LUTS after basic management. Furthermore, pressure-flow studies were recommended prior to invasive therapy, unless the maximum flow rate on noninvasive flow recording is <10 mL/s. Previous studies have likewise suggested that a flow rate <8 mL/s is highly

predictive of BOO [7]. Optional tests include imaging of the prostate with transabdominal or transrectal ultrasound, upper urinary tract imaging with ultrasound or intravenous urography, and endoscopy of the lower urinary tract.

The AUA Guideline Panel on the Management of BPH also made recommendations regarding the treatment of LUTS in men [4]. As a standard, the Panel recommended a strategy of watchful waiting for men with mild symptoms (AUASS < 7) and men with moderate or severe symptoms (AUASS > 8) whose symptoms do not interfere with activities of daily living. For men with bothersome moderate to severe symptoms of BPH (AUASS > 8), therapeutic options include watchful waiting and medical, minimally invasive, or surgical therapies. Over the last decade, the use of surgical intervention for BPH has steadily declined, while medical therapy with alpha-adrenergic antagonists (α-blockers) and 5-alpha reductase inhibitors (5-ARIs) has become the most popular option in clinical practice [8]. However, for men developing AUR, UTIs, signs of upper tract compromise, and failure or dissatisfaction with more conservative therapy, surgery remains an important component of the treatment algorithm. Data has confirmed that even if men with AUR successfully pass a trial of voiding, they are still at an increased risk of requiring surgery within the next year [9–11].

Surgical Management of BPH

Surgical intervention is an appropriate treatment alternative for patients with moderate to severe LUTS and for patients who have developed AUR or other BPH-related complications [4]. By definition, surgery is the most invasive option for BPH management and, generally, patients will have failed medical therapy before proceeding with surgery. However, medical therapy should not be viewed as a prerequisite to surgery, as some patients may opt to pursue surgical therapy as a primary treatment if their symptoms are particularly bothersome.

Transurethral Resection of the Prostate

Transurethral resection of the prostate (TURP) is considered the gold standard for surgical treatment because its efficacy is supported by the most data [4]. TURP is usually performed under general or spinal anesthesia and involves the surgical removal of the prostate's inner portion via a cystoscopic resection with a monopolar loop [4]. One unique complication of TURP is TUR syndrome, a dilutional hyponatremia that occurs when irrigant solution is absorbed through prostatic sinuses into the bloodstream. An update of MEDLINE literature regarding TURP complications compared recent results (2000–2005) with early results (1979–1994) [12]. Technological improvements such as video TUR have helped to reduce perioperative complications (recent vs. early) such as transfusion rate (0.4 % vs. 7.1 %), TUR syndrome (0 % vs. 1.1 %), clot retention (2 % vs. 5 %), and UTI (1.7 % vs. 8.2 %). Late iatrogenic stress urinary incontinence was rare (<0.5 %). Despite the age of men undergoing TURP increasing in the recent time period, the associated morbidity remained <1 % with a mortality rate of 0–2.5 %. The major late complications were development of urethral strictures (2.2–9.8 %) and bladder neck contractures (0.3–9.2 %). The retreatment rate was 3–14.5 % after 5 years. Bipolar resection of the prostate utilizes a specialized resectoscope loop that incorporates both the active and the return electrodes and the bipolar loop can be used to resect tissue as well as coagulate and vaporize tissue [4]. This design limits the dispersal of the current flow in the body which theoretically reduces the deleterious effects of the stray current. Furthermore, because the bipolar resectoscope uses 0.9 % sodium chloride solution as irrigation fluid, the risk of TUR syndrome is eliminated. The AUA Guidelines Panel classified TURP as an *option* and as an appropriate and effective primary alternative for surgical therapy in men with moderate to severe LUTS and/or those who are significantly bothered by these symptoms [4]. A recent review of the literature by Mamoulakis

et al. concluded that bipolar TURP shares similar efficacy with monopolar TURP and that the urethral stricture rates were not significantly different between the monopolar and bipolar arms [13]. The AUA Panel suggested that the choice of a monopolar or bipolar approach should be based on the patient's presentation and anatomy, the surgeon's experience, and discussion of the potential risks and likely benefits [4].

Open Prostatectomy

Open prostatectomy, or surgical enucleation of the inner prostate, was deemed an *option* by the AUA Guidelines Panel and was found to be an appropriate and effective treatment alternative for men with moderate to severe LUTS and/or those with significant symptom bother [4]. The choice of approach should be based on the patient's individual presentation and anatomy, the surgeon's experience, and discussion of the potential benefit and risks for complications. The Panel noted that there is usually a longer hospital stay and a larger loss of blood associated with open procedures. The Panel noted that open prostatectomies may be needed only for men with very enlarged prostate glands and for men with bladder diverticula or stones [4].

Laser-Assisted Therapy

Alternative technologies such as laser-assisted TURP were reported to offer lower morbidities but were typically still performed in the operating room setting and require anesthesia [4]. Current surgical options for BPH management include transurethral holmium laser ablation of the prostate (HoLAP), transurethral holmium laser enucleation of the prostate (HoLEP), holmium laser resection of the prostate (HoLRP), photoselective vaporization of the prostate (PVP), transurethral incision of the prostate (TUIP), and transurethral vaporization of the prostate (TUVP).

The holmium laser has a wavelength of 2140 nm that is strongly absorbed by water. The laser has a relatively shallow depth of penetration

(0.4 mm) that results in precise tissue vaporization. This also minimizes deep coagulation or char effect. HoLEP involves transurethrally enucleating the lobes of the prostate with an end-firing laser and then removing the floating lobes with a transurethral morcellator. In a review of over 5,000 men undergoing HoLEP, Kuntz cited longer operative times than the TURP, but lower intraoperative blood loss and shorter hospitalization and urethral catheterization times in favor of HoLEP [14]. Despite durable results obtained with HoLEP at 3- and 4-year follow-up, this procedure may have a steep learning curve which may limit its routine adoption [15, 16]. HoLAP with a 100-W laser may have a shorter learning curve owing to its side-firing laser. PVP uses an 80-W potassium titanyl phosphate ("green light") laser that emits a 532-nm wavelength that is selectively absorbed by hemoglobin. The depth of penetration is 2–4 mm, which may be associated with a transient dysuria [17]. Malek et al. also reported durable improvements in AUASS, quality of life (QoL) score, maximum flow rate (Q_{max}), and PVR for up to 5 years [17].

In a recent systematic literature review, Lourenco et al. identified 45 randomized, controlled trials (RCTs) encompassing nearly 4,000 patients that included TURP as one of the treatment arms [18]. None of the newer technologies resulted in significantly greater improvements in symptoms than TURP at 12 months, although a trend suggested a better outcome with HoLEP and worse outcome with laser vaporization. Improvements in secondary measures such as Q_{max} were consistent with change in symptoms. Blood transfusion rates were higher for TURP than for the newer methods (4.8 % vs. 0.7 %) and hospital stay was up to 1 day shorter for the newer methods.

After review of the literature, the AUA Panel deemed the following laser therapies as an *option*: HoLRP, HoLEP, HoLAP, and PVP [4]. These are appropriate and effective treatment alternatives to TURP and open prostatectomy in men with moderate to severe LUTS and/or those who are significantly bothered by these symptoms. The choice of approach should be based on the patient's presentation and anatomy, the surgeon's level of training and experience, and a discussion of the potential benefit and risks for complications.

Generally, transurethral laser approaches have been associated with shorter catheterization time and length of stay, with comparable improvements in LUTS [4]. There is a decreased risk of perioperative TUR syndrome. Information concerning certain outcomes, including retreatment rates and incidence of postoperative urethral strictures, is limited due to short follow-up. The Panel cautioned that, as with all new devices, comparison of outcomes between studies should be considered carefully given the rapid evolution in technologies and power levels. Emerging evidence suggests a possible role of transurethral enucleation and laser vaporization as options for men with very large prostates (>100 g) [4].

Other Surgical Options

In the TUIP procedure, one or two cuts are made in the prostate and prostatic capsule, reducing constriction of the urethra [4]. Lourenco et al. performed a systematic review to evaluate the comparative effectiveness of this procedure and the TURP [19]. The review included data from 795 randomized patients across ten RCTs of moderate to poor quality. There was no statistical difference in the degree of symptomatic improvement between the two procedures, while TURP was associated with higher Q_{max} and higher rates of transfusion and TUR syndrome. Rates of AUR, UTI, incontinence, and urethral stricture formation did not differ between the two approaches. The AUA Panel characterized TUIP as an *option* and an appropriate and effective treatment alternative in men with moderate to severe LUTS and/or who are significantly bothered by these symptoms when prostate size is less than 30 mL [4]. Likewise, TUVP with a rollerball electrode was characterized as an *option* for men with moderate to severe symptoms and/or significant bother [4]. Compared to TURP, TUVP resulted in equivalent, short-term improvements in AUASS, Q_{max}, and QoL indices [4]. There is a decreased risk of TUR syndrome compared with traditional monopolar TURP. However, the rates of postoperative storage and voiding symptoms, dysuria, and AUR, as well as the need for unplanned secondary catheterization, appear to be higher after TUVP. Reoperation rates were also higher with TUVP than with TURP. Long-term comparative trials are currently lacking.

Minimally Invasive Technology

Minimally invasive therapies include transurethral needle ablation (TUNA) and transurethral microwave thermotherapy (TUMT). During a TUNA procedure, radiofrequency energy is used to treat the prostatic tissue. Selected literature has suggested that this modality may be most suitable for men with mild to moderate symptoms and prostate volumes <60 mL [20]. While morbidity may be low, TUNA may be associated with a retreatment rate that exceeds 80 % at 10 years [21]. Bouza et al. performed a meta-analysis on TUNA therapy that included 35 studies [22]. TUNA improved AUASS and QoL scores by 50–60 % from baseline and provided a 30–35 % improvement in objective parameters (PVR and Q_{max}). The retreatment rate of men undergoing TUNA was 7.44 times higher than that of those men undergoing TURP; however, the complication rates after TUNA were significantly lower than after TURP. Hoffman et al. performed a meta-analysis comparing TUMT with TURP [23]. The pooled mean AUASS decreased by 65 % after TUMT and by 77 % after TURP, while Q_{max} increased by 70 % after TUMT and 119 % after TURP. Complications such as retrograde ejaculation, transfusion rate, and treatment of strictures were all significantly higher after TURP. The retreatment rate, however, was significantly higher after TUMT. The AUA Guidelines Panel classified both TUNA and TUMT as an *option*, as both were found to be effective in partially relieving LUTS secondary to BPH and may be considered in men with moderate or severe symptoms [4].

Primary Bladder Neck Obstruction

Primary bladder neck obstruction (PBNO) is an infrequently diagnosed cause of lower urinary tract dysfunction that is mainly found in men younger than 50 years of age. In PBNO, the bladder neck fails to open adequately during voiding, in the absence of other anatomic obstruction [24]. Complaints may range from urinary storage symptoms, such as urinary urgency, frequency, and nocturia, to voiding symptoms, such as hesitancy, intermittency, and decreased force of stream. Men may also present with AUR and its sequelae, such as bladder stones and diverticula, UTIs, and upper tract compromise. It is this wide spectrum of symptoms that makes the diagnosis of PBNO challenging. Furthermore, the correct diagnosis is frequently delayed by ineffective treatment with antibiotics and anti-inflammatory medications [24]. Several theories have been proposed to elucidate the etiology of PBNO. Structural changes at the bladder neck have been attributed to fibrous narrowing or hyperplasia [25], faulty dissolution of bladder neck mesenchyme [26], and abnormal morphologic arrangement of detrusor/trigonal musculature [27]. Neurological theories proposed by Awad et al. and Crowe et al. have focused on variations in the sympathetic innervation of the bladder neck [28, 29]. Today, PBNO is a video-urodynamic diagnosis consisting of high voiding detrusor pressure, low uroflow, radiographic evidence of obstruction at the bladder neck, relaxation (quiescence) of the external sphincter during voiding, and absence of obstruction distal to the bladder neck [24].

While watchful waiting is a potential therapeutic option for men with low symptom bother and absence of upper tract changes, α-blockers are the mainstay of therapy due to their inhibitory effects on the bladder neck smooth muscle. Surgical intervention involves transurethral incision of the bladder neck (TUIBN). While various techniques and modifications have been reported [30], the most common variant of this procedure involves incising the bladder neck with a Collins knife at the 5 and/or 7 o'clock positions. The incisions begin distal to each ureteral orifice and extend just proximal to the verumontanum until fat is reached [31]. Bilateral incision has been associated with an 80–90 % subjective success rate and a significant improvement in Q_{max} [32, 33]. The most concerning adverse event after TUIBN is retrograde ejaculation, which may be especially worrisome in young men and those requiring future fertility.

While bilateral incision has been associated with variable degrees of retrograde ejaculation [32–34], unilateral incision may achieve similar subjective and objective outcomes while preserving antegrade ejaculation [35].

Conclusions

While medical therapy is the mainstay for treatment of men with bothersome BPH/LUTS, a role remains for surgical treatment of medical failures or men with AUR, UTIs, or signs of upper tract compromise. TURP is the "gold standard" against which all other surgical procedures are compared and is associated with durable improvements in Q_{max}, PVR, AUASS, and QoL scores. Novel technology such as the bipolar electrode have decreased or eliminated significant complications, such as bleeding and TUR syndrome. Laser-assisted technologies have also decreased the incidence of serious complications but may be associated with a significant learning curve. While long-term outcomes are thus far absent in the literature, initial comparisons with the TURP are promising. Minimally invasive procedures such as TUNA and TUMT may be performed in the office setting and may also be considered for men with bothersome LUTS. TUIBN is the surgical procedure of choice in men with PBNO, and unilateral incision may significantly decrease the incidence of retrograde ejaculation.

References

1. Roehrborn CG. Benign prostatic hyperplasia: an overview. Rev Urol. 2005;7 Suppl 9:S3–14.
2. Jacobsen SJ, Girman CJ, Jacobson DJ, et al. Long-term (92-month) natural history of changes in lower urinary tract symptom severity. J Urol. 2000;163 Suppl 4:248–9.
3. McConnell JD, Roehrborn CG, Bautista OM, et al. The long-term effect of doxazosin, finasteride, and combination therapy on the clinical progression of benign prostatic hyperplasia. N Engl J Med. 2003;349:2387–98.
4. McVary KT, Roehrborn CG, Avins AL, et al. American Urological Association guideline: management of benign prostatic hyperplasia (BPH). Linthicum, MD: American Urological Association, Education and Research, Inc.; 2010.
5. Barry MJ, Fowler Jr FJ, O'Leary MP, et al. The American Urological Association symptom index for benign prostatic hyperplasia. The Measurement Committee of the American Urological Association. J Urol. 1992;148:1549–57.
6. Abrams P, Chapple C, Khoury S, Roehrborn C, de la Rosette J. Evaluation and treatment of lower urinary tract symptoms in older men. J Urol. 2008;181: 1779–87.
7. Ockrim JL, Laniado ME, Patel A, Tubaro A, St Clair Carter S. A probability based system for combining simple office parameters as a predictor of bladder outflow obstruction. J Urol. 2001;166:2221–5.
8. Sarma AV, Jacobson DJ, McGree ME, Roberts RO, Lieber MM, Jacobsen SJ. A population based study of incidence and treatment of benign prostatic hyperplasia among residents of Olmstead County, Minnesota: 1987 to 1997. J Urol. 2005;173:2048–53.
9. Pickard R, Emberton M, Neal DE. The management of men with acute urinary retention. Br J Urol. 1998; 81:712–20.
10. Choong S, Emberton M. Acute urinary retention. BJU Int. 2000;85:186–201.
11. Desgrandchamps F, de la Taille A, Doublet JD. The management of acute urinary retention in France: a cross-sectional survey in 2618 men with benign prostatic hyperplasia. BJU Int. 2006;97:727–33.
12. Rassweiler J, Teber D, Kuntz R, Hofmann R. Complications of transurethral resection of the prostate (TURP)—incidence, management, and prevention. Eur Urol. 2006;50:969–80.
13. Mamoulakis C, Trompetter M, de la Rosette J. Bipolar transurethral resection of the prostate: the 'golden standard' reclaims its leading position. Curr Opin Urol. 2009;19:26–32.
14. Kuntz RM. Current role of lasers in the treatment of benign prostatic hyperplasia (BPH). Eur Urol. 2006; 49:961–9.
15. Ahyai SA, Lehrich K, Kuntz RM. Holmium laser enucleation versus transurethral resection of the prostate: 3-year follow-up results of a randomized clinical trial. Eur Urol. 2007;52:1456–63.
16. Westenberg A, Gilling P, Kennett K, Frampton C, Fraundorfer M. Holmium laser resection of the prostate versus transurethral resection of the prostate: results of a randomized trial with 4-year minimum long-term followup. J Urol. 2004;172:616–9.
17. Malek RS, Kuntzman RS, Barrett DM. Photoselective potassium-titanyl-phosphate laser vaporization of the benign obstructive prostate: observations on long-term outcomes. J Urol. 2005;174:1344–8.
18. Lourenco T, Pickard R, Vale L, et al. Alternative approaches to endoscopic ablation for benign enlargement of the prostate: systematic review of randomised controlled trials. BMJ. 2008;337:a449.
19. Lourenco T, Shaw M, Fraser C, MacLennan G, N'Dow J, Pickard R. The clinical effectiveness of transurethral incision of the prostate: a systematic review of randomised controlled trials. World J Urol. 2010;28:23–32.

20. Roehrborn CG, Issa M, Bruskewitz RC, et al. Transurethral needle ablation for benign prostatic hyperplasia: 12-month results of a prospective, multicenter U.S. study. Urology. 1998;51:415–21.

21. Rosario DJ, Phillips JT, Chapple CR. Durability and cost-effectiveness of transurethral needle ablation of the prostate as an alternative to transurethral resection when alpha-adrenergic antagonist therapy fails. J Urol. 2007;177:1047–51.

22. Bouza C, Lopez T, Magro A, Navalpotro L, Amate JM. Systematic review and meta-analysis of transurethral needle ablation in symptomatic benign prostatic hyperplasia. BMC Urol. 2006;6:14.

23. Hoffman RM, MacDonald R, Monga M, Wilt TJ. Transurethral microwave thermotherapy vs transurethral resection for treating benign prostatic hyperplasia: a systematic review. BJU Int. 2004;94:1031–6.

24. Huckabay C, Nitti VW. Diagnosis and treatment of primary bladder neck obstruction in men. Curr Bladder Dysfunct Rep. 2006;1:47–51.

25. Marion G. Surgery of the neck of the bladder. Br J Urol. 1933;5:351–7.

26. Leadbetter Jr GW, Leadbetter WF. Diagnosis and treatment of congenital bladder-neck obstruction in children. N Engl J Med. 1959;260:633–7.

27. Turner-Warwick R, Whiteside CG, Worth PH, Milroy EJ, Bates CP. A urodynamic view of the clinical problems associated with bladder neck dysfunction and its treatment by endoscopic incision and trans-trigonal posterior prostatectomy. Br J Urol. 1973;45:44–59.

28. Awad SA, Downie JW, Lywood DW, Young RA, Jarzylo SV. Sympathetic activity in the proximal urethra in patients with urinary obstruction. J Urol. 1976;115:545–7.

29. Crowe R, Noble J, Robson T, Soediono P, Milroy EJ, Burnstock G. An increase in neuropeptide Y but not nitric acid synthase-immunoreactive nerves in the bladder neck from male patients with bladder neck dyssynergia. J Urol. 1995;154:1231–6.

30. Kraus SP, Smith CP, Boone TB. Primary bladder neck obstruction in the male. AUA Update Series. Linthicum, MD: American Urological Association, Education and Research; 2000; Vol. XIX: Lesson 8.

31. Sirls LT, Ganabathi K, Zimmern PE, Roskamp DA, Wolde-Tsadik G, Leach GE. Transurethral incision of the prostate: an objective and subjective evaluation of long-term efficacy. J Urol. 1993;150:1615–21.

32. Christensen MG, Nordling J, Anderson JT, Hald T. Functional bladder neck obstruction results of endoscopic bladder neck incision in 131 consecutive patients. Br J Urol. 1985;57:60–2.

33. Norlen LJ, Blaivas JG. Unsuspected proximal urethral obstruction in young and middle-aged men. J Urol. 1986;135:972–6.

34. Trockman BA, Gerspach J, Dmochowski R, Haab F, Zimmern PE, Leach GE. Primary bladder neck obstruction in men: urodynamic findings and treatment results in 36 men. J Urol. 1996;156:1418–20.

35. Kaplan SA, Te AE, Jacobz BZ. Urodynamic evidence of vesical neck obstruction in men with misdiagnosed chronic nonbacterial prostatitis and the therapeutic role of endoscopic incision of the bladder neck. J Urol. 1994;152:2063–5.

Alex Gomelsky and Roger R. Dmochowski

Pathophysiology of Stress Urinary Incontinence

Stress urinary incontinence (SUI) is defined by the International Continence Society as the involuntary loss of urine through an intact urethra in response to a sudden increase in intra-abdominal pressure, in the absence of a detrusor contraction or an overdistended bladder [1]. It is accepted that continence depends on the interaction of urethral and bladder neck support, intrinsic urethral properties, urethral sphincter mechanism, and pelvic floor musculature. At rest, a "mucosal" seal composed of submucosal connective tissue and luminal secretions from the periurethral glands forms a watertight closure by compressing mucosal urethral folds. During stress maneuvers, a reflex contraction of the levator ani musculature and urogenital diaphragm elevates suburethral supporting tissue and compresses the proximal urethra ("hammock hypothesis") [2]. Additionally, the urethropelvic ligaments augment the muscular closure of the pelvic floor by enveloping the proximal urethra and bladder neck medially and

A. Gomelsky, M.D.
Department of Urology, LSU Health—Shreveport, Shreveport, LA, USA

R.R. Dmochowski, M.D., M.M.H.C. (✉)
Department of Urologic Surgery, Vanderbilt University Medical Center, A1302 Medical Center North, Nashville, TN 37232-2765, USA
e-mail: roger.dmochowski@vanderbilt.edu

inserting laterally onto the arcus tendineus fascia pelvis. Finally, striated muscles in the urethrovaginal sphincter and compressor urethrae compress the urethra during stress maneuvers. The net effect of these changes is equal transmission of abdominal pressure to the bladder and urethra, leading to increased outlet resistance and continence. Conversely, in women with loss of anatomic support, the proximal urethra descends during stress maneuvers and rotates inferiorly and anteriorly.

A novel continence mechanism proposed by Petros and Ulmsten suggested that the mid-urethra, rather than the bladder neck, may be the linchpin for urinary continence [3]. Their "integral theory" proposed that contraction of the pubococcygeus muscle pulls the anterior vaginal wall forward and closes off the urethra during an increase in intra-abdominal pressure. This response is contingent on an intact attachment between the anterior vaginal wall and the pubo-urethral ligaments, which act as a fulcrum at the mid-urethra. Laxity in the pubourethral ligaments contributes to incontinence during increases in intra-abdominal pressure.

The purpose of anti-incontinence surgery is to prevent involuntary urine loss during periods of increased intra-abdominal pressure. Procedures can be broadly divided into several classes, based on the mechanism they address. Buttress operations, such as anterior colporrhaphy and Kelly plication, support the urethrovesical junction by plicating the pubocervical fascia. Bladder neck suspensions (retropubic needle suspensions (RBNS) and transvaginal needle suspensions (TNS)) provide support by suspending and elevating tissues on either side of the urethra. Slings placed at the bladder neck (PVS) not only replace and augment normal lateral urethral support structures but also buttress the bladder neck to prevent descent and funneling during stress maneuvers. Mid-urethral slings (MUS; retropubic (RP) and transobturator (TO)) support the mid-urethra in a tension-free fashion to prevent SUI. Finally, urethral bulking procedures augment the "mucosal seal" mechanism to aid effective apposition of the urethra in a watertight fashion.

Outcomes of Surgical Procedures for SUI

A Cochrane review summarized the outcomes of ten trials encompassing 1,012 women, of whom 385 underwent anterior vaginal repair (AR) [4]. In eight trials comparing AR to RBNS, the subjective failure rates were lower for women undergoing RBNS at all follow-up periods: short term (10 % vs. 19 %), medium term (16 % vs. 36 %), and long term (28 % vs. 53 %). Objective cure rates were likewise lower for women undergoing RBNS at all follow-up periods: short term (10 % vs. 25 %), medium term (19 % vs. 44 %), and long term (26 % vs. 54 %). In six trials comparing AR with Burch colposuspension in women with concomitant pelvic organ prolapse (POP), women undergoing Burch had lower medium-term and long-term subjective failure rates than women undergoing AR. More women who underwent AR (23 %) required repeat anti-incontinence surgery when compared with women undergoing Burch (2 %). In three trials, women undergoing AR (35 %) and TNS (32 %) had similar subjective incontinence rates after 1 year; however, these trials may have been underpowered to detect a statistical difference. There were no trials comparing AR with sham procedure, lap RBNS, PVS, or MUS. At this time, AR is not considered a standard for the treatment of SUI in women.

TNS procedures include the Gittes, Pereyra, Stamey, and Raz suspensions. Additionally, some surgeons have modified these operations by varying the site of initial approach (abdominal vs. vaginal) and incorporating spacers or sheaths. A Cochrane database evaluating the efficacy of TNS included ten trials encompassing 864 women, 375 of whom underwent one of six different TNS procedures [5]. There were no studies comparing TNS with a sham procedure or conservative intervention. TNS was compared with RBNS in seven trials, and fewer women did not achieve subjective cure after RBNS (10.8 %) than after TNS (15.3 %) in short-term follow-up [5, 6]. A similar relationship was seen in medium-term (13.7 % vs. 22.7 %) and long-term (18.2 % vs. 56.7 %) follow-up. Likewise, fewer women did not achieve objective cure after RBNS than after TNS in short-term (8.7 % vs. 14.4 %), medium-term (12.9 % vs. 21 %), and long-term follow-up (18.2 % vs. 56.7 %). A single study comparing TNS and PVS was underpowered to detect a statistical difference. As with AR, TNS are not currently considered a standard for surgical treatment of SUI in women.

RBNS have been evaluated extensively in another Cochrane review that encompassed 39 trials and 3,301 women [6]. In two small trials, women undergoing RBNS had higher subjective and objective cure rates than women undergoing pelvic floor muscle training. In the Cochrane review, RBNS was compared to sling procedures in 12 trials encompassing 945 women [6]. Seven trials compared RBNS to the tension-free vaginal tape (TVT), while five trials compared RBNS to a PVS constructed from different materials. In three of these trials with short-term follow-up, there was no significant difference in subjective failure between RBNS and a sling procedure. Likewise, in three different trials with medium-term follow-up, there was no significant difference in subjective failure rates between RBNS and slings. Objective failure rates between RBNS and slings were not significantly different in short-term and medium-term follow-up periods. Two trials have reported long-term outcomes comparing Burch colposuspension and slings [7, 8]. In a small trial of 28 women, objective cure rates were not statistically different (84.6 % vs. 100 %) for Burch and polytetrafluoroethylene (PTFE) sling, respectively [7]. In a large, high-quality trial, Ward and Hilton reported no significant difference in objective SUI cure between women undergoing TVT (81 %) and Burch (90 %) at a 5-year follow-up [8]. Recently, investigators of the Urinary Incontinence Treatment Network evaluated 655 women who underwent either Burch or autologous rectus fascia (ARF) PVS. [9] At 24 months of follow-up, 520 women (79 %) completed the outcome assessment. Overall success rates were significantly higher for women in the sling group (47 % vs. 38 %), as were SUI-specific success rates (66 % vs. 49 %). Results of a recent trial comparing TO MUS and Burch revealed similar subjective and objective cure rates at 1 and 2 years of follow-up [10]. A recent meta-analysis by Tan et al. encompassing 16 studies and 1,807 women revealed similar cure rates between RBNS and laparoscopic RBNS at 2 years of follow-up [11].

In eight trials, there was no statistically significant difference in the reported subjective cure rates between laparoscopic RBNS and MUS within 18 months [12]. Objective cure rates (according to micturition diary, pad testing, or urodynamics) assessed in all but one study were higher for women after MUS when compared with laparoscopic RBNS. The inclusion of data from two recent trials, one comparing laparoscopic RBNS with MUS (SPARC, AMS) and another comparing laparoscopic RBNS with TVT, did not change the conclusions of the analysis [13, 14].

Traditional PVS placed at the bladder neck have been evaluated in yet another Cochrane database [15]. Thirteen trials including 760 women were identified, of whom 627 underwent PVS. In the single small trial comparing porcine dermis PVS with TNS, there were no differences in cure rates at 3 and 24 months [16]. Five trials compared one type of PVS against an autologous PVS constructed from rectus fascia or fascia lata [15]. Failure rates were similar both in short-term and long-term follow-up. In a recent meta-analysis, Novara et al. identified five RCTs comparing PVS to TVT [17]. TVT and PVS showed similar continence rates by any definition

of continence, and similar results were obtained when only autologous slings were considered. Further sensitivity analyses limited to RCTs with >12 months of follow-up did not significantly change the aforementioned conclusions. Two additional trials comparing PVS with MUS have since been identified. In a trial randomizing 100 women to TVT and ARF PVS, 61 women completed 12-month follow-up [18]. There was no significant difference in objective cure rate between the two procedures. In the second trial, 139 women were randomized to cadaver fascia lata (CFL) PVS or IVS, a multifilament polypropylene MUS. [19] In short-term follow-up, the overall success rates of the two procedures were not significantly different.

To date, one multicenter prospective RCT has compared MUS to no treatment. Campeau et al. randomized women over 70 years of age to undergo immediate TVT or to wait 6 months to undergo the same surgery (control group) [20]. Although continence was not an endpoint, quality of life indices were significantly higher in the immediate surgery group. There are no comparisons of MUS with AR or TNS. Although the results of the Cochrane database evaluating MUS outcomes are not yet mature, Novara et al. published a systematic review of RCTs after MUS surgery [17]. Four RCTs compared TVT to SPARC, a monofilament polypropylene RP MUS with characteristics similar to the TVT [17]. With regard to continence rates, TVT was better than SPARC in terms of subjective and objective cure rate by multiple definitions. However, the comparison data were significantly influenced by the findings from a single study [21]. Lord et al. enrolled almost half of the analyzed patients, and the women were evaluated at only 2 months of follow-up. If this RCT is excluded from analysis, only a non-statistically significant trend in favor of TVT was identified considering objective cure rates. Although the TO MUS is a relatively novel procedure, a number of RCTs have compared it with the RP MUS. A systematic review by Sung et al. revealed six RCTs and 11 cohort studies comparing the two types of procedures [22]. The authors found insufficient evidence in objective outcomes to support one approach over another. Likewise, there was no difference in subjective failure between the two approaches after pooling data from RCTs.

Novara et al. also assessed 14 RCTs comparing various RP and TO MUS, with half of the trials comparing TVT and TVT-O [17]. The data revealed that women randomized to RP or TO MUS yielded similar postoperative objective, subjective, and overall continence rates. Since the meta-analysis, several additional RCTs totaling 1,166 women have been published comparing RP and TO MUS [23–29]. In six of the trials, there was no significant difference in subjective or objective cure rates between RP and TO MUS. In the trial by Araco et al., women with intrinsic sphincter deficiency were significantly more likely to achieve cure after TVT than the TVT-O [23]. Three RCTs comparing the TVT-O to the Monarc revealed no significant difference in success rates at 4–12 months of follow-up [30–32].

Conclusions

Although there is a multitude of publications evaluating surgical options for female SUI, RCTs are relatively uncommon. Additionally, the quality of the RCTs may be questionable due to inadequate randomization or blinding, underpowering, short follow-up periods, and inconsistent definitions of cure. Despite these observations, several conclusions may be drawn from the RCT literature. The evidence supporting the use of AR for primary SUI in women is limited and, typically, of low quality. Limited evidence indicates that TNS are less effective than RBNS, while current evidence suggests that RBNS, especially the Burch colposuspension, is an effective treatment modality for SUI. Within the first year of treatment, the overall continence rate approaches 90 % and may be near 70 % 5 years after treatment. Despite laparoscopy being a relatively novel technique, eight of the ten trials comparing lap RBNS and RBNS were of good quality. Subjective outcomes between RBNS and lap RBNS are similar; however, objective cure rates may be lower in the laparoscopic group.

Although the number of RCTs involving bladder neck PVS is limited, the bulk of the short- and medium-term outcomes suggest that this therapy is as effective as RBNS and MUS. However, a recent, large, high-quality trial from the UITN has demonstrated significantly better success rates for the ARF PVS compared to the Burch. Mid-urethral slings appear to have similar efficacy in short- and medium-term follow-up as the Burch. There is also some evidence that the TVT may be associated with better results than the SPARC. However, the latter conclusion is based on a study with a 2-month follow-up. At this time, the retropubic and transobturator approaches are associated with similar short- and medium-term outcomes, although women with more intact intrinsic urethral function may have better outcomes after RP MUS than TO MUS. At this time, the inside-out and outside-in TO approaches appear to yield similar results.

Surgery for Pelvic Organ Prolapse

POP is a prevalent condition. An analysis of women who participated in the 2005–2006 National Health and Nutrition Examination Survey (NHANES) cited a weighted overall prevalence of POP to be 2.9 % [33]. The prevalence increased from 1.6 % in women ages 20–39 years to 4.1 % in women ages 80 years or older. Using recent population projections from the US Census Bureau, Wu et al. estimated that the number of women with POP will increase by 46 % from 3.3 to 4.9 million from the years 2010 to 2050 [34]. As the demand for POP surgery will only increase in the ensuing decades, more scrutiny is being given to the efficacy and complication rates of currently available surgical options. The following is a brief review of surgical treatment of POP.

Anatomy of Pelvic Prolapse

The pelvic organs are held in position by connections between the bony pelvis, musculature, and extensive connective tissue. When evaluating vaginal support cephalad to caudad, the cardinal ligaments anchor the upper vagina and cervix to the pelvic sidewall (Level I support) [35].

In the mid-vagina, the vesicopelvic ligament extends from the arcus tendineus fasciae pelvis (ATFP) to support the bladder base and the anterior vaginal wall (Level II support) while the posterior vaginal wall is attached laterally to the fascia overlying the levator ani muscle. In the anterior vagina, Level III support is due to the urethropelvic ligaments providing support to the urethra. In the posterior compartment, the vagina is separated from the rectum by the rectovaginal septum [36]. The septum is fused distally with the urogenital diaphragm and perineal body (Level III support) and is attached laterally to the arcus tendineus fasciae rectovaginalis in the distal one-third of the vagina and to the ATFP in the proximal two-thirds [35, 37]. Proximally, the septum fuses with the uterosacral ligaments laterally and the pericervical ring centrally.

Anterior compartment prolapse arises when the bladder and urethra herniate through a weak pubocervical fascia into the potential space of the vagina [38]. Loss of urethral support may result in SUI, while loss of bladder support may be classified as central, lateral, or combined. A central anterior compartment defect (cystocele) results from an attenuated pubocervical fascia while the lateral attachment of the vesicopelvic ligament to the ATFP is intact. Lateral defects result from an intact pubocervical fascia and disrupted attachment of the vesicopelvic ligament to the ATFP. Central defects are often associated with loss of Level I support at the cardinal ligaments, and patients may present with a concomitant enterocele. Traditional repair of a central defect cystocele has involved a plication of the pubocervical fascia in the midline (anterior colporrhaphy), while a lateral defect cystocele is repaired with reattachment of the vesicopelvic ligament to the pelvic sidewall (paravaginal repair). Graft augmentation may address central and lateral defects concomitantly.

As in the anterior compartment, a posterior compartment defect (rectocele) in the rectovaginal septum may be central or lateral. Likewise, proximal detachment of the rectovaginal septum from the uterosacral ligaments may be associated with an enterocele, while disruption of the distal attachment to the perineal body may result in weakening of the perineal body. Reapproximation of the perineal body (perineorrhaphy) repairs a perineal weakness while a plication of the rectovaginal fascia (posterior colporrhaphy) repairs a rectocele. A "site-specific" approach repairs discrete rents in the rectovaginal fascia instead of a midline plication [39]. Graft augmentation in this compartment may also address all types of rectoceles. Additionally, suspension from the sacral promontory, uterosacral or sacrospinous ligaments, or the iliococcygeus fascia may be performed to repair concomitant apical compartment defects (vault prolapse).

Outcomes of Standard POP Repair

The reports of success after cystocele repair have been inconsistent. While some reports cite long-term recurrence rates under 5 % after anterior colporrhaphy [40], most authors cite anterior compartment recurrence rates that exceed 40 % [41–43]. Although no long-term prospective trials have been performed, anatomic cure rates after isolated rectocele repair typically exceed 85 % [44–47]. These findings should be interpreted cautiously as published outcomes are often difficult to compare due to variations in patient populations and surgical technique, definitions of success and failure, and indications for repair. Nevertheless, these data suggest that traditional plication-type repairs, especially in the anterior compartment, may be associated with significant recurrence rates.

In the apical compartment, abdominal sacral colpopexy (ASC) is considered the gold standard for its low recurrence rate at the apex; however, transvaginal vault suspensions also have durable outcomes. Nygaard and members of the Pelvic Floor Disorders Network performed a MEDLINE review assessing ASC literature from 1966 to 2004 [48]. Follow-up duration for most studies ranged from 6 months to 3 years. The success rate, when defined as lack of apical prolapse postoperatively, ranged from 78 to 100 % and, when defined as no postoperative POP, from 58 to 100 %. The median reoperation rate for POP and in the studies that reported these outcomes was 4.4 % (range: 0–18.2 %). In a 2010 Cochrane review, ASC was better than sacrospinous ligament fixation (SSLF) in terms of a lower rate of recurrent vault prolapse and less dyspareunia; however, there was no statistically significant difference in reoperation rates for prolapse [49]. However, SSLF was quicker and cheaper to perform and women had an earlier return to activities of daily living. In a review of MEDLINE literature from 1996 to 2010, Petri and Ashok confirmed that the SSLF provides good long-term objective and subjective outcomes and improves QoL of women with POP [50]. The complication rates of SSLF were comparable to ASC and were much less than transvaginal mesh procedures. Finally, Maher et al. randomly assigned 95 women to undergo ASC or SSLF. [51] At a mean of 2 years, the subjective success rate was 94 % and 91 % in the ASC and SSLF groups, respectively, while the objective success rate was 76 % and 69 % in the ASC and SSLF groups, respectively. As already mentioned, the ASC was associated with a significantly longer operating time, a slower return to activities of daily living, and a greater cost than the SSLF. Both surgeries significantly improved the patients' QoL.

Outcomes of Graft Augmentation

As plicating potentially weak tissue has been associated with suboptimal outcomes, supplementing traditional plication-type repairs with interposition grafts has become a common practice. Theoretically, grafts have several advantages over plication-type repairs. One graft may address both central and lateral compartment defects simultaneously, and a graft may be anchored to an apical landmark or placed suburethrally to provide concomitant Level I and Level III support, respectively. To date, numerous allografts, xenografts, and synthetics have been described for repair of anterior compartment and posterior compartment defects, with short-term anatomic cure rates approaching 90 % [52]. However, cure rates after augmentation with some biologics appeared to wane with longer follow-up.

Several studies have compared standard and augmented repairs. A 2010 Cochrane review evaluated anterior colporrhaphy vs. anterior

compartment repair with mesh reinforcement [49]. Standard anterior repair was associated with more recurrent cystoceles than when supplemented with a polyglactin mesh or porcine dermis inlay. Standard anterior repair was also associated with more anterior compartment failures on examination than for polypropylene mesh repair as an overlay or armed transobturator mesh. Guerette et al. determined that the anatomic success rate at 2 years of follow-up was similar in women undergoing bovine pericardium interposition and colporrhaphy alone [53]. At 12 months of follow-up, Carey et al. observed anatomic success rates of 81 % of women undergoing polypropylene mesh augmentation vs. 65.6 % in the no-mesh group [54]. A high level of satisfaction and improvements in QoL indices were observed vs. baseline in both groups. Finally, a meta-analysis encompassing 49 studies and over 4,500 women determined that nonabsorbable synthetic mesh had a significantly lower objective anterior compartment recurrence rate (8.8 %) than absorbable synthetic mesh (23.1 %) and biological graft (17.9 %) [55].

There are few RCTs comparing standard posterior colporrhaphy with graft-augmented repair. Sand et al. determined that posterior compartment recurrence was similar after colporrhaphy with or without polyglactin mesh reinforcement [49, 56]. In another trial, Paraiso et al. stated that the addition of porcine small intestinal submucosa did not necessarily improve anatomic outcomes of standard posterior colporrhaphy or site-specific repair [49, 57]. After 1 year, women undergoing graft augmentation had a significantly greater anatomic failure rate than those who underwent posterior colporrhaphy. However, there were no differences in subjective prolapse symptoms.

Commercial Prolapse Repair Kits

Prolapse repair "kits" have become an appealing method to perform graft-augmented repairs. The kit is "all-inclusive" and contains the graft (monofilament, polypropylene synthetic mesh in most cases), trocars/tunnelers, and standardized directions for placement of the graft using bony and ligamentous landmarks through a vaginal approach. Currently, several variations of kits are available to address either Level II support or Level I and II support simultaneously, either through an anterior or posterior compartment approach [52].

The anatomic outcomes after transvaginal kit repairs have been promising in the short term. A recent meta-analysis encompassing 30 studies with 2,653 patients calculated the objective success rates to be 87–95 % for different kits [58]. RCTs comparing outcomes after a mesh kit procedure and standard anterior colporrhaphy are emerging. Nguyen and Burchette cited a significantly higher anatomic success rate (89 %) 12 months after Perigee (AMS Inc., Minnetonka, MN) compared to 55 % after anterior colporrhaphy [59]. QoL indices were improved in both groups. More recently, Altman et al. randomly assigned 389 women to undergo anterior repair with a mesh kit or traditional colporrhaphy [60]. At 1 year, the primary outcome (anatomical stage 0–1 per the POP quantification system and the subjective absence of symptoms of vaginal bulging) was significantly more common in the women treated with transvaginal mesh repair (60.8 %) than in those who underwent colporrhaphy (34.5 %). Additionally, in a 2010 Cochrane database review, standard anterior repair was associated with more anterior compartment failures on examination than for polypropylene mesh repair as an overlay or armed transobturator mesh [49]. However, the review also emphasized that there were no differences in subjective outcomes, QoL data, de novo dyspareunia, SUI, reoperation rates for prolapse, or incontinence, although some of these data were limited.

Complications of POP Repairs

All POP repairs are associated with varying, but mostly minimal, degrees of significant intraoperative bleeding and inadvertent pelvic organ injury. The incorporation of synthetic grafts, and kit use in particular, may be associated with additional and unique complications. A recent meta-analysis of over 70 studies and case reports evaluated the rates and spectrum of adverse events associated with graft use [61]. These adverse events included bleeding (0–3 %), visceral injury (1–4 %), urinary tract infection (0–19 %), graft extrusion (0–30 %), and fistula formation (1 %). There were insufficient data regarding dyspareunia, sexual, voiding, or defecatory dysfunction. Vaginal mesh extrusion was cited in 10 % of the patients in the Cochrane review [61], compared with a 3.4 % incidence of mesh erosion after ASC [48].

As the use of synthetic mesh for POP repair has increased, the reporting of complications has been closely scrutinized. In the last few years, the French Health Authorities, the Society of Gynecologic Surgeons Systematic Review Group, and the US Food and Drug Administration have all issued warnings regarding the unique complications associated with mesh use in the pelvis [52]. In July 2011, the FDA released an update to their 2008 warning in response to the reporting of more complications associated with transvaginal mesh [62]. Although the issue is currently under investigation, transvaginal mesh may ultimately undergo device reclassification and require additional post-market surveillance.

Conclusions

Several conclusions can be drawn regarding the available literature on POP repair. First, grafting of any type in the anterior compartment significantly improves anatomic success in the short term. However, subjective outcomes are not significantly different between augmented and standard anterior repairs, and QoL is improved regardless of approach. Second, nonabsorbable synthetic mesh is associated with significantly lower recurrence rates than other grafts. Third, standard posterior compartment repairs have a low incidence of POP recurrence, and, currently, there is insufficient information to support graft augmentation in the posterior compartment. Fourth, ASC may provide superior apical support to transvaginal approaches, but the abdominal approach takes longer to perform and is more expensive, and patients take longer to return to activities of daily living. Fifth, mesh extrusion and complications from percutaneous trocar passage add significant morbidity to the procedure. Adequate surgeon experience and judicious patient selection prior to any repair is paramount to surgical success.

References

1. Abrams P, Cardozo L, Fall M, et al. Standardization of terminology of lower urinary tract function: Report from the standardization sub-committee of the International Continence Society. Neurourol Urodyn. 2002;21:167–78.
2. DeLancey JOL. Structural support of the urethra as it relates to stress urinary incontinence: the hammock hypothesis. Am J Obstet Gynecol. 1994;170:1713–23.
3. Petros PE, Ulmsten U. An integral theory of female urinary incontinence. Acta Obstet Gynecol Scand. 1990;69(Suppl):7–31.
4. Glazener CM, Cooper K. Anterior vaginal repair for urinary incontinence in women. Cochrane Database Syst Rev. 2001;1, CD001755.
5. Glazener CM, Cooper K. Bladder neck needle suspension for urinary incontinence in women. Cochrane Database Syst Rev. 2004;2, CD003636.
6. Lapitan MC, Cody DJ, Grant AM. Open retropubic colposuspension for urinary incontinence in women. Cochrane Database Syst Rev. 2005;3, CD002912.
7. Culligan PJ, Goldberg RP, Sand PK. A randomized controlled trial comparing a modified Burch procedure and a suburethral sling: long-term follow-up. Int Urogynecol J Pelvic Floor Dysfunct. 2003;14:229–33.
8. Ward KL, Hilton P. Tension-free vaginal tape versus colposuspension for primary urodynamic stress incontinence: 5-year follow-up. BJOG. 2008;115:226–33.
9. Albo ME, Richter HE, Brubaker L, et al. Burch colposuspension versus fascial sling to reduce urinary stress incontinence. N Engl J Med. 2007;356:2143–55.
10. Sivaslioglu AA, Caliskan E, Dolen I, Haberal A. A randomized comparison of transobturator tape and Burch colposuspension in the treatment of female stress urinary incontinence. Int Urogynecol J Pelvic Floor Dysfunct. 2007;18:1015–9.
11. Tan E, Tekkis PP, Cornish J, Teoh TG, Darzi AW, Khullar V. Laparoscopic versus open colposuspension for urodynamic stress incontinence. Neurourol Urodyn. 2007;26:158–69.
12. Dean NM, Ellis G, Wilson PD, Herbison GP. Laparoscopic colposuspension for urinary incontinence in women. Cochrane Database Syst Rev. 2006;3, CD002239.
13. Foote AJ, Maughan V, Carne C. Laparoscopic colposuspension versus vaginal suburethral slingplasty: a randomised prospective trial. Aust N Z J Obstet Gynaecol. 2006;46:517–20.
14. Jelovsek JE, Barber MD, Karram MM, Walters MD, Paraiso MF. Randomised trial of laparoscopic Burch colposuspension versus tension-free vaginal tape: long-term follow up. BJOG. 2008;115:219–25.
15. Bezerra CA, Bruschini H, Cody DJ. Traditional suburethral sling operations for urinary incontinence in women. Cochrane Database Syst Rev. 2005;3, CD001754.
16. Hilton P. A clinical and urodynamic study comparing the Stamey bladder neck suspension and suburethral sling procedures in the treatment of genuine stress incontinence. Br J Obstet Gynaecol. 1989;96:213–20.
17. Novara G, Ficarra V, Boscolo-Berto R, Secco S, Cavalleri S, Artibani W. Tension-free midurethral slings in the treatment of female stress urinary incontinence: a systematic review and meta-analysis of randomized controlled trials of effectiveness. Eur Urol. 2007;52:663–78.
18. Sharifiaghdas F, Mortazavi N. Tension-free vaginal tape and autologous rectus fascia pubovaginal sling for the treatment of urinary stress incontinence: a medium-term follow-up. Med Princ Pract. 2008;17:209–14.
19. Basok EK, Yildirim A, Atsu N, Basaran A, Tokuc R. Cadaveric fascia lata versus intravaginal slingplasty for the pubovaginal sling: surgical outcome, overall success and patient satisfaction rates. Urol Int. 2008;80:46–51.
20. Campeau L, Tu LM, Lemieux MC, et al. A multicenter, prospective, randomized clinical trial comparing tension-free vaginal tape surgery and no treatment for the management of stress urinary incontinence in elderly women. Neurourol Urodyn. 2007;26:990–4.
21. Lord HE, Taylor JD, Finn JC, et al. A randomized controlled equivalence trial of short-term complications and efficacy of tension-free vaginal tape and suprapubic urethral support sling for treating stress incontinence. BJU Int. 2006;98:367–76.
22. Sung VW, Schleinitz MD, Rardin CR, Ward RM, Myers DL. Comparison of retropubic versus transobturator approach to midurethral slings: a systematic review and meta-analysis. Am J Obstet Gynecol. 2007;197:3–11.
23. Araco F, Gravante G, Sorge R, et al. TVT-O vs TVT: a randomized trial in patients with different degrees of urinary stress incontinence. Int Urogynecol J Pelvic Floor Dysfunct. 2008;19:917–26.
24. Wang AC, Lin YH, Tseng LH, Chih SY, Lee CJ. Prospective randomized comparison of transobturator suburethral sling (Monarc) vs suprapubic arc (Sparc) sling procedures for female urodynamic stress incontinence. Int Urogynecol J Pelvic Floor Dysfunct. 2006;17:439–43.
25. Barber MD, Kleeman S, Karram MM, et al. Transobturator tape compared with tension-free vaginal tape for the treatment of stress urinary incontinence: a randomized controlled trial. Obstet Gynecol. 2008;111:611–21.
26. Barry C, Lim YN, Muller R, et al. A multi-centre, randomised clinical control trial comparing the retropubic (RP) approach versus the transobturator approach (TO) for tension-free, suburethral sling treatment of urodynamic stress incontinence: the TORP study. Int Urogynecol J Pelvic Floor Dysfunct. 2008;19:171–8.

27. Porena M, Costantini E, Frea B, et al. Tension-free vaginal tape versus transobturator tape as surgery for stress urinary incontinence: results of a multicentre randomised trial. Eur Urol. 2007;52:1481–90.

28. Palva K, Rinne K, Aukee P, et al. A randomized trial comparing tension-free vaginal tape with tension-free vaginal tape-obturator: 36-month results. Int Urogynecol J Pelvic Floor Dysfunct. 2010;21:1049–55.

29. Zhu L, Lang J, Hai N, Wong F. Comparing vaginal tape and transobturator tape for the treatment of mild and moderate stress incontinence. Int J Gynaecol Obstet. 2007;99:14–7.

30. Debodinance P. Trans-obturator urethral sling for surgical correction of female stress urinary incontinence: outside-in (Monarc) versus inside-out (TVT-O). Are both ways safe? J Gynecol Obstet. Biol Reprod. 2006;35:571–7.

31. But I, Faganelj M. Complications and short-term results of two different transobturator techniques for surgical treatment of women with urinary incontinence: a randomized study. Int Urogynecol J Pelvic Floor Dysfunct. 2008;19:857–61.

32. Liapis A, Bakas P, Creatsas G. Monarc vs TVT-O for the treatment of primary stress incontinence: a randomized study. Int Urogynecol J Pelvic Floor Dysfunct. 2008;19:185–90.

33. Nygaard I, Barber MD, Burgio KL, et al., for the Pelvic Floor Disorders Network. Prevalence of symptomatic pelvic floor disorders in US women. JAMA. 2008;300:1311–16.

34. Wu JM, Hundley AF, Fulton RG, Myers ER. Forecasting the prevalence of pelvic floor disorders in U.S. women: 2010 to 2050. Obstet Gynecol. 2009; 114:1278–83.

35. Delancey JOL. Anatomic aspects of vaginal eversion after hysterectomy. Am J Obstet Gynecol. 1992;166: 1717–24.

36. Zimmerman CW. Pelvic organ prolapse. In: Rock JA, Jones HW, editors. TeLinde's operative gynecology. 9th ed. Philadelphia: Lippincott Williams & Wilkins; 2003. p. 927–48.

37. Leffler KS, Thompson JR, Cundiff GW, Buller JL, Burrows LJ, Schön Ybarra MA. Attachment of the rectovaginal septum to the pelvic sidewall. Am J Obstet Gynecol. 2001;185:41–3.

38. Dmochowski RR, Gomelsky A. Cystocele and anterior vaginal prolapse. In: Graham SD, Glenn JF, Keane TE, editors. Glenn's Urologic Surgery. 6th ed. Philadelphia: Lippincott Williams & Wilkins; 2004. p. 339–48.

39. Cundiff GW, Weidner AC, Visco AG, Addision WA, Bump RC. An anatomic and functional assessment of the discrete defect rectocele repair. Am J Obstet Gynecol. 1998;179:1451–6.

40. Beck RP, McCormick S, Nordstrum L. A 25 year experience with 519 anterior colporrhaphy procedures. Obstet Gynecol. 1991;78:1011–4.

41. Paraiso MF, Ballard LA, Walters MD, Lee JC, Mitchinson AR. Pelvic support defects and visceral and sexual function in women treated with sacrospinous ligament suspension and pelvic reconstruction. Am J Obstet Gynecol. 1996;175:1423–31.

42. Shull BL, Capen CV, Riggs MW, Kuehl TJ. Preoperative and postoperative analysis of site-specific pelvic support defects in 81 women treated with sacrospinous ligament suspension and pelvic reconstruction. Am J Obstet Gynecol. 1992;166:1764–71.

43. Maher C, Baessler K. Surgical management of anterior vaginal wall prolapse: an evidence based literature review. Int Urogynecol J Pelvic Floor Dysfunct. 2006;17:195–201.

44. Singh K, Cortes E, Reid WM. Evaluation of the fascial technique for surgical repair of the isolated posterior vaginal wall prolapse. Obstet Gynecol. 2003;101: 320–4.

45. Maher CF, Qatawneh A, Baessler K, Schluter PJ. Midline rectovaginal fascial plication for repair of rectocele and obstructed defecation. Obstet Gynecol. 2004;104:685–9.

46. Kenton K, Shott S, Brubaker L. Outcome after rectovaginal fascia reattachment for rectocele repair. Am J Obstet Gynecol. 1999;181:1360–3.

47. Cundiff GW, Weidner AC, Visco AG, Addison WA, Bump RC. An anatomic and functional assessment of the discrete defect rectocele repair. Am J Obstet Gynecol. 1998;179:1451–6.

48. Nygaard IE, McCreery R, Brubaker L, et al.; Pelvic Floor Disorders Network. Abdominal sacrocolpopexy: a comprehensive review. Obstet Gynecol. 2004; 104:805–23.

49. Maher C, Feiner B, Baessler K, Adams EJ, Hagen S, Glazener CM. Surgical management of pelvic organ prolapse in women. Cochrane Database Syst Rev. 2010;4, CD004014.

50. Petri E, Ashok K. Sacrospinous vaginal fixation—current status. Acta Obstet Gynecol Scand. 2011;90: 429–36.

51. Maher CF, Qatawneh AM, Dwyer PL, Carey MP, Cornish A, Schluter PJ. Abdominal sacral colpopexy or vaginal sacrospinous colpopexy for vaginal vault prolapse: a prospective randomized study. Am J Obstet Gynecol. 2004;190:20–6.

52. Gomelsky A, Penson DF, Dmochowski RR. Pelvic organ prolapse (POP) surgery: the evidence for the repairs. BJU Int. 2011;107:1704–19.

53. Guerette NL, Peterson TV, Aguirre OA, Vandrie DM, Biller DH, Davila GW. Anterior repair with or without collagen matrix reinforcement: a randomized controlled trial. Obstet Gynecol. 2009;114:59–65.

54. Carey M, Higgs P, Goh J, et al. Vaginal repair with mesh versus colporrhaphy for prolapse: a randomized controlled trial. BJOG. 2009;116:1380–6.

55. Jia X, Glazener C, Mowatt G, et al. Efficacy and safety of using mesh or grafts in surgery for anterior and/or posterior vaginal wall prolapse: systematic review and meta-analysis. BJOG. 2008;115:1350–61.

56. Sand PK, Koduri S, Lobel RW, et al. Prospective randomized trial of polyglactin 910 mesh to prevent recurrence of cystoceles and rectoceles. Am J Obstet Gynecol. 2001;184:1357–62.

57. Paraiso MF, Barber MD, Muir TW, Walters MD. Rectocele repair: a randomized trial of three surgical techniques including graft augmentation. Am J Obstet Gynecol. 2006;195:1762–71.

58. Feiner B, Jelovsek JE, Maher C. Efficacy and safety of transvaginal mesh kits in the treatment of prolapse of the vaginal apex: a systematic review. BJOG. 2009; 116:15–24.

59. Nguyen JN, Burchette RJ. Outcome after anterior vaginal prolapse repair: a randomized controlled trial. Obstet Gynecol. 2008;111:891–8.

60. Altman D, Väyrynen T, Engh ME, Axelsen S, Falconer C, Nordic Transvaginal Mesh Group. Anterior colporrhaphy versus transvaginal mesh for pelvic-organ prolapse. N Engl J Med. 2011;364: 1826–36.

61. Sung VW, Rogers RG, Schaffer JI, et al; Society of Gynecologic Surgeons Systematic Review Group. Graft use in transvaginal pelvic organ prolapse repair: a systematic review. Obstet Gynecol. 2008;112: 1131–42.

62. http://www.fda.gov/MedicalDevices/Safety/ AlertsandNotices/ucm262435.htm

Surgery for Neuropathic Bladder Dysfunction

17

Alex Gomelsky and Roger R. Dmochowski

Surgery for Neuropathic Bladder Dysfunction

The primary objective in managing the lower urinary tract of any patient with neuropathic bladder dysfunction is protecting the upper urinary tracts. McGuire et al., studying patients with spina bifida, have shown that when bladder storage pressures exceed 40 cmH$_2$O, intervention may be required to protect against potential renal damage and failure [1]. Renal compromise in the face of spinal cord injury (SCI) is common. It has been shown in one study that 7 % of men sustaining SCI and performing clean intermittent catheterization (CIC) had developed upper tract complications, such as hydronephrosis, febrile urinary tract infections (UTI), urolithiasis, or vesicoureteral reflux (VUR) [2]. Additional research has since confirmed that all methods of bladder management, including indwelling urethral catheterization, may be associated with upper tract compromise [3, 4]. Secondary objectives include maintaining social continence, minimizing UTIs, and establishing independence in bladder

A. Gomelsky, M.D.
Department of Urology, LSU Health—Shreveport, Shreveport, LA, USA

R.R. Dmochowski, M.D., M.M.H.C. (✉)
Department of Urologic Surgery, Vanderbilt University Medical Center, A1302 Medical Center North, Nashville, TN 37232-2765, USA
e-mail: roger.dmochowski@vanderbilt.edu

management and are no less important. The optimal lower urinary tract management method is one which optimally achieves the primary and secondary objectives. The method needs to be individualized according to the patient's wishes, their level of injury and manual dexterity, and available assistance or presence of caregivers. While it is clear that one method does not fit every patient scenario, certain options are less invasive than others and may be attempted first. However, in patients where primary methods have failed, a role for surgical management of the lower urinary tract remains. In 2006, the Consortium for Spinal Cord Medicine published guidelines for bladder management of the patient with SCI based on a systematic review of the literature after 1993 [5]. The surgical options included in the guideline are discussed in detail.

Augmentation Cystoplasty (Bladder Augmentation)

Traditionally, bladder augmentation has been one of the most common surgeries performed in patients with SCI. Common reasons to undergo bladder augmentation include elevated bladder storage pressures and leakage of urine between intermittent catheterizations despite appropriate treatment with muscarinic receptor antagonists [6]. This procedure increases bladder capacity, reduces reflex contractility, and improves autonomic dysreflexia in patients with cervical and upper thoracic SCI. Additional benefits in certain

A.J. Wein et al. (eds.), *Bladder Dysfunction in the Adult: The Basis for Clinical Management*, Current Clinical Urology, DOI 10.1007/978-1-4939-0853-0_17, © Springer Science+Business Media New York 2014

patients potentially include a decrease in the incidence of UTIs and VUR. The Panel noted that for a bladder augmentation to be successful, the patient must have the ability and motivation to perform CIC [5].

While augmentation may be performed with the stomach and small or large intestine, the ileum is the segment most commonly employed (ileocystoplasty). The advantages of this bowel segment include abundant quantity of material, reliable blood supply, mobility, and ease of handling [7]. Additionally, the ileum is the most compliant segment of bowel; produces less mucus than the colon; is associated with less severe metabolic complications compared with the stomach, jejunum, or colon; and is associated with fewer gastrointestinal complications than the cecum [7]. Briefly, the procedure is as follows [7]. A segment of the ileum 20–30 cm long and located at a minimum of 15 cm proximal to the ileocecal valve is isolated and detubularized. After bowel continuity is reestablished, the ileum is reconfigured into a U, S, or W shape depending on the length of the segment. The bowel is then sewn together with delayed absorbable sutures to create a cup patch, which is then sewn to a bladder that has been bivalved in a "clam shell" fashion. Ginsberg has suggested using an "extraperitoneal" approach when possible, by creating a small peritoneotomy to harvest the ileal segment to be used for augmentation [6]. This technique would theoretically minimize potential ileus for this class of patients who may already be afflicted with neurogenic bowel [8].

There have been numerous studies documenting the long-term efficacy and complications of bladder augmentation. Flood et al. reported on 106 SCI patients with long-term follow-up [9]. Mean bladder capacity increased from 108 mL preoperatively to 438 mL postoperatively, and 75 % were reported to have "excellent" results. Complications included bladder calculi (21 %), reoperation for revision (15 %), postoperative incontinence (13 %), pyelonephritis (11 %), and small bowel obstruction (4 %). In a large series, Venn and Mundy reported on 267 patients, of whom 152 had neuropathic bladder dysfunction [10]. At a minimum follow-up of 3 years, urodynamic parameters were improved and 78 % were continent with augmentation alone. At 8 years of follow-up, Quek and Ginsberg demonstrated durable improvement in bladder capacity and mean maximum detrusor pressure in 26 patients [11]. More recently, Gurung et al. reported outcomes in 19 patients with suprasacral SCI at a mean follow-up of 14.7 years (range: 10.5–20.3 years) [12]. Twelve of 19 were male and the mean period from injury to surgery was 4.5 years (range: 0.3–22 years). CMG showed a significant improvement in bladder capacity and a decrease in intravesical pressures. Long-term complications included bladder stones ($N=4$), urosepsis (2), VUR (2), neurogenic detrusor overactivity (NDO; 1), and laparotomy for bowel obstruction (1). Surveillance cystoscopies did not detect any bladder neoplasms. Thirteen of 14 patients responding to a validated questionnaire were satisfied with the operation such that they would consider it again or recommend it to a friend. No patient reported any significant changes in either bowel habit or sexual function.

Continent Urinary Diversion

Creation of a continent lower urinary tract reconstruction to the skin may be an option for patients unable to perform CIC through the native urethra. The majority of the orthotopic continent diversions (e.g., Koch, Indiana, Mainz, T-pouch) and their modifications have been mainly used for bladder substitution following cystectomy for bladder cancer. All of the procedures involve detubularizing various lengths of the small and large intestines, fashioning a catheterizable stoma, and constructing a continence mechanism by creating anti-leakage valves using bowel segments. Additionally, a continent cutaneous catheterizable channel may be created using appendix (Mitrofanoff) or detubularized ileum (Monti). These latter procedures employ a minimal amount of small bowel in reconstruction and may be created in concert with a native or augmented bladder. However, the success of these procedures may be limited by absence of appendix and body habitus. While all of these procedures have potential advantages and disadvantages, none of the techniques may be superior to another, and the surgery should be performed according to surgeon experience [6]. The Panel had several recommendations regarding the use of continent urinary diversion in patients with SCI [5]. This procedure should be considered in patients with intractable DO in whom it is not feasible to augment the native bladder or access the native urethra because of congenital abnormalities, spasticity, obesity, contracture, tetraplegia, or because closure of an incompetent bladder neck is required. It may also be a way of treating women with tetraplegia in whom a chronic indwelling urethral catheter has caused urethral erosion or men with SCI with unsalvageable bladders secondary to urethral fistula and sacral pressure ulcers [5, 13].

Incontinent Urinary Diversion

Urinary diversion into a collecting device is occasionally performed for patients with neuropathic bladder dysfunction. While any segment of the small or large intestine could theoretically be brought out to the skin as a stoma, the most popular option is a segment of terminal ileum. Since the introduction of the technique by Bricker in 1950, the procedure has changed very little [14]. Briefly, a 10–15 cm segment of terminal ileum at least 15 cm proximal to the ileocecal valve is isolated on its mesentery and bowel continuity is reestablished. The ureters are divided as distally as possible and mobilized, with the left ureter tunneled retroperitoneally behind the sigmoid mesocolon and into the right lower quadrant. A uretero-ileal anastomosis is performed at the proximal end of the ileal loop, while the distal end is brought out to the skin as a stoma. The Panel felt that this method of urinary diversion may be preferable to continent diversion in patients who have poor hand function [5]. The Panel also recommended considering this form of diversion in those patients with cannot perform CIC and have urethrocutaneous fistulas, perineal pressure ulcers, a devastated urethra, or other urinary complications secondary to a longstanding indwelling urethral catheter [5].

The incidence of complications following an ileal conduit increases with each year of follow-up. Of 131 patients with 5-year follow-up in the series by Madersbacher et al., 66 % suffered a long-term complication [15]. This rate increased to 94 % in 18 patients who were followed for 15 years. However, the incidence of complications appears to be lower in the long term than in those patients undergoing continent cutaneous urinary diversion [16]. A prolonged ileus is the most common early postoperative complication, occurring in up to 18 % of patients [17]. Stomal stenosis is reported in 3–6 % of patients following ileal conduit, and the rate appears to be lower in patients with the Turnbull type of stoma as compared with the Brooke version [17]. Obstruction at the level of the uretero-ileal anastomosis occurs in 5–10 % and is most commonly attributed to stricturing of the distal ureter due to devascularization [17]. Bowel complications such as fistulas between the urinary and gastrointestinal tracts are rare. While metabolic derangements are possible any time urine comes into contact with the intestine, these fluctuations are relatively infrequent after ileal conduit. The ileum has less absorptive capacity than the jejunum, and conduits minimize the amount of surface area and time over which urine is in contact with the bowel [17]. Infectious complications are common and can range from asymptomatic to urosepsis. Of the 131 patients in the series of Madersbacher et al., 23 % developed infectious complications in the long term [15]. Urolithiasis is another potential long-term complication. In Dretler's review of 740 patients who underwent an ileal conduit over a 16-year period, stones were found in 4.8 % of the patients [18]. Infection, hyperchloremic acidosis, and high conduit residual volumes were identified as risk factors for stone formation [18].

Cutaneous Ileovesicostomy

Cutaneous ileovesicostomy was first described in 1957 by Cordonnier in children with myelomeningocele [19]. This procedure involves the creation of an ileal conduit and suturing the proximal end to the bladder dome with delayed absorbable suture. The distal end is brought out to the skin as an incontinent stoma, and the urine collects into an appliance. Zimmerman and Santucci proposed three situations to consider an ileovesicostomy in patients with a neuropathic bladder: (1) patients wishing to avoid the long-term complications of chronic indwelling suprapubic or urethral catheter drainage, who are unwilling to use CIC or a continent catheterizable stoma; (2) patients with intractable lower urinary tract obstruction (e.g., bladder neck contracture) who are unable or unwilling to have an alternate suprapubic diversion (e.g., suprapubic tube or continent catheterizable stoma); and (3) patients with urethrocutaneous fistula that drains into a decubitus ulcer [20]. Likewise, the Panel recommended that this procedure be considered for SCI patients with normal ureterovesical junctions who require urinary diversion [5]. As patients with an incompetent bladder outlet may also have a problem storing urine, the Panel noted that it may be necessary to perform a concomitant procedure to prevent urethral incontinence [5, 21, 22].

Outcomes of ileovesicostomy have been reported in several series. Leng et al. reported that in the long term, 93 % of their 41 patients maintained detrusor leak point pressures >40 cmH$_2$O [23]. Likewise, at a mean follow-up of 45 months, Schwartz et al. reported that 21 of their 23 SCI patients were maintaining bladder pressures <20 cmH$_2$O [22]. Additionally, Tan et al. reported resolution of incontinence after ileovesicostomy in 72 % of their 50 patients at a mean follow-up of 26 months [24]. Despite the promising functional outcomes, these procedures are not without complications. Zimmerman and Santucci compiled a summary of complications associated with ileovesicostomy, and they are as follows: urethral incontinence (16–88 %), UTIs (16 %), urinary fistula (32 %), wound infection (7–34 %), hematuria (18 %), stomal stenosis (7–16 %), ileovesicostomy obstruction (12 %), fascial stenosis (12 %), and small bowel obstruction/ileus (15 %) [20]. Patients being considered for cutaneous ileovesicostomy should be evaluated for concomitant urinary incontinence due to an incompetent bladder outlet. If this condition is diagnosed, the patient may continue to have urinary incontinence unless they undergo a simultaneous outlet procedure such as bladder neck closure or an obstructing pubo-urethral sling.

Conclusions

Multiple therapeutic options are available for the patient with neuropathic storage or emptying dysfunction. The goals of therapy are individualized: protect the upper tracts, maintain continence, minimize UTIs, and facilitate bladder emptying. Nonsurgical measures, such as CIC and pharmaceutical therapy with muscarinic receptor antagonists, are a preferred initial method. While this option provides many SCI patients with independence and fulfills the goals of therapy, some patients may ultimately require surgical intervention to stabilize their lower urinary tracts. Surgical manipulation of the lower urinary tract ranges in complexity and may be associated with significant long-term complications. The surgical choice depends on the surgeon's experience and patient-related details, such as level of SCI, body habitus, and presence of complicating factors like fistulae or decubitus ulcers. Ultimately, the motivation and ability to perform CIC long term may be the most important factor in choosing the type of surgical management of the neuropathic bladder.

References

1. McGuire EJ, Woodside JR, Borden TA, Weiss RM. Prognostic value of urodynamic testing in myelodysplastic patients. J Urol. 1981;2:205–9.
2. Killorin W, Gray M, Bennett JK, Green BG. The value of urodynamics and bladder management in predicting upper urinary tract complications in male spinal cord injury patients. Paraplegia. 1992;30:437–41.
3. Weld KJ, Wall BM, Mangold TA, Steere EL, Dmochowski RR. Influences on renal function in chronic spinal cord injured patients. J Urol. 2000; 164:1490–3.
4. Drake MJ, Cortina-Borja M, Savic G, Charlifue SW, Gardner BP. Prospective evaluation of urological effects of aging in chronic spinal cord injury by method of bladder management. Neurourol Urodyn. 2005;24:111–6.

5. Consortium for Spinal Cord Medicine. Bladder management for adults with spinal cord injury: a clinical practice guideline for health-care providers. J Spinal Cord Med. 2006;29:527–73.

6. Ginsberg DA. Management of neurogenic voiding dysfunction in the male patient. Curr Bladder Dysfunct Rep. 2007;2:173–9.

7. Colvert III JR, Kropp BP, Cheng EY. Bladder augmentation: current and future techniques. AUA Update Series. Linthicum, MD: American Urological Association, Education and Research; 2003; Vol. XXII: Lesson 32.

8. Albo M, Raz S, Dupont MC. Anterior flap extraperitoneal cystoplasty. J Urol. 1997;157:2095–8.

9. Flood HD, Malhotra SJ, O'Connell HE, Ritchey MJ, Bloom DA, McGuire EJ. Long-term results and complications using augmentation cystoplasty in reconstructive urology. Neurourol Urodyn. 1995;14: 297–309.

10. Venn SN, Mundy AR. Long-term results of augmentation cystoplasty. Eur Urol. 1998;34(Suppl):40–2.

11. Quek ML, Ginsberg DA. Long-term urodynamics follow-up of bladder augmentation for neurogenic bladder. J Urol. 2003;169:195–8.

12. Gurung PM, Attar KH, Abdul-Rahman A, Morris T, Hamid R, Shah PJ. Long-term outcomes of augmentation ileocystoplasty in patients with spinal cord injury: a minimum of 10 years of follow-up. BJU Int. 2012;109(8):1236–42.

13. Linsenmeyer TA. Update on bladder evaluation recommendations and bladder management guideline in patients with spinal cord injury. Curr Bladder Dysfunct Rep. 2007;2:134–40.

14. Bricker EM. Bladder substitution after pelvic evisceration. Surg Clin North Am. 1950;30:1511–21.

15. Madersbacher S, Schmidt J, Eberle JM, et al. Long-term outcome of ileal conduit diversion. J Urol. 2003;169:985–90.

16. Frazier HA, Robertson JE, Paulson DF. Complications of radical cystectomy and urinary diversion: a retrospective review of 675 cases in 2 decades. J Urol. 1992;148:1401–5.

17. Novak TE, Schoenberg M. A new look at the ileal conduit. AUA Update Series. Linthicum, MD: American Urological Association, Education and Research; 2006; Vol. 25: Lesson 8.

18. Dretler SP. The pathogenesis of urinary tract calculi occurring after ileal conduit diversion: I. Clinical study. II. Conduit study. 3. Prevention. J Urol. 1973; 109:204–9.

19. Cordonnier JJ. Ileocystostomy for neurogenic bladder. J Urol. 1957;78:605–10.

20. Zimmerman WB, Santucci RA. Ileovesicostomy: an update. Arch Esp Urol. 2011;64:207–17.

21. Bennett JK, Gray M, Green BG, Foote JE. Continent diversion and bladder augmentation in spinal cord-injured patients. Semin Urol. 1992;10:121–32.

22. Schwartz SL, Kennelly MJ, McGuire EJ, Faerber GJ. Incontinent ileo-vesicostomy urinary diversion in the treatment of lower urinary tract dysfunction. J Urol. 1994;152:99–102.

23. Leng WW, Faerber G, Del Terzo M, McGuire EJ. Long-term outcome of incontinent ileovesicostomy management of severe lower urinary tract dysfunction. J Urol. 1999;161:1803–6.

24. Tan HJ, Stoffel J, Daignault S, McGuire EJ, Latini JM. Ileovesicostomy for adults with neurogenic bladders: complications and potential risk factors for adverse outcomes. Neurourol Urodyn. 2008;27: 238–43.

Urinary Diversion

18

Jonathan J. Aning and Hashim Hashim

Introduction

Patients with dysfunctional and unsafe native bladders may require urinary diversion if alternative options fail. Although the oncological rationale for urinary diversion is easily comprehensible, the benign indications for urinary diversion, congenital urological anatomical abnormalities, neuropathic bladder, refractory detrusor overactivity and chronic pelvic pain syndromes, are equally important. Significant improvement in patient quality of life from these debilitating conditions may be achieved with a successful urinary diversion.

Principles of Urinary Diversion

The 'normal' lower urinary tract stores urine in the bladder at low pressure, has a mechanism which provides continence (the external urethral sphincter) and a conduit for expelling urine outside the body (the urethra) regulated by the brain and the spinal cord. The aim of urinary diversion

surgery is to approximate the normal urinary tract within the constraints of the patient's wishes, their perceived ability to manage the choice of urinary diversion after surgery and their underlying medical condition and prognosis. The goals of urinary diversion surgery are to improve quality of life, preserve renal function by providing a low-pressure reservoir, allow control of voiding, minimise urinary tract infections and avoid immediate or late postoperative complications.

The majority of urinary diversions are formed by incorporating reconfigured bowel segments into the urinary tract. It is important to consider three factors when planning any urinary diversion: firstly, how the ureters will be connected to the diversion/reservoir; secondly, what reservoir the ureters will be connected to; and thirdly, how the reservoir will be emptied. Comprehensive knowledge of the blood supply to the gastrointestinal tract is mandatory for surgeons performing urinary tract reconstruction, as virtually any segment may be used to form the reservoir. Urinary diversions may be classified broadly by whether they achieve continence and how the urine is expelled. The broad categories are incontinent cutaneous diversion, continent cutaneous reservoir, continent rectal reservoir and orthotopic neobladder. Continent urinary reservoirs or neobladders avoid the need for external urine collection appliances. These categories will be discussed in greater detail later in the chapter.

Rarely, the patient's own bladder may be left in situ and a supra vesical diversion performed. It is imperative to follow such patients up and

18

18

18

J.J. Aning, D.M., F.R.C.S. (Urol.) • H. Hashim, M.B.B.S., M.R.C.S. (Eng.), M.D., F.E.B.U., F.R.C.S. (Urol.) (✉)
Southmead Hospital, Bristol Urological Institute, Southmead Road, Bristol BS10 5NB, UK
e-mail: h.hashim@gmail.com

A.J. Wein et al. (eds.), *Bladder Dysfunction in the Adult: The Basis for Clinical Management*, Current Clinical Urology, DOI 10.1007/978-1-4939-0853-0_18, © Springer Science+Business Media New York 2014

for urologists to be aware of the common complications of the native bladder remaining in situ: pyocystis, bleeding and pain.

Preoperative Preparation

All patients considered suitable for urinary diversion must be counselled appropriately regarding the risks and the benefits of each procedure. Those considering continent diversions, especially an orthotopic neobladder, must have realistic expectations and be screened for relative contraindications to this method of diversion (Table 18.1).

A thorough preoperative assessment pathway should include baseline blood tests and an appointment with the stoma nurse to ensure a suitable urostomy site is chosen and marked. Patients may also find it helpful to have the opportunity to speak or meet patients who have already had this procedure performed, in order to gain a perspective of routine perioperative care, ongoing bowel function and psychosexual issues. The evolution of enhanced recovery protocols and greater understanding of perioperative physiology has demonstrated that it is not necessary to give patients bowel preparation prior to diversion surgery. The only group of patients who may require bowel preparation are patients with neuropathic bladders suffering from severe constipation such as those with spina bifida.

Table 18.1 Contraindications to continent diversion formation

Impaired renal function
Impaired liver function
History of bowel tumour
Inflammatory bowel disease
Previous bowel surgery
Diverticulitis
Previous radiotherapy
Poor functional status
Inadequate intellectual capacity
Inadequate dexterity
Patients not likely to comply with follow-up

A description of all the variations of surgical techniques to construct urinary diversions is beyond the scope of this chapter; however, examples of common methods employed are reviewed.

Incontinent Cutaneous Diversions

Incontinent cutaneous diversions allow urine to be continuously expelled via the skin. Conduits are the most well-known form of this diversion.

Conduit diversion principle: The ureters are anastomosed to a segment of bowel (the conduit) which is brought out through the abdominal wall to form a stoma, known as a urostomy. Intraoperatively, the segment of the bowel is chosen and isolated, retaining its mesentery as a blood supply, and the continuity of the remaining bowel re-established. The conduit must be long enough to traverse the abdominal wall and form a spout which allows urine drained to be collected in a stoma bag without causing skin damage. Excessive conduit length is avoided, to facilitate drainage and reduce the surface area of bowel in contact with urine, so as to minimise metabolic complications. Ureteric catheters are temporarily sited across the ureteric anastomoses at surgery to protect the anastomoses.

Conduits: Ileal conduits are the commonest type of urinary diversion; the ileal segment is taken at least 15–20 cm from the ileo-caecal valve to avoid removing the terminal ileum where vitamin B12 and bile salt absorption takes place. The colon is also suitable for conduit formation; the transverse colon or sigmoid colon may be particularly useful in patients who have previously had pelvic irradiation or have short ureters. Colonic conduits permit the construction of a non-refluxing ureteral–intestinal anastomosis. The jejunum is rarely used as a conduit because of greater risk of metabolic complications.

Other examples of incontinent diversions: In circumstances when a bowel conduit cannot be constructed, the ureters may be anastomosed directly to the abdominal skin surface, forming a cutaneous ureterostomy. This may be associated with a high ureteric stenosis rate in the long term. Permanent percutaneous nephrostomy is an alternative method of achieving urinary diversion in frail patients. Permanent nephrostomies are limiting for patients because their lifestyle must be adapted to avoid pulling out the nephrostomy inadvertently and they are committed to lifelong regular nephrostomy changes.

Continent Urinary Diversion: Principles of Reconstruction

Generally accepted key principles of reconstruction are that the bowel used to form the urinary reservoir is detubularised and cross-folded to form a spherical reservoir.

Detubularisation is a process where bowel is opened on its antimesenteric border and then resutured in a different configuration. Detubularisation eliminates coordinated contractions from bowel peristalsis, which facilitates the formation of a low-pressure reservoir.

Spheroidal shape allows the maximum radius of the reconstructed reservoir to be achieved. Laplace's law (pressure=tension/radius) dictates that this creates a lower filling pressure. Current evidence suggests that spheroidal reservoirs ensure maximum volume to surface area with minimal resorptive surface area, thus also minimising metabolic complications. Spherical reservoirs formed from detubularised bowel may be shaped in many configurations such as W, M, Z or a cross-folded U; their functional outcomes appear to be equivalent. The pioneers of the various techniques advised the specific length of bowel required for their reconstruction. The temptation to take a longer segment of bowel to create a larger capacity reservoir at surgery must be resisted because, although early continence may ensue, there is more chance of creating a flaccid poorly emptying reservoir that then holds chronically infected urine and requires intermittent catheterisation.

The advantages of detubularisation include larger reservoir capacity and reduction in pressure generated by bowel contractions. This means that there is a quicker achievement of day-time continence with longer voiding intervals and better night-time continence. However, detubularisation does cause a higher incidence of urinary retention.

Anti-reflux techniques may be employed to connect the ureters to the reconstruction to prevent reflux nephropathy. However, published series demonstrate that these may be associated with a higher anastomotic stricture rate, which may itself lead to renal damage.

Continent Rectal Reservoirs

Continent rectal reservoirs allow urine diverted to the reservoir to be stored and voided rectally by the patient. Ureterosigmoidostomy is the most well-known example of this type of diversion.

Ureterosigmoidostomy principle: The ureters are implanted directly into the colon using anti-reflux techniques. Urine and faeces are then retained together in the rectum and voluntarily emptied when the patient senses the rectum is full. Preoperatively, patients have to demonstrate their ability to retain a watery and solid enema solution, in an upright position, to confirm an intact rectal sphincter. Ureteric catheters are temporarily sited across the ureteric anastomoses at surgery to protect the anastomoses and in addition to a rectal catheter.

Ureterosigmoidostomy was one of the earliest forms of continent urinary diversion and was the primary method of urinary diversion in the early twentieth century. The procedure fell out of vogue however because a significant number of patients suffered complications including incontinence post-surgery (especially at night), electrolyte disturbances, renal function deterioration, urinary tract calculi and pyelonephritis. A team at the University of Mainz developed a modification of the conventional ureterosigmoidostomy technique, the Mainz II, to address the complication rate. Instead of simply anastomosing the ureters directly to the sigmoid colon, the sigmoid colon and rectum are detubularised.

The reconstruction was in an inverted U shape. The Mainz II has been associated with a lower complication rate than its predecessor. Contraindications to ureterosigmoidostomy include previous pelvic irradiation because this may have compromised the sigmoid colon, impaired renal function or gross hydronephrosis due to the risks of reflux and associated renal unit damage and hepatic dysfunction, because ammonia may be absorbed across the bowel surface – leading to increased risk of hyperammonaemic encephalopathy. This method of urinary diversion is not commonly employed in patients with neuropathic bladder dysfunction, because of likely associated functional bowel abnormalities. Ureterosigmoidostomy is associated with development of adenocarcinoma at the site where the ureters are implanted. All patients undergoing the procedure should have annual surveillance flexible sigmoidoscopies from 5 years post surgery and be advised to seek urgent review if they suffer rectal bleeding or a change in bowel habit.

Continent Cutaneous Reservoirs

Continent cutaneous reservoirs allow urine diverted to a reservoir to be stored and emptied regularly using clean intermittent self-catheterisation (CISC) of an abdominal wall stoma.

Continent cutaneous reservoir principle: The ureters are anastomosed to the reservoir reconstructed from bowel. A conduit to the abdominal wall skin is formed using either a piece of bowel such as the appendix (Mitrofanoff) or ileum (Monti) and anastomosed to the reservoir. The conduit is fashioned to maintain continence unless catheterised. The stoma is usually sited at the umbilicus or lower abdominal wall. Ureteric catheters are sited across the ureteric anastomoses at surgery to protect the anastomoses and may be removed after 7 days.

Continent cutaneous reservoir examples: The Indiana pouch is a commonly used example of a continent cutaneous reservoir. The reservoir is created out of detubularised ascending colon, and

a portion of ileum is used as the catheterisable stoma, brought through the abdominal wall. The ileo-caecal valve, which is preserved in the reconstruction, forms an anti-reflux mechanism to maintain continence. The Kock pouch is an alternative urinary diversion which uses ileum alone to construct the reservoir; an intussuscepted nipple is created using staples at both the efferent and afferent locations in the reservoir, to act as the anti-reflux mechanism to maintain continence. The Kock pouch is technically more difficult to construct, and nipple failure resulting in loss of continence is the most common complication. The use of staples in this diversion is associated with a slightly higher reported incidence of stones when compared to other urinary diversions. The appendix is generally avoided as a potential conduit in continent cutaneous diversion reconstructions because it has a small luminal diameter. Intestinal reservoirs may produce a lot of mucus; the unaltered appendix generally allows 12 or 14 Fr catheterisation only, making irrigation and emptying of the reservoir difficult. The appendix may also be absent or of insufficient length.

Orthotopic Neobladder

Orthotopic neobladders allow urine diverted to a reservoir to be stored and voided urethrally. They are a desirable method of diversion because they offer a better cosmetic outcome and can significantly improve patient quality of life, approximating 'normality'. Although surgical technique is important, the best outcomes are achieved in highly motivated patients who are compliant with follow-up.

Orthotopic neobladder principle: The ureters are anastomosed to a reservoir constructed from bowel. The reservoir is anastomosed directly to the urethra. For optimal continence outcomes, it is essential to preserve the urethral sphincter mechanism by adopting a nerve-sparing approach when performing the cystectomy and neobladder reconstruction and to preserve urethral length. This also minimises the chance of long-term erectile dysfunction.

Patients void by relaxing their pelvic floor, followed by slight abdominal straining, aided by gentle hand pressure on the abdomen, and bending and flexing their torso. CISC is used to drain the residual urine. The initial neobladder capacity may be small. However, through patient education and postoperative training, a capacity of 500 mL may be achieved. Ureteric catheters are temporarily sited across the ureteric anastomoses at surgery to protect the anastomoses.

Orthotopic neobladder examples: The Studer neobladder is an established example of a neobladder constructed from ileum. A 54 cm segment of ileum is used to construct the neobladder. Both ends of the ileal segment are oversewn and a 40 cm opening made in the distal end of the ileal segment along its antimesenteric border to detubularise the segment. The ureters are spatulated and anastomosed end to side to the paramedian antimesenteric side of the intact tubular afferent ileal segment (a single chimney). The reservoir is reconstructed in a U shape, a 1 cm hole is made in the reservoir at the most caudal point at the bottom of the U. This forms the outlet of the neobladder, which is anastomosed to the urethra. Care is taken to ensure that the reservoir lies flat at the urethral anastomosis. This prevents kinking of the reservoir outlet which may impair voiding. A suprapubic catheter and urethral catheter are left in situ postoperatively. The catheters are flushed 6 hourly to prevent catheter blockages, which could rupture the neobladder. Professor Studer's unit performs a cystogram at 8–10 days, and if there is no leak, the suprapubic catheter is removed. Some centres may not perform a cystogram and merely leave the catheters in situ for a longer period of time. The urethral catheter may be removed 48 h after the suprapubic catheter has been removed. Close attention is paid to the patient's acid–base, hydration and nutrition status postoperatively. Patients are advised to void initially whilst seated, 2 hourly during the day and 3 hourly at night. An alarm clock is useful in supporting this regimen overnight. CISC is used initially post-voiding to empty the neobladder and measure post-

micturition residuals. The neobladder capacity increase is monitored and the duration between voiding gradually increased, CISC is continued if appropriate.

The Hautmann neobladder is a commonly employed alternative technique. The neobladder is constructed out of 60–80 cm of detubularised ileum in a W configuration. The W configuration allows the ureters to be anastomosed to separate chimneys, and the urethral plate of the reservoir may be wider. There appears to be no significant difference in functional outcome.

Other pouches include the Mansoura pouch, Padua pouch and Z-pouch.

Complications of Urinary Diversions

Patients undergoing reconstructive urinary tract surgery may suffer complications. In addition to general postoperative complications, early complications specific to urinary diversion include bowel leak, ileus, urinoma, urinary tract sepsis and metabolic complications.

Metabolic complications are caused primarily by the interaction between the bowel segment used in the reconstruction and urine. The purpose of the gastrointestinal tract is to absorb fluids and nutrients. The type and length of bowel used in the reconstruction in addition to the contact time between urine and bowel determine the metabolic consequences. Pre-existing renal failure may potentiate the susceptibility to patient compromise. Clinically, patients may be asymptomatic. However, most exhibit general malaise, lethargy, nausea, vomiting and anorexia. The metabolic abnormalities seen with each bowel segment are summarised in Table 18.2. All patients who undergo reconstruction must be monitored for biochemical abnormalities postoperatively, and clinicians must be aware that patients may present late. Chronic acidosis affects bone metabolism, and if not recognised, late complications include osteomalacia or osteoporosis. Once diagnosed, early management involves monitoring serum biochemistry with regular venous blood gas analysis and sodium bicarbonate supplementation.

Table 18.2 Metabolic abnormalities exhibited by bowel segments used in reconstruction

Bowel segment	Ions secreted into bowel segment	Ions absorbed by bowel segment	Metabolic abnormality
Ileum	Na, Cl	H, K	Hyponatraemic, hyperchloraemic, hyperkalaemic acidosis
Jejunum	Na, Cl	H, K	Hyponatraemic, hyperkalaemic acidosis
Colon	HCO_3	Na, Cl	Hyperchloraemic acidosis
Stomach	H, Cl		Hyponatraemic hypochloraemic, hypokalaemic alkalosis

Most patients do not require supplementation for more than 3 months.

Stoma complications in the form of stenosis, retraction, prolapse and parastomal hernia may significantly affect patient quality of life and require revision. Change in bowel habit is not unusual post-surgery, though certain types of diarrhoea may be treatable.

Ileal resection may be associated with fat malabsorption and steatorrhoea due to large amounts of bile salts reaching the colon and causing decreased water absorption. This may compromise absorption of fat soluble vitamins A and D. Cholestyramine may be used to treat bile salt diarrhoea. Vitamin B12 deficiency may also occur late because stores may last for years. Clinically, this may present as megaloblastic anaemia or peripheral nerve paraesthesias and is treated by vitamin supplementation. Reconstructions which remove the ileo-caecal valve may reduce bowel transit time. Urinary tract calculi are also a common late complication. Certain patients, especially with continent reservoirs, may suffer from recurrent urinary tract infections and 'pouchitis'. This can be treated with antibiotics.

Follow-Up of Patients After Urinary Diversion

Patients undergoing urinary diversion for benign disease must be followed up attentively to pick up complications and to monitor and maintain

Table 18.3 A follow-up regime after urinary diversion

	3	6	12	24	36	48	60
Examination	X	X	X	X	X	X	X
Urine dipstick	X	X	X	X	X	X	X
Weight and blood pressure	X		X	X	X	X	X
Blood tests (full blood count, renal function, bicarbonate, chloride)	X	X	X	X	X	X	X
Folic acid and Vitamin B12				X		X	
Ultrasound scan of renal tract			X	X	X	X	X	X
Post-micturition residual	X	X	X	X	X	X	X

function. Although there are no consensus guidelines regarding follow-up of patients undergoing reconstruction, Table 18.3 illustrates an example follow-up regime.

Conclusion

Urinary diversion is a valuable treatment option for patients with dysfunctional bladder symptoms that have not responded to conservative treatment. Continent diversions offer significant benefits in terms of quality of life. However, patients considering these options must be motivated and compliant with follow-up to ensure long-term success.

Suggested Reading

1. Wein AJ, Kavoussi LR, Novick AC, Partin AW, Peters CA, editors. Campbell—Walsh urology. 10th ed. Philadelphia: Elsevier Saunders; 2007.
2. Thurairaja R, Burkhard FC, Studer UE. The orthotopic neobladder. BJU Int. 2008;102:1307–13.
3. Arumainayagam N, McGrath J, Jefferson KP, Gillatt DA. Introduction of an enhanced recovery protocol for radical cystectomy. BJU Int. 2008;101: 698–701.
4. Gerharz EW, Mansson A, Hunt S, Skinner EC. Quality of life after cystectomy and urinary diversion: an evidence based analysis. J Urol. 2005;174: 1729–36.

Tissue Engineering for Neurogenic Bladder

19

Alex Gomelsky and Roger R. Dmochowski

Introduction

Neurogenic bladder (NGB) consists of any number of conditions that have their origin in the central or peripheral nervous system and impact the ability of the bladder to store or empty urine. For the purpose of this chapter, NGB will refer to the conditions of impaired urinary storage, resulting in decreased bladder compliance or detrusor overactivity. Traditionally, these disorders have been addressed with pharmacologic interventions (e.g., muscarinic receptor antagonists) and, when those failed, augmentation cystoplasty [1]. More recently, β-3 adrenergic agonists, various neuromodulation approaches, and intradetrusor injection of botulinum toxin A (onabotulinumtoxinA) have found a place in the treatment algorithm, seemingly diminishing the current role of augmentation cystoplasty. These modalities have been welcome additions, as cystoplasty is an often morbid procedure, potentially resulting in metabolic abnormalities, infections, urolithiasis, and, rarely, malignancy [2, 3]. The chief concern regarding the use of enteric segments for urological

A. Gomelsky, M.D.
Department of Urology, LSU Health—Shreveport, Shreveport, LA, USA

R.R. Dmochowski, M.D., M.M.H.C. (✉)
Department of Urologic Surgery, Vanderbilt University Medical Center, A1302 Medical Center North, Nashville, TN 37232-2765, USA
e-mail: roger.dmochowski@vanderbilt.edu

reconstruction is that these tissues are not created for urinary storage and, thus, not optimal substrates for that purpose. Hence, the concept of bladder augmentation (autoaugmentation and ureterocystoplasty) or substitution with similar tissue is very appealing [4, 5]. The introduction of tissue engineering strategies by incorporating scaffolds and cell cultures has the potential to remediate the deficiencies seen in enteric segments. Furthermore, this technology may, in theory, optimize the bladder's ability to regenerate and restore its original structure and function [6]. This chapter will explore the approaches to tissue engineering for NGB, with a focus on the advantages and disadvantages of each approach, as well as the currently available literature detailing the progress of the field.

The "Basics" of Engineered Tissue

Tissue engineering of the urinary bladder may be most easily divided into an acellular and cellular approach [7]. In the acellular approach, natural or synthetic scaffolds assist in directing new tissue growth and optimize the ability of the bladder to repair itself. In the cellular approach, the scaffold may be seeded with donor cells (cell-seeded scaffold), with the cells being autologous, allogeneic, or xenogeneic. Conversely, donor cells may be used alone (stem cell approach). Thus, the primary requirements for producing an engineered tissue are the presence of adequate stem cells or progenitor cells, an appropriate extracellular matrix (ECM), an adequate blood supply, and the presence of regulatory signals [7]. While the chapter will predominantly focus on various sources of scaffolding and cells, the presence of a viable blood supply cannot be overstated. In the absence of such, even an optimal combination of cells and scaffold may fail.

The choice of biomaterial is critical for the proper development of a reconstructed bladder. The material must be capable of controlling the structure and function of engineered tissue in a predesigned manner by interacting with host or transplanted cells [8]. As with materials for surgical correction of hernias, stress urinary incontinence (SUI), and pelvic organ prolapse (POP), the ideal biomaterial for bladder reconstruction should be strong and noncarcinogenic and should incite a minimal, if any, inflammatory response [9–11]. In the case of the bladder, the biomaterial should be strong enough to withstand the stress on the bladder from abdominal and pelvic pressures and should retain strength until the engineered bladder can withstand those forces on its own [8, 12]. The ideal biomaterial for bladder reconstruction should be biodegradable and bioresorbable, with acceptable rates of degradation and degradation products in the tissues [8, 13]. As a scaffold must support the expansion of both urothelial and smooth muscle cells (SMCs), the ideal biomaterial should also regulate cell activities such as adhesion, proliferation, migration, and differentiation [8, 14, 15]. Finally, the biomaterial should possess the ability to be sculpted into a hollow, spherical configuration that is optimal for urinary storage [8].

Biomaterials for Scaffold Construction

There is a rich history of implementing allografts, xenografts, and synthetic polymers in the surgical correction of female SUI and POP [11]. Similarly, three classes of biomaterials have been used for engineering of genitourinary tissues, naturally derived materials, acellular tissue matrices, and synthetic polymers, with each having the common goal of providing the proper orientation and direction for cell growth [8].

While scaffolds for SUI and POP serve predominantly as a framework for native tissue ingrowth and stabilization of weak support structures, scaffolds or matrices for bladder regeneration must also support reconstitution of both the smooth muscle component to restore organ contractile function and the urothelium to reestablish barrier function [16]. Each class of biomaterials has unique advantages and detractors and will be discussed in more detail.

Naturally Derived Materials

This class of biomaterials includes collagen, the most abundant protein found in mammals, and alginate, a polysaccharide isolated from seaweed. Collagen may be extracted from both allogeneic and xenogeneic sources after a variety of decellularization treatments with enzymes or acid/base solutions [17]. It may be further cross-linked by various chemical or physical methods to retard its degradation by the body's enzymes [16]. Furthermore, collagen may contain cell-adhesion domain sequences [e.g., Arg-Gly-Asp (RGD)] that exhibit specific cellular interactions, which may help retain the phenotype and activity of cells such as fibroblasts and chondrocytes [8, 18, 19]. Due to alginate's biocompatibility and simple gelation with divalent cations, it has been used for encapsulation, cell delivery, and cell immobilization [20].

Acellular Tissue Matrices

Matrices derived from decellularized tissues have included small intestinal submucosa (SIS) or bladder acellular submucosa matrix (BAM). These matrices slowly degrade upon implantation and are replaced and remodeled by new ECM proteins synthesized and secreted by transplanted or ingrowing host cells [21]. While both types of matrices have been associated with release of endogenous growth factors that optimize bladder healing in animal models [22–24], unpredictable mechanical integrity has been shown to result in graft fibrosis, contracture, and calcification [25–27].

To overcome the significant variations in microarchitecture and inconsistent results, several groups have introduced hybrid biologic/synthetic matrices with varying outcomes. Horst et al. developed a bilayered hybrid scaffold by electrospinning poly(lactic-co-glycolic) acid (PLGA) microfibers directly onto the abluminal surface of a BAM in a rat bladder model [28]. The electrospinning process allows parameters such as high porosity and ratio of surface area to volume, thought to be desirable qualities for a scaffold, to be varied quickly [21]. Histological analysis of the resulting three-dimensional framework in vivo at 4 and 8 weeks after implantation revealed regeneration of bladder urothelium, smooth muscle, and collagen-rich layers infiltrated with host cells and microvasculature. Furthermore, these hybrid scaffolds maintained normal bladder capacity. Mondalek et al. introduced PLGA nanoparticles (NPs) to SIS with the intent of decreasing the heterogeneity and improving the consistency of this biomaterial [29]. The NPs loaded in the SIS did not change the tensile properties of the unmodified SIS or alter pH values in a cell culture. Finally, Roth et al. incorporated hyaluronic acid (HA) into porcine SIS through PLGA NPs to improve the consistency of the biomaterial in a beagle augmentation model [30]. Histological assessment showed improved smooth muscle regeneration in the HA-PLGA-modified SIS group, but for both groups of dogs, urodynamic assessment and graft measurements showed ~40 % reduction in bladder capacity and graft size from pre-augmentation to post-regeneration measurements. Application of a novel scoring system created to evaluate gross and histological presentations of regenerative bladders and subsequent statistical analysis failed to show a significant difference between the groups. At present, additional research into the role and long-term benefits of NPs and HA is needed.

Synthetic Polymers

Synthetic materials for bladder reconstruction such as polyglycolic acid (PGA), a delayed absorbable fabric used extensively in surgical sutures, can have their structural and mechanical properties specifically tailored to match the target tissue of interest and offer an advantage over biologic materials [31]. In the case of regenerating the bladder, these matrices should be able to support the de novo formation of both smooth muscle and urothelium, and this has already been supported by clinical trials [32]. Conversely, as with synthetic implants in other parts of the body, matrices constructed from PGA may elicit a chronic inflammatory infiltrate that may lead to foreign body reaction and poor graft integration [33]. The authors suggested that inhibiting components that amplify the alternative pathway of the complement cascade (e.g., C5a) may limit the inflammation associated with PGA implantation. Additional polyesters of naturally occurring α-hydroxy acids are polylactic acid (PLA) and PLGA.

Another synthetic material that has been assayed for bladder reconstruction is silk fibroin. This material is derived from the *Bombyx mori* silkworm cocoons, and through the process of gel spinning, the resultant multi-laminate matrices can be produced with tailored pore size and architecture [34]. This material has been shown to have lower antigenicity at 70 days in a murine bladder augmentation model than both SIS and PGA, which revealed fibrosis and chronic inflammation, respectively [35, 36]. Furthermore, this material has been shown to possess significant mechanical stability and a favorable biodegradability profile [37–39]. Mauney et al. recently reported on a prototype acellular gel spun silk matrix that supported bladder regeneration in a rodent augment model [35]. While this material resulted in organized urothelial and smooth muscle compartments, along with increased bladder capacity, increased voided volumes, and stable compliance, the design exhibited a relatively slow rate of degradation over the 70-day postimplantation. Numata et al. demonstrated that silk fibroin may be susceptible to biodegradation by proteolytic enzymes such as chymotrypsin, actinase, and carboxylase [40].

The rate of degradation is key in the success of any biomaterial for bladder regeneration, as the material must be present long enough to support tissue ingrowth while providing strength and structure to the construct in the early postimplant period.

Rapid degradation may result in biomaterial collapse and necrosis at the defect site [41], while slow degradation can increase the possibility of urinary stone formation on the graft and delay the integration of host tissue [42]. Researchers have recently shown that rates of silk resorption are dependent on many factors, including the type of solvent used in processing, implantation site, and the animal model used [38, 39, 43, 44], and that manipulating these factors can enhance the degradation rate of silk scaffolds [45].

In an effort to improve on the performance of biologic scaffolds under vascular stresses, Lee et al. employed electrospinning to develop a durable vascular scaffold composed of poly (epsilon-caprolactone) (PCL) and collagen [46, 47]. The PCL/collagen composite scaffolds possessed appropriate tensile strength and elasticity, with a greater burst pressure than that of the PCL-only scaffolds and native vessels. When seeded with bovine endothelial cells (bECs) and smooth muscle cells (bSMCs), the composite scaffolds showed the formation of a confluent layer of bECs on the lumen and bSMCs on the outer surface of the scaffold.

Cell Sources

As discussed previously, unseeded matrices in tissue engineering have several shortcomings and have been replaced in favor of seeded matrices, biologic or synthetic scaffolds that are seeded with stem or progenitor cells and then implanted into the host. An advantage of the seeded approach is that cells may be autologous and rejection is a possible sequela. Donor tissue may be removed from the host and then implanted directly back into the host or attached to a support matrix after expansion in tissue culture. In an ideal situation, this approach would allow for tissue function to be restored or with limited complications [8]. Cells for implantation may be obtained from several sources and are discussed below [48].

Native Progenitor Cells

Autologous progenitor cells are an ideal option for seeding of matrices for several reasons. A progenitor cell is like a stem cell in that it has a tendency to differentiate into a specific type of cell but is already more specific than a stem cell and is pushed to differentiate into its target cell. They are referred to as unipotent, as these cells have the capacity to differentiate into only one cell type and can be found in many organs in the body. The most important difference between stem cells and progenitor cells is that stem cells can replicate indefinitely, whereas progenitor cells can divide only a limited number of times. Likewise, since these cells are autologous, their use is not associated with inflammatory reactions and rejection that is observed with nonself donor tissue. Furthermore, there are no ethical concerns regarding the use of progenitor cells, and they do not show any malignant potential when implanted.

A limitation of applying cell-based regenerative medicine techniques to organ replacement has been the challenge of growing certain human cell types in large quantities [8, 21]. Urothelial cells have traditionally been one of these cell types; however, techniques to improve cell expansion in vitro have been standardized. Cilento et al. developed a simple method for harvesting urothelial cells from surgical specimens to generate strains of normal, human urothelial cells that could be reproducibly cultivated, passaged, and extensively expanded in a serum-free medium [49]. Immunostaining of the bladder epithelial cells with antibodies reacting to cytokeratin 7, a transitional cell marker, indicated that they expressed a stable epithelial phenotype with serial passage. Immunostaining for E-cadherin and an anti-vimentin antibody indicated that the uroepithelial cells express a nonbarrier-forming phenotype under these culture conditions. However, when the urothelial cells were seeded onto biodegradable synthetic polymers and implanted subcutaneously into athymic mice, they formed multilayered structures, suggesting that they retain the capability to differentiate in a living host. Additionally, cytogenetic analysis indicated that urothelial cells cultured for six passages possessed a normal chromosomal complement. Additional studies have further demonstrated the techniques that keep undifferentiated cells in an undifferentiated state during their growth phase and that are able to expand an urothelial strain exponentially from a single specimen [49–54].

These results demonstrated that primary cultures of autologous human bladder epithelial cells can be extensively expanded in vitro and, consequently, might be used in cell transplantation strategies for genitourinary reconstruction [49]. However, a theoretical concern regarding the use of autologous progenitor cells has been the possibility of inferior cell quality procured from a diseased organ. Lin et al. compared primary cultures of SMCs from patients with a neuropathic bladder and a normal bladder [55]. The authors found that while normal and neuropathic SMCs showed similar morphology in culture and similar patterns of SM marker protein expression (alpha-SM actin and SM myosin), the number of neuropathic SMCs was 170 % more than normal SMCs. Additionally, in response to angiotensin II, neuropathic SMCs reached 54 % of maximal growth capacity vs. 30 % for normal SMCs ($p < 0.01$). Furthermore, neuropathic SMCs contracted significantly less by in vitro contractility assays and had significantly fewer adherent cells than normal SMCs following enzymatic treatment. Fortunately, studies have shown that genetically normal progenitor cells may be present in diseased organs. Lai et al. grew, expanded, and seeded onto polymer scaffolds human SMCs derived from patients with functionally normal bladders and functionally abnormal exstrophic and neuropathic bladders [56]. Human bladder cells showed similar expression of alpha-actin and myosin in vitro and after 2 months in vivo, regardless of their origin, and all scaffolds showed similar muscle formation in vivo. The cell-seeded scaffolds demonstrated the typical "contraction–relaxation" response to supramaximal electrical field and carbachol stimulation, and there were no statistical differences among the experimental groups (normal, exstrophic,

neurogenic). Thus, normal progenitors will develop into to normal tissue regardless of the quality of the organ of origin.

Stem Cells

While a complete discussion of human stem cells is beyond the limits of this chapter, it is important to mention several aspects of this potentially vital technology. Stem cells may be useful for organ regeneration for three reasons [7, 21, 57]. They have the capacity for self-renewal (i.e., proliferating in an undifferentiated but pluripotent state), have the ability to differentiate into most of the specialized cell types in the body, and have the ability to form clonal populations. Stem cells can be obtained from several different sources, including early embryonic, fetal, postnatal, and adult sources. Embryonic stem cells (ESCs) can be isolated from the embryo as early as 5 days after fertilization and have been shown to differentiate into cells from all three embryonic germ layers in vitro (ectoderm, mesoderm, endoderm) [57]. While the ethical considerations regarding harvesting of ESCs make the use of these cells today entirely a theoretical issue, the tumorigenic potential of this cell type further limits its use. As these cells are pluripotent, ESCs can form embryoid bodies, which are cell aggregations that contain all three embryonic germ layers while in culture, and can form teratomas in vivo [21, 58]. At present, the use of human ESCs is banned in the USA [21].

Additional sources of stem cells exist. Adult stem cells or mesenchymal stem cells (MSCs), specifically those harvested from bone marrow, are among the best studied. While there is no ethical issue regarding their use, some questions have been raised regarding some of the adult cells being present in small numbers and having low proliferative capacity in vitro [59, 60]. Adipose-derived stem cells obtained through liposuction have been shown to differentiate into endothelial cells and SMCs [61, 62]. Amniotic fluid- and placental-derived stem cells can be induced to differentiate into cells representing each embryonic germ layer, with differentiation into kidney tissue reported [8, 63].

Additionally, De Coppi et al. showed that while MSCs from rat amniotic fluid or bone marrow injected into cryo-injured rat bladder walls had a limited effect on SMC regeneration, they appeared to prevent cryo-injury induced hypertrophy of surviving SMCs, possibly via a paracrine mechanism [64]. Furthermore, these cells do not appear to be tumorigenic in vivo.

Outcomes of Bladder Regeneration

Unseeded Matrices

While one of the advantages of using unseeded matrices is that the relative antigenicity of these constructs is low, the outcomes in animal studies have been unpredictable. Kanematsu et al. loaded basic fibroblast growth factor (bFGF) protein in a lyophilized BAM and implanted it into a rat augmentation model [65]. The authors observed a sustained release of bFGF from BAM in vitro and in vivo, with in vivo biological activity of bFGF in BAM preserved for more than 3 weeks. In the bladder augmentation model, angiogenesis into the matrix was promoted, and graft shrinkage was significantly inhibited by incorporated bFGF in a dose-dependent manner at 4 weeks. Kropp et al. also demonstrated bladder regeneration using an unseeded SIS matrix, with the distal ileum being preferable for SIS harvest [66]. One of the disadvantages of using unseeded matrices is that, while the urothelium appeared to regenerate in a normal fashion, the smooth muscle layer either did not develop or developed incompletely [67–69]. This finding may be associated with significant graft contraction [70, 71]. Additionally, Landman et al. reported that 1 year after hemicystectomy, no advantage in bladder capacity or compliance was seen compared to primary bladder closure [71].

Cell-Seeded Matrices

Tissue engineering techniques have already been employed in the construction of a male urethra and male and female reproductive organs [21]. Likewise, bladder substitutes have been constructed from cell-seeded matrices. Yoo et al. cultured SMCs from canine native bladder biopsies and seeded them onto bladder-shaped polymer matrices [67, 72]. The native bladders were subsequently excised from canine donors and replaced with the tissue-engineered neo-organs. In functional evaluations for up to 11 months, the bladder neo-organs demonstrated a normal capacity to retain urine, normal elastic properties, and histological architecture. The bladders augmented with cell-seeded scaffolds showed a significant increase in capacity when compared with unseeded scaffolds. Additional studies have confirmed these outcomes in the long-term, in terms of both efficacy and safety [73–75].

Atala et al. initially reported on the development of a system for the harvest, delivery, and growth of rabbit urothelium in vivo using biodegradable polymers [76]. The authors then expanded and adapted this system for the harvest and in vivo implantation of human bladder urothelial and muscle cells [77]. Rabbit uroepithelial cells seeded on a PGA scaffold were implanted into athymic host animals. PGA supported the proliferation of rabbit urothelial cells in situ, and human urothelial cells and bladder muscle cells, when implanted on PGA, formed new urological structures in vivo composed of both cell types. As previously mentioned, clinical outcomes using both unseeded and cell-seeded SIS have shown graft contraction in some canine studies [29].

Clinical outcomes in humans are novel. Atala et al. obtained a bladder biopsy from seven patients with myelomeningocele and high-pressure or poorly compliant bladders [32]. Urothelial and SMCs were grown in culture and seeded on a biodegradable bladder-shaped scaffold made of collagen or a composite of collagen and PGA. Approximately 7 weeks after biopsy, the engineered bladders were used for cystoplasty with or without an omental wrap. At a mean follow-up of 46 months, the mean bladder leak point pressure decreased at capacity, and the volume and compliance increase was greatest in the composite-engineered bladders with an omental wrap. No metabolic consequences were noted and renal function was preserved. Furthermore, the engineered bladder biopsies showed an adequate structural architecture and phenotype.

Conclusions

The prospect of regenerating a bladder capable of efficient urinary storage for patients with NGB is appealing and quite tangible. Research into matrices and cells capable of forming functional bladder urothelium and smooth muscle continues to progress at an exponential pace. At present, several conclusions can be made based on the available data. First, acellular tissue matrices may be associated with graft fibrosis and contracture in vivo while synthetic polymers may be associated with inflammation and foreign body reaction. Composite scaffolds can be tailored to maximize the benefits of each option and minimize the potential adverse sequelae. Second, cell-seeded matrices perform better than unseeded matrices. Third, urothelium, likely owing to its high reparative capacity, is easier to regenerate than smooth muscle. Fourth, SMCs obtained from a neuropathic bladder showed the same properties as the tissues engineered with normal cells. Finally, stem cell research in bladder regeneration may eventually yield multiple effective options for cell seeding, but at the present time, progenitor cells are the primary cells available for normal cell differentiation. While promising, these advances are not yet ready for widespread use, and clinical outcomes in humans are limited.

References

1. Niknead KG, Atala A. Bladder augmentation techniques in women. Int Urogynecol J Pelvic Floor Dysfunct. 2000;11:156–69.
2. Hensle TW, Gilbert SM. A review of metabolic consequences and long-term complications of enterocystoplasty in children. Curr Urol Rep. 2007;8:157–62.
3. Somani BK, et al. Bowel dysfunction after transposition of intestinal segments into the urinary tract: 8-year prospective cohort study. J Urol. 2007; 177:1793–8.
4. Cartwright PC, Snow BW. Bladder autoaugmentation: partial detrusor excision to augment the bladder without use of bowel. J Urol. 1989;142:1050–3.
5. Bellinger MF. Ureterocystoplasty: a unique method for vesical augmentation in children. J Urol. 1993; 149:811–3.
6. Bartold PM, Xiao Y, Lyngstaadas SP, Paine ML, Snead ML. Principles and application of cell delivery systems for periodontal regeneration. Periodontology. 2006;41:123–35.
7. Petrovic V, Stankovic J, Stefanovic V. Tissue engineering of the urinary bladder: current concepts and future perspectives. Sci World J. 2011;11:1479–88.
8. Atala A. Tissue engineering of human bladder. Br Med Bull. 2011;97:81–104.
9. Cumberland VH. A preliminary report on the use of prefabricated nylon weave in the repair of ventral hernia. Med J Aust. 1952;1:143.
10. Scales JT. Materials for hernia repair. Proc R Soc Med. 1953;46:647.
11. Gomelsky A, Dmochowski RR. Biocompatibility assessment of synthetic sling materials for female stress urinary incontinence. J Urol. 2007;178:1171–81.
12. Atala A. Engineering tissues, organs, and cells. J Tissue Eng Regen Med. 2007;1:83–96.
13. Bergsma JE, Rozema FR, Bos RR, et al. In vivo degradation and biocompatibility study of in vitro, predegraded as-polymerized polyactide particles. Biomaterials. 1995;16:267–74.
14. Barrera DA, Zylstra E, Lansbury PT, et al. Synthesis and RGD peptide modification of a new biodegradable copolymer poly (lactic acid-co-lysine). J Am Chem Soc. 1993;115:11010–1.
15. Cook AD, Hrkach JS, Gao NN, et al. Characterization and development of RGD peptide-modified poly (lactic acid-co-lysine) as an interactive, resorbable biomaterial. J Biomed Mater Res. 1997;35:213–23.
16. Roth CC, Kropp BP. Recent advances in urologic tissue engineering. Curr Urol Rep. 2009;10:119–25.
17. Li ST. Biologic biomaterials: tissue derived biomaterials (collagen). In: Brozino JD, editor. The biomedical engineering handbook. Boca Raton, FL: CRS Press; 1995. p. 627–47.
18. Silver FH, Pins G. Cell growth on collagen: a review of tissue engineering using scaffolds containing extracellular matrix. J Long Term Eff Med Implants. 1992;2:67–80.
19. Sams AE, Nixon AJ. Chondrocyte-laden collagen scaffolds for resurfacing extensive articular cartilage defects. Osteoarthritis Cartilage. 1995;3:47–59.
20. Smidsrod O, Skjak-Braek G. Alginate as immobilization matrix for cells. Trends Biotechnol. 1990;8:71–8.
21. Atala A. Tissue engineering of reproductive tissues and organs. Fertil Steril. 2012;98:21–9.
22. Kropp BP. Small-intestinal submucosa for bladder augmentation: a review of preclinical studies. World J Urol. 1998;16:262–7.
23. Yang B, Zhang Y, Zhou L, Sun Z, Zheng J, Chen Y, et al. Development of a porcine bladder acellular

matrix with well-preserved extracellular bioactive factors for tissue engineering. Tissue Eng Part C. 2010;16:1201–11.

24. Sharma AK, Bury MI, Marks AJ, Fuller NJ, Meisner JW, Tapaskar N, et al. A non-human primate model for urinary bladder regeneration utilizing autologous sources of bone marrow derived mesenchymal stem cells. Stem Cells. 2011;29:241–50.

25. Chung SY, Krivorov NP, Rausei V, Thomas L, Frantzen M, Landsittel D, et al. Bladder reconstitution with bone marrow derived stem cells seeded on small intestinal submucosa improves morphological and molecular composition. J Urol. 2005;174:353–9.

26. Ashley RA, Roth CC, Palmer BW, Kibar Y, Routh JC, Fung KM, et al. Regional variations in small intestinal submucosa evoke differences in inflammation with subsequent impact on tissue regeneration in the rat bladder augmentation model. BJU Int. 2010; 105:1462–8.

27. Zhang Y, Frimberger D, Cheng EY, Lin HK, Kropp BP. Challenges in a larger bladder replacement with cell-seeded and unseeded small intestinal submucosa grafts in a subtotal cystectomy model. BJU Int. 2006;98:1100–5.

28. Horst M, Madduri S, Milleret V, Sulser T, Gobet R, Eberli D. A bilayered hybrid microfibrous PLGA—acellular matrix scaffold for hollow organ tissue engineering. Biomaterials. 2013;34:1537–45.

29. Mondalek FG, Lawrence BJ, Kropp BP, Grady BP, Fung KM, Madihally SV, Lin HK. The incorporation of poly(lactic-co-glycolic) acid nanoparticles into porcine small intestinal submucosa biomaterials. Biomaterials. 2008;29:1159–66.

30. Roth CC, Mondalek FG, Kibar Y, Ashley RA, Bell CH, Califano JA, Madihally SV, Frimberger D, Lin HK, Kropp BP. Bladder regeneration in a canine model using hyaluronic acid-poly(lactic-co-glycolic-acid) nanoparticle modified porcine small intestinal submucosa. BJU Int. 2011;108:148–55.

31. Yang S, Leong KF, Du Z, Chua CK. The design of scaffolds for use in tissue engineering. Part I. Traditional factors. Tissue Eng. 2001;7:679–89.

32. Atala A, Bauer SB, Soker S, Yoo JJ, Retik AB. Tissue-engineered autologous bladders for patients needing cystoplasty. Lancet. 2006;367:1241–6.

33. Ceonzo K, Gaynor A, Shaffer L, Kojima K, Vacanti CA, Stahl GL. Polyglycolic acid-induced inflammation: role of hydrolysis and resulting complement activation. Tissue Eng. 2006;12:301–8.

34. Lovett ML, Cannizzaro CM, Vunjak-Novakovic G, Kaplan DL. Gel spinning of silk tubes for tissue engineering. Biomaterials. 2008;29:4650–7.

35. Mauney JR, Cannon GM, Lovett ML, Gong EM, Di Vizio D, Gomez 3rd P, Kaplan DL, Adam RM, Estrada Jr CR. Evaluation of gel spun silk-based biomaterials in a murine model of bladder augmentation. Biomaterials. 2011;32:808–18.

36. Meinel L, Hofmann S, Karageorgiou V, Kirker-Head C, McCool J, Gronowicz G, et al. The inflammatory

responses to silk films in vitro and in vivo. Biomaterials. 2005;26:147–55.

37. Shao Z, Vollrath F. Surprising strength of silkworm silk. Nature. 2002;418:741.

38. Kim UJ, Park J, Kim HJ, Wada M, Kaplan DL. Three-dimensional aqueous-derived biomaterial scaffolds from silk fibroin. Biomaterials. 2005;26:2775–85.

39. Wang Y, Rudym DD, Walsh A, Abrahamsen L, Kim HJ, Kim HS, et al. In vivo degradation of three-dimensional silk fibroin scaffolds. Biomaterials. 2008;29:3415–28.

40. Numata K, Cebe P, Kaplan DL. Mechanism of enzymatic degradation of beta-sheet crystals. Biomaterials. 2010;31:2926–33.

41. Sanz-Herrera JA, Garcia-Aznar JM, Doblare M. On scaffold designing for bone regeneration: a computational multiscale approach. Acta Biomater. 2009;5:219–29.

42. Su ST, Huang HF, Chang SF. Encrusted bladder stone on non-absorbable sutures after a cesarean section: a case report. JTUA. 2009;20:143–5.

43. Altman GH, Diaz F, Jakuba C, Calabro T, Horan RL, Chen J, et al. Silk-based biomaterials. Biomaterials. 2003;24:401–16.

44. Tu DD, Seth A, Gil ES, Kaplan DL, Mauney JR, Estrada Jr CR. Evaluation of biomaterials for bladder augmentation using cystometric analyses in various rodent models. J Vis Exp. 2012;(66)pii: 3981.

45. Gomez 3rd P, Gil ES, Lovett ML, Rockwood DN, Di Vizio D, Kaplan DL, Adam RM, Estrada Jr CR, Mauney JR. The effect of manipulation of silk scaffold fabrication parameters on matrix performance in a murine model of bladder augmentation. Biomaterials. 2011;32:7562–70.

46. Lee SJ, Liu J, Oh SH, Soker S, Atala A, Yoo JJ. Development of a composite vascular scaffolding system that withstands physiological vascular conditions. Biomaterials. 2008;29:2891–8.

47. Lee SJ, Oh SH, Liu J, Soker S, Atala A, Yoo JJ. The use of thermal treatments to enhance the mechanical properties of electrospun poly(epsiloncaprolectone) scaffolds. Biomaterials. 2008;29:1422–30.

48. Aboushwareb T, Atala A. Stem cells in urology. Nat Clin Pract Urol. 2008;5:621–31.

49. Cilento BG, Freeman MR, Schneck FX, Retik AB, Atala A. Phenotypic and cytogenetic characterization of human bladder urothelia expanded in vitro. J Urol. 1994;152:665–70.

50. Scriven SD, Booth C, Thomas DF, Trejdosiewicz LK, Southgate J. Reconstitution of human urothelium from monolayer cultures. J Urol. 1997;158:1147–52.

51. Liebert M, Hubbel A, Chung M, Wedemeyer G, Lomax MI, Hegeman A, et al. Expression of mal is associated with urothelial differentiation in vitro: identification by differential display reverse-transcriptase polymerase chain reaction. Differentiation. 1997;61:177–85.

52. Liebert M, Wedemeyer G, Abruzzo LV, Kunkel SL, Hammerberg C, Cooper KD, et al. Stimulated urothelial

cells produce cytokines and express an activated cell surface antigenic phenotype. Semin Urol. 1991;9:124–30.

53. Puthenveettil JA, Burger MS, Reznikoff CA. Replicative senescence in human uroepithelial cells. Adv Exp Med Biol. 1999;462:83–91.

54. Nguyen HT, Park JM, Peters CA, Adam RM, Orsola A, Atala A, et al. Cell-specific activation of the HB-EGF and ErbB1 genes by stretch in primary human bladder cells. In Vitro Cell Dev Biol Anim. 1999;35:371–5.

55. Lin HK, Cowan R, Moore P, Zhang Y, Yang Q, Peterson Jr JA, Tomasek JJ, Kropp BP, Cheng E. Characterization of neuropathic bladder smooth muscle cells in culture. J Urol. 2004;171:1348–52.

56. Lai JY, Yoon CY, Yoo JJ, Wulf T, Atala A. Phenotypic and functional characterization of in vivo tissue engineered smooth muscle from normal and pathological bladders. J Urol. 2002;168:1853–7.

57. Brivanlou AH, Gage FH, Jaenisch R, Jessell T, Melton D, Rossant J. Stem cells. Setting standards for human embryonic stem cells. Science. 2003;300:913–6.

58. Itskovitz-Eldor J, Schuldiner M, Karsenti D, Eden A, Yanuka O, Amit M, et al. Differentiation of human embryonic stem cells into embryoid bodies compromising the three embryonic germ layers. Mol Med. 2000;6:88–95.

59. Mimeault M, Batra SK. Recent progress on tissue-resident adult stem cell biology and their therapeutic implications. Stem Cell Rev. 2008;4:27–49.

60. Hristov M, Zernecke A, Schober A, et al. Adult progenitor cells in vascular remodeling during atherosclerosis. Biol Chem. 2008;389:837–44.

61. Jumabay M, Zhang R, Yao Y, Goldhaber JI, Boström KI. Spontaneously beating cardiomyocytes derived from white mature adipocytes. Cardiovasc Res. 2010;85:17–27.

62. Scholz T, Sumarto A, Krichevsky A, Evans GR. Neuronal differentiation of human adipose tissue-derived stem cells for peripheral nerve regeneration in vivo. Arch Surg. 2011;146:666–74.

63. Perin L, Giuliani S, Jin D, et al. Renal differentiation of amniotic fluid stem cells. Cell Prolif. 2007; 40:936–48.

64. De Coppi P, Callegari A, Chiavegato A, et al. Amniotic fluid and bone marrow derived mesenchymal stem cells can be converted to smooth muscle cells in the cryo-injured rat bladder and prevent compensatory hypertrophy of surviving smooth muscle cells. J Urol. 2007;177:369–76.

65. Kanematsu A, Yamamoto S, Noguchi T, Ozeki M, Tabata Y, Ogawa O. Bladder regeneration by bladder acellular matrix combined with sustained release of exogenous growth factor. J Urol. 2003;170:1633–8.

66. Kropp BP, Cheng EY, Lin HK, Zhang Y. Reliable and reproducible bladder regeneration using unseeded distal small intestinal submucosa. J Urol. 2004;172:1710–3.

67. Yoo JJ, Meng J, Oberpenning F, Atala A. Bladder augmentation using allogenic bladder submucosa seeded with cells. Urology. 1998;51:221–5.

68. Probst M, Dahiya R, Carrier S, Tanagho EA. Reproduction of functional smooth muscle tissue and partial bladder replacement. Br J Urol. 1997;79:505–15.

69. Kropp BP, Rippy MK, Badylak SF, Adams MC, Keating MA, Rink RC, Thor KB. Regenerative urinary bladder augmentation using small intestinal submucosa: urodynamic and histopathologic assessment in long-term canine bladder augmentations. J Urol. 1996;155:2098–104.

70. Portis AJ, Elbahnasy AM, Shalhav AL, Brewer A, Humphrey P, McDougall EM, Clayman RV. Laparoscopic augmentation cystoplasty with different biodegradable grafts in an animal model. J Urol. 2000;164:1405–11.

71. Landman J, Olweny E, Sundaram CP, Andreoni C, Collyer WC, Rehman J, Jerde TJ, Lin K, Lee DI, Nunlist EH, Humphrey PA, Nakada SY, Clayman RV. Laparoscopic mid sagittal hemicystectomy and bladder reconstruction with small intestinal submucosa and reimplantation of ureter into small intestinal submucosa: 1-year followup. J Urol. 2004;171:2450–5.

72. Oberpenning F, Meng J, Yoo JJ, Atala A. De novo reconstitution of a functional mammalian urinary bladder by tissue engineering. Nat Biotechnol. 1999;17:149–55.

73. Jayo MJ, Jain D, Wagner BJ, et al. Early cellular and stromal responses in regeneration versus repair of a mammalian bladder using autologous cell and biodegradable scaffold technologies. J Urol. 2008;180:392–7.

74. Jayo MJ, Jain D, Ludlow JW, et al. Long-term durability, tissue regeneration and neo-organ growth during skeletal maturation with a neo-bladder augmentation construct. Regen Med. 2008;3:671–82.

75. Kwon TG, Yoo JJ, Atala A. Local and systemic effects of a tissue engineered neobladder in a canine cystoplasty model. J Urol. 2008;179:2035–41.

76. Atala A, Vacanti JP, Peters CA, Mandell J, Retik AB, Freeman MR. Formation of urothelial structures in vivo from dissociated cells attached to biodegradable polymer scaffolds in vitro. J Urol. 1992;148:658–62.

77. Atala A, Freeman MR, Vacanti JP, Shepard J, Retik AB. Implantation in vivo and retrieval of artificial structures consisting of rabbit and human urothelium and human bladder muscle. J Urol. 1993;150:608–12.

Part V

Other Considerations

Emily J. Henderson

A Conceptual Framework

In the 1960s, Sir Bernard Isaacs identified incontinence, along with immobility, instability and intellectual impairment, as the "giants" of geriatric medicine [1]. Multiple pathological and physiological factors converge and finally manifest as these common syndromes. Each syndrome should not be considered in isolation. The syndromes share common risk factors and all are associated with increased risk of functional decline. As such, older age, baseline functional impairment, impaired mobility and baseline cognitive impairment are risk factors not only for incontinence but also for pressure ulcers, falls, functional decline and delirium [2]. An overarching concept of "frailty" unifies these findings. Frailty is the notion that accumulated impairments, in multiple systems, contribute to a state of increased vulnerability to poor outcomes, namely, disability, dependence and death [2].

Understanding incontinence within the concept of frailty is key to approaching the assessment and management of UI in frail older people. Rather than a single pathology, exerting a direct

E.J. Henderson, M.B., Ch.B., M.R.C.P. (✉)
School of Social and Community Medicine,
University of Bristol, 39 Whatley Road, Clifton,
Bristol BS8 2PS, UK
e-mail: Emily.Henderson@bristol.ac.uk

effect on the lower urinary tract incontinence in frail older people results from complex interactions of multiple pathologies in different organ systems. These "anatomically remote" determinants of continence include mobility, cognitive function, environmental factors, medications and comorbid medical illness.

Older people are a heterogeneous population and have been historically mostly excluded from clinical trials. Whilst evidence-based interventions and guidelines for the treatment of incontinence in older people do exist [3], there remains a relative lack of substantial, good quality evidence to guide clinical decision making in this population. Whilst interventions with proven efficacy in younger populations can be extrapolated to the "independent and active" cohort, frail older people require a more individualized approach. Specific aspects of assessment and management of factors that contribute to incontinence in frail older people form the focus of this chapter.

Epidemiology and Impact

Urinary incontinence is the complaint of any involuntary leakage of urine [4]. The prevalence of UI increases with age. Estimates vary widely because of different definitions and methodology employed in studies. Using the 2002 International Continence Society (ICS) definitions, the EPIC study found lower urinary tract symptoms (LUTS) to be highly prevalent in men and women with 10.4 % of men and 19.3 % of women over the age of 60 reporting UI [5]. Within older people those living in institutional care have particularly high prevalence with results from a cross-national database reporting rates between 43 and 65 % in women [6]. With an increasingly ageing population, the number of older people with UI is set to increase.

UI is associated with an increased risk of hospitalization and nursing home placement, falls and fractures and excess mortality when associated with stroke [7–9]. The negative impact of UI on all aspects of quality of life can often exceed that of other conditions with which it is associated [10]. The high prevalence of UI, coupled with associated direct (management related) costs and indirect (provision of care related) costs, leads to a significant economic burden.

Continence

Normal voiding requires intact neurological and muscle function of the lower urinary tract and pelvic floor. Continence additionally requires adequate and intact cognitive function to react appropriately to bladder filling as well as dexterity and mobility to toilet. Incontinence can occur when any of these mechanisms are disrupted.

The investigation of the incontinent patient requires a detailed history and thorough examination, with appropriate use of relevant investigations. Assessment should be targeted to identify factors that may be amenable to intervention. The choice of appropriate management strategies is aided if the type of incontinence can be determined (Table 20.1). Furthermore, assessment of indirect factors such as cognition, comorbidities, medications and mobility is considered in more detail as these are particularly pertinent in frail older people.

It is important to establish and regularly review the goal of therapy. In older people assessing the effect on quality of life is vital and should always inform treatment decisions. This should involve consideration of prognosis, life expectancy, compliance with therapy, degree of symptom "bother" as well as feasibility and burden in respect to carers who are involved. The treatment preferences of

Table 20.1 2002 ICS definitions [4]

Term	Definition
Nocturia	The complaint that the individual has to wake at night one or more times to void
Urinary incontinence	The complaint of any involuntary leakage of urine
Stress urinary incontinence	The complaint of involuntary leakage on effort or exertion or on sneezing or coughing
Urge urinary incontinence	The complaint of involuntary leakage accompanied by or immediately preceded by urgency
Mixed urinary incontinence	Involuntary leakage associated with urgency and also with exertion, effort, sneezing or coughing

the patient often differ to that of their carers and/or family members and this should be explored [11]. Goals of therapy can range from complete resolution of symptoms with a single intervention or ongoing therapy to containment with pads, appliances and catheters [12].

Cognitive Function

The presence of cognitive impairment may directly affect a person's ability sufficiently to plan, organize and regulate their behaviour to toilet effectively, as well as their ability to comply with behavioural interventions. Susceptibility to adverse cognitive effects is conferred by underlying conditions such as Parkinson's disease, stroke, dementia and mild cognitive impairment as well as concomitant medications with high anticholinergic burden such as tricyclic antidepressants and antihistamines. Vulnerability to cognitive impairment must be assessed when considering treatments such as antimuscarinic drugs for overactive bladder or surgical options with the associated risk of post-operative delirium.

Whilst antimuscarinics are effective for overactive bladder in older people, specific consideration should be given to the choice of drug [13]. Cognitive testing should detect impairment at baseline and monitor any change. Many studies looking at UI and antimuscarinics have used the Mini-Mental State Examination (MMSE) to test cognition. Whilst the MMSE is familiar, it may not be adequately sensitive to detect subtle change. It does not measure the domain of executive function (which confers an ability to multitask, plan and organize) which is frequently affected by white matter lesions disrupting frontal-subcortical circuits. As an alternative, the CLOX test is a clock drawing test that is easily administered and is associated with cognitive test scores but specifically taps executive function [14]. Despite being a valid and potentially better choice than the MMSE, it is not yet in widespread use.

White matter lesions are common neuroradiological findings in older people, manifest as hyperintensities on magnetic resonance imaging and indicate damage to brain parenchyma. The prevalence and severity of white matter lesions increase with age. The finding of white matter lesions is common to many geriatric syndromes including falls, cognitive impairment, depression and urge UI, postulated to result from hyper-reflexic uninhibited detrusor muscle [15]. Once labelled as "silent" it is now evident that disruption of frontal-subcortical circuits contributes to the common clinical presentations of older people.

In respect to incontinence, urodynamic evidence of detrusor overactivity has been associated with white matter hyperintensities (WMH) as well as cognitive and gait dysfunction. Higher grades of lesions were associated with increasing severity of all three dysfunctions. Investigation of the anatomy of the lesions showed that the burden of WMH within the cingulate gyrus predicted UI symptoms with severity. WMH in the anterior corona radiata were related to "bother" associated with UI [16]. With this established association, targeting the risk factors for the development of WMH may prove a novel way to tackle incontinence and other geriatric syndromes associated with these lesions.

Mobility

Any cause of impaired mobility can lead to difficulty accessing and using toilet facilities. The relationship between mobility impairment and incontinence appears to be bidirectional. A meta-analysis of the relationship between falls and urinary incontinence, in a community dwelling population, demonstrated that the presence of UI increased the chance of falling with a greater risk with urge rather than stress incontinence [17, 18]. This intuitively makes sense if people rush to get to the toilet. Whilst interventions to tackle incontinence feature in some multifactorial falls assessment and prevention programmes, evidence to suggest that treating incontinence alone prevents falls is lacking. Inactivity is associated with UI and strategies that have sought to improve mobility with walking have shown positive results for incontinence, as well as strategies employing physical training and toileting skills [19–21].

Assessment of mobility can be performed in clinic using the "timed up and go test". It involves standing up, walking 3 m, turning 180°, walking back and sitting down and should be completed within 12 s [22]. People who take longer are more likely to have functional and mobility impairment which can be effectively targeted with mobility aids, exercise programmes and physiotherapy input.

Medication Review

Drugs prescribed for comorbid conditions may influence continence directly or indirectly. It is unclear whether adjustment of culprit drugs alters incontinence or whether LUTS result from the drug or underlying condition for which it is prescribed. A pragmatic approach however dictates sensible consideration of drugs that affect voiding.

A study that sought to establish the relationship between self-reported urinary difficulties and urologically active medications reported diuretics, anticholinergics and benzodiazepines as the most prevalent subclasses of implicated drugs [23]. Benzodiazepines may directly affect pelvic floor musculature, interfere with afferent bladder sensory messages or negatively affect cognition. Data from Italy has demonstrated a 44 % increased risk of UI with benzodiazepine use [24]. Alternatively benzodiazepines, along with other psychotropic drugs, and opiates may mediate their effect centrally though altered cognition.

Diuretics are often cited by patients as a contributive factor to LUTS and review of their use has been advocated. However, evidence as to their role is conflicting [25]. Cholinesterase inhibitors have been linked to incontinence and are purported to exert influence on the lower urinary tract by increasing cholinergic transmission at muscarinic receptors in the bladder wall thereby augmenting detrusor contractility. This is supported by two studies that both found 7 % of patients started on a cholinesterase inhibitor developed new or worsening UI [26, 27]. Furthermore, a retrospective cohort study identified that patients prescribed with a cholinesterase inhibitor for dementia were then more likely to be prescribed with an anticholinergic drug for incontinence [28].

Comorbid Conditions

Whilst it is not known whether treatment of conditions associated with UI improves outcomes, potentially remediable conditions should be addressed. Patient preference and the degree to which the underlying condition is treatable will tend to dictate the appropriate approach.

Polyuria can contribute to UI. A common scenario is polyuria secondary to hyperglycaemia in diabetes mellitus. Tight control of blood sugar levels may be warranted but should be carefully balanced against the risk of hypoglycaemia and the burden of testing. Other causes of polyuria to explore include hypercalcaemia, diabetes insipidus and drugs including diuretics, caffeine and alcohol.

Sleep apnoea can cause nocturia; the associated hypoxaemia causes the release of brain type natriuretic peptide from the heart, increasing secretion of sodium and water as a result of vasodilatation and inhibition of aldosterone. Treatment of the underlying condition with continuous positive airway pressure has been shown to decrease the number of nocturic episodes [29].

Peripheral oedema results from low protein states, heart failure, liver failure and kidney failure and is a common side effect of drugs such as calcium channel blockers and nonsteroidal anti-inflammatories. It can cause nocturnal diuresis, as fluid is resorbed in the supine position. In some cases an appropriately timed dose of a diuretic can be of benefit [30]

Stress incontinence may be worsened by cough resulting from respiratory disease or angiotensin-converting enzyme inhibitors. If associated with the latter, it can remit on discontinuation of the drug [31].

Constipation is extremely common in older people and associated with retention of urine and LUTS. Digital rectal examination (DRE) will identify faecal loading and allow assessment of the prostate. This is particularly relevant in care homes where there may be a lack of clinicians who are able to perform this task [32].

Conclusion

UI is common in frail older people and can cause profound suffering. Consideration of factors beyond the lower urinary tract warrants particular consideration. This fits within the concept of frailty whereby incontinence along with other geriatric syndromes is the end result of complex interplay of factors often distant from the presenting complaint. A collaborative approach from a multidisciplinary team that includes experts in geriatric medicine and urology will facilitate the delivery of a high standard of care to older people. The future poses many challenges and opportunities to improve the care we provide to the particularly vulnerable and expanding population of older people.

References

1. Isaacs B. An introduction to geriatrics. London: Williams & Wilkins Co.; 1965.
2. Inouye SK, et al. Geriatric syndromes: clinical, research, and policy implications of a core geriatric concept. J Am Geriatr Soc. 2007;55(5):780–91.
3. DuBeau CE, et al. Incontinence in the Frail Elderly: report from the 4th international consultation on incontinence. Neurourol Urodyn. 2010;29(1):165–78.
4. Abrams P, et al. The standardisation of terminology of lower urinary tract function: report from the

standardisation subcommittee of the international continence society. Neurourol Urodyn. 2002;21(2):167–78.

5. Irwin DE, et al. Population-based survey of urinary incontinence, overactive bladder, and other lower urinary tract symptoms in five countries: results of the EPIC study. Eur Urol. 2006;50(6):1306–15.

6. Sgadari A, et al. Urinary incontinence in nursing home residents: a cross-national comparison. Age Ageing. 1997;26 Suppl 2:49.

7. Thom DH, Haan MN, Van den Eeden SK. Medically recognized urinary incontinence and risks of hospitalization, nursing home admission and mortality. Age Ageing. 1997;26(5):367.

8. Baztan JJ, et al. New-onset urinary incontinence and rehabilitation outcomes in frail older patients. Age Ageing. 2005;34(2):172.

9. Wagner TH, et al. Health-related consequences of overactive bladder. Am J Manag Care. 2002;8(19 Supp):598–607.

10. Holroyd Leduc JM, Mehta KM, Covinsky KE. Urinary incontinence and its association with death, nursing home admission, and functional decline. J Am Geriatr Soc. 2004;52(5):712–8.

11. Pfisterer MHD, et al. Geriatric patients' preferences for treatment of urinary incontinence: a study of hospitalized, cognitively competent adults aged 80 and older. J Am Geriatr Soc. 2007;55(12):2016–22.

12. Fonda D, DuBeau CE, Harari D, et al. Incontinence in the frail elderly. In: Abrams P, Cardozo L, Khoury S, Wein A, editors. Incontinence, vols 1 and 2: vol 1: basics & evaluation—vol 2: management. Plymouth: Health Publications; 2005. p. 1163–239.

13. Wagg A, Verdejo C, Molander U. Review of cognitive impairment with antimuscarinic agents in elderly patients with overactive bladder. Int J Clin Pract. 2010;64(9):1279–86.

14. Royall DR, Cordes JA, Polk M. CLOX: an executive clock drawing task. J Neurol Neurosurg Psychiatry. 1998;64(5):588.

15. Kuo HK, Lipsitz LA. Cerebral white matter changes and geriatric syndromes: is there a link? J Gerontol A Biol Sci Med Sci. 2004;59(8):M818.

16. Kuchel GA, et al. Localization of brain white matter hyperintensities and urinary incontinence in community-dwelling older adults. J Gerontol A Biol Sci Med Sci. 2009;64(8):902.

17. Chiarelli PE, Mackenzie LA, Osmotherly PG. Urinary incontinence is associated with an increase in falls: a systematic review. Aust J Physiother. 2009;55(2):89–95.

18. Brown J, et al. Urinary incontinence: does it increase risk for falls and fractures? Study of osteoporotic fractures research group. J Am Geriatr Soc. 2000; 48(7):721.

19. Kikuchi A, et al. Association between physical activity and urinary incontinence in a community-based elderly population aged 70 years and over. Eur Urol. 2007;52(3):868–75.

20. Jirovec MM. The impact of daily exercise on the mobility, balance and urine control of cognitively impaired nursing home residents. Int J Nurs Stud. 1991;28(2):145–51.

21. Van Houten P, Achterberg W, Ribbe M. Urinary incontinence in disabled elderly women: a randomized clinical trial on the effect of training mobility and toileting skills to achieve independent toileting. Gerontology. 2007;53(4):205.

22. Bischoff HA, et al. Identifying a cut off point for normal mobility: a comparison of the timed 'up and go' test in community dwelling and institutionalised elderly women. Age Ageing. 2003;32(3):315.

23. Ruby CM, et al. Medication use and control of urination among community-dwelling older adults. J Aging Health. 2005;17(5):661.

24. Landi F, et al. Benzodiazepines and the risk of urinary incontinence in frail older persons living in the community. Clin Pharmacol Ther. 2002;72(6):729–34.

25. Tannenbaum C. Medications that contribute to LUTS in the elderly: a review. Br J Urol. 2011;5(5 Suppl 2):S139–42.

26. Starr JM. Cholinesterase inhibitor treatment and urinary incontinence in Alzheimer's disease. J Am Geriatr Soc. 2007;55(5):800–1.

27. Hashimoto M, et al. Urinary incontinence: an unrecognised adverse effect with donepezil. Lancet. 2000;356(9229):568.

28. Gill SS, et al. A prescribing cascade involving cholinesterase inhibitors and anticholinergic drugs. Arch Intern Med. 2005;165(7):808.

29. Margel D, et al. Continuous positive airway pressure reduces nocturia in patients with obstructive sleep apnea. Urology. 2006;67(5):974–7.

30. Reynard J, et al. A novel therapy for nocturnal polyuria: a double-blind randomized trial of furosemide against placebo. Br J Urol. 1998;81:215–8.

31. Casanova J. Incontinence after use of enalapril. J Urol. 1990;143(6):1237.

32. Wagg A, et al. National Audit of Continence Care. London: Royal College of Physicians; 2010.

Adolescent Urology and Transitional Care

21

Andrew D. Baird

Introduction

The ability to follow the progress of young patients as they grow and develop is paramount to understanding the long-term outcomes of treatments inflicted upon them. The only way to achieve this is to establish and manage good-quality longitudinal care in carefully followed populations of patients as they leave paediatric practice and enter adult healthcare. There is also a need to report health-related outcomes in the contemporary medical literature. The inevitable long lead time in completing such population-based outcome studies must be considered, and detail can easily be lost within the longevity of follow-up. Continuity through transitional care, robust methods of ongoing follow-up and reliable access to help when there are problems are the cornerstones of building a trusting and long-lasting professional relationship [1].

Adolescence and Adolescent Urology

During the formative years of teenage development, we expect to see our patients develop their own identity and to integrate that with how they

perceive their functional role in their extended peer group and local society. Theoretical models of adolescent development describe a biological onset at puberty with a subsequent series of complex social transactions heralding its completion [2, 3]. Social relationships and interactions develop whilst boundaries of behavioural acceptability are sometimes explored, and it is well recognised that risk-taking behaviour becomes a significant problem in some adolescent groups [4–6]. Adolescents have a strong sense of self-worth and strive for independence, whilst often regarding the opinions of their peers as highly important and that of their parents somewhat questionable. Exploration of sexuality follows [7], and the transition into young adulthood is inevitable. It is important to recognise and accept these changes in our patients and help the more vulnerable individuals through this sometimes rapid period of turbulent change.

The prevalence of chronic illness in adolescent populations is difficult to quantify, but data from a number of epidemiological studies seem to suggest that 10–15 % of adolescents suffer from a chronic condition which arose during earlier childhood [8, 9]. Some chronic childhood conditions may have a self-limiting course (e.g. childhood asthma and other atopic conditions) but others persist into and beyond young adulthood. As human pubertal growth is accompanied by major changes in physical condition and brain maturation, adolescence has profound consequences for future health and well-being. The management of a chronic condition in adolescence

A.D. Baird, M.B., Ch.B., F.R.C.S. (Urol.) (✉)
Paediatric, Adolescent and Reconstructive Urology,
Alder Hey Children's Hospital, Eaton Road,
Liverpool, Merseyside L12 2AP, UK
e-mail: andrew.baird@alderhey.nhs.uk

A.J. Wein et al. (eds.), *Bladder Dysfunction in the Adult: The Basis for Clinical Management*, Current
Clinical Urology, DOI 10.1007/978-1-4939-0853-0_21, © Springer Science+Business Media New York 2014

is a major challenge for the patient and family, their contemporaries and the healthcare professionals involved.

Adolescent urology as a concept is not new and exists in different forms at the interface between paediatric and adult urology. Pathways and methods of transition vary between centres but have the common goal of delivering quality healthcare to adolescent patients as their follow-up moves into the domain of the adult hospital.

An adolescent urology service should be capable of handling all aspects of urology which may occur in the adolescent population, including 'core' urology (e.g. endoscopic and peno-scrotal surgery), as well as more complex interventions such as stone management, renal surgery and lower urinary tract reconstructive surgery including urethral reconstruction and a comprehensive range of diagnostic skills. Close integration with relevant specialities (particularly neurosurgery, orthopaedics, nephrology, endocrinology and gynaecology) is key to the successful implementation of an adolescent urology service.

At the authors' institution, a structured and fully integrated adolescent and reconstructive urology service has developed which oversees the care of all suitable urology patients before, during and after the transition of their care to adult services. The lead consultant provides outpatient, diagnostic and surgical sessions at the regional Children's Hospital and continues to care for patients in adult urology within the city. Age boundaries in the clinic are flexibly applied, with adolescent urological care being tailored to the maturity, readiness and awareness of the individual patient, ranging from 11 to 19 years old. Independent thinking is encouraged and the patient is at the centre of decision-making wherever possible. The author believes that this approach helps to improve future compliance with follow-up and builds good long-term relationships with patients and their families.

Concepts in Transitional Care

Transition planning at the interface of transfer between paediatric and adult care is a vital process in ensuring that an appropriate level of care is provided to meet individual requirements. In planning services for ongoing healthcare for adolescents with chronic health needs, treatment of the medical condition must be paralleled by a focus on prevention of ill health, promotion of healthy lifestyles and access to adequate support, e.g. sexual healthcare services [10]. Each young person can expect the right to be treated with respect and as an individual, be involved in decisions about their care and receive communication (verbal or written), which is appropriate for their level of development and understanding [11].

Transitional care practice has been a focus of recent development in paediatric services [2, 12–15], yet many barriers remain. There is a risk that services may fail to manage this transition effectively, with the result that the health and well-being of these young people is compromised and their potential unrealised.

The UK Department of Health document entitled 'Transition: Moving on Well' [13] emphasises not only the input of the patient but also their family and recognises the importance of identifying potential problem areas early, treating transition as a process rather than an isolated event. A multidisciplinary approach is vital in addressing the entire package of care requirements for individuals with often very complex health and social needs [16] and the implementation of transition clinics is advocated [17, 18].

There are good examples of transitional care practice in areas of adolescent chronic health such as renal disease [18, 19], cystic fibrosis [20], diabetes [21] and inflammatory bowel disease [22, 23], from which models of care can be emulated. However, the development of health services for young adults with complex conditions such as spina bifida has lagged behind those for adults with chronic health needs, even though the need for comprehensive specialist health provision may be even more critical [15].

It is helpful whilst considering transitional care to distinguish between the terms *transition* and *transfer*. Moving healthcare delivery from paediatric to adult services usually involves a change of geographical place and specialist medical practitioner and usually a change in emphasis from a family-centred approach to one where discussions and decisions are undertaken between doctor and patient with less input from parent or guardian. The term *transition* can be used to describe the preparation and support given before, during and after the process of *transfer* of service delivery [24]. This includes the appropriate transfer of health information.

One of the major difficulties with managing transition in healthcare is compliance or adherence to plans and treatments. Each young patient has the right to be treated as a respected individual, but behavioural difficulties sometimes arise [4–6] and can be the source of emotional difficulty and conflict during adolescence—particularly in females [25]. Even though adjustment to the emotional and psychological aspects of long-term illness or disability often occurs quickly for children [26], ill adolescents are more likely to develop behavioural or psychological disorders than their healthy contemporaries. They are also more likely to miss important periods of time at school [27], which may have affected their educational development. Any of these factors can influence the adherence of the adolescent patient to treatments or clinical management plans. Agreeing such treatments and plans in partnership with the patient and discussing longer-term strategies and goals may help in increasing compliance and reducing non-attendance. The involvement of an independent advocate can be useful, perhaps recruiting the input of a representative from a charitable organisation or patient-centred group [28].

A number of issues may be considered during the implementation of transitional care, and addressing each of the following helps to build a meaningful health and social care plan for young adult patients where adherence may be improved:
- Does an overriding strategy for all young people exist in the local area?
- Do policies for different conditions link with multi-agency strategy protocol/policy?
- Have policies/strategy been developed in partnership?
- Do young people know they are entering a period of transition?
- Are young people treated as partners in the transition process—enabled to participate and express their views?
- Does the primary care provider have a strategic lead for transition?

Transitional Care in Urology

The majority of cases suitable for careful transition in urological practice are those with 'congenital' urological conditions. Examples include neuropathic bladder requiring ongoing careful monitoring (whether or not any reconstructive surgery has taken place), posterior urethral valves, hypospadias, exstrophy/epispadias, sacral agenesis and anorectal malformations, urogenital sinus abnormalities, abnormalities of female sexual development [29] and abnormalities of upper urinary tract development.

At the authors' clinic, the transition service is based upon the following plan:
- Identify early those who need guidance through transition.
- List some clearly defined goals and objectives.
- Multidisciplinary involvement.
- Develop a 'person-centred health plan'.
- Make transition to adult services smooth and seamless.
- Review and improve the service as necessary; this involves listening to the comments of the users.

The philosophy of transitional care is centred around helping to prepare young people and their families for the significant uncertainties and changes which accompany the move to adult healthcare. The wider sphere of urology encompasses potentially complex areas such as sexual health, fertility, relationships, future paternity, pregnancy tests, obstetric care, contraception, taking risks, 'letting go' issues, etc.

Education should ideally form part of the transition process. Teenagers with long-term urological conditions should be educated about their anatomy, urinary tract dysfunction and the reasons for needing to take medications, catheterise, wash out the bladder, care for the bowel and take part in a scheduled follow-up plan. The medical consequences of a patient with such needs being lost in follow-up are potentially serious and often difficult to rectify when considerable time has elapsed since the patient was last seen [1].

Areas of Development in Transitional Care

Services aimed at patients with complex needs work most effectively when the process is reviewed, improved and implemented whenever necessary. In the authors' service, the following areas are considered important in attempts to improve and develop:

- What should effective transition be like?
- Should transitional care be provider driven or consumer driven?
- What are the necessary pathways and partnerships involved and do they integrate well?
- Who directs the ownership of the service, and who monitors the outcome?
- How do we adapt the process for the variety of complex conditions we see?
- Will the service become increasingly technology dependent?
- Are young patients likely to opt out of follow-up if they perceive transition to have failed them and how can we prevent this?
- How can we continue to encourage dialogue, patient involvement and choice and greater inclusivity (i.e. involve more patients, and make the service available to whoever needs it)?

Conclusions

The ideas and concepts in this chapter offer an overview of how the development of a transitional care service might be approached. Each service development project should aim to provide a bespoke care pathway to safely deliver any individual adolescent patient through the process of transfer and transition of their care to the adult health sector. Any transition service needs to be flexible and changeable to meet individual needs and should be reviewed periodically to determine whether there are any areas requiring revision. Obtaining the backing and support from both primary care and secondary care providers is essential. Enlisting the involvement of a multidisciplinary team of healthcare professionals from all relevant speciality areas should be part of the early development process. Listening to the views of the users, i.e. young people and their careers, will ensure that any transition service meets its targets and delivers effective care.

References

1. Borer JB. Current approaches to the urologic care of children with spina bifida. Curr Urol Rep. 2008;9:151–57.
2. Patten GC, Viner R. Pubertal transitions in health. Lancet. 2007;369:1130–39.
3. Lerner RM. Concepts and theories of human development. 2nd ed. New York: Academic; 1986.
4. Parsons JT, Siegel AW, Cousins JH. Late adolescent risk-taking: Effects of perceived benefits and perceived risks on behavioural intentions and behavioural change. J Adolesc. 1997;20(4):381–92.
5. Siegel JT. Dying for romance: risk taking as purposive behavior. Psychol Health Med. 2011;16(6):719–26.
6. Romer D, Betancourt LM, Brodsky NL, et al. Does adolescent risk taking imply weak executive function? A prospective study of relations between working memory performance, impulsivity and risk taking in early adolescence. Dev Sci. 2011;14(5):1119–33.
7. Burack R. Teenage sexual behaviour: attitudes towards and declared sexual activity. Br J Fam Plann. 1999;24(4):145–8.
8. Newacheck P, Stoddard J. Prevalence and impact of multiple childhood chronic illnesses. J Paediatr. 1994;124:40–8.
9. Suris JC, Michaud PA, Viner R. The adolescent with a chronic condition. Part 1: developmental issues. Arch Dis Child. 2004;89:938–42.
10. Michaud PA, Suris JC, Viner R. The adolescent with a chronic condition. Part 2: healthcare provision. Arch Dis Child. 2004;89:943–49.
11. Department of Health. Getting the right start: National Service Framework for children. Standard for hospital services. London: Department of Health; 2003.
12. Care Services Improvement Partnership. Briefing note: children's services transitions. London: CSIP; 2003.
13. Transition: Moving On Well www.dh.gov.uk/publications ref 284732.
14. Care Services Improvement Partnership (2007) Compendium of (transition) good practice. http://kc.csip.org.uk/viewdocument.php?action=viewdox&pid=0&doc=36506&grp=1
15. Sawyer SM, Macnee S. Transition to adult health care for adolescents with spina bifida: research issues. Dev Disabil Res Rev. 2010;16:60–5.

16. Binks JA, Barden WS, Burke TA, et al. What do we really know about the transition to adult-centred health care? A focus on cerebral palsy and spina bifida. Arch Phys Med Rehabil. 2007; 88:1064–73.
17. McLone DG. Commentary: an interdisciplinary approach. J Padiatr Rehabil Med. 2008;1:283–4.
18. Chaturvedi S, Jones C, Walker R, et al. The transition of kidney transplant recipients: a work in progress. Pediatr Nephrol. 2009;24:1055–60.
19. Bell L. Adolescents with renal disease in an adult world: meeting the challenge of transition of care. Nephrol Dial Transplant. 2007;22(4):988–91.
20. Kraynack NC, McBride JT. Improving care at cystic fibrosis centers through quality improvement. Semin Respir Crit Care Med. 2009;30:547–58.
21. Datta J. Moving up with diabetes. The transition from paediatric to adult care. London: National Children's Bureau; 2003.
22. Leung Y, Heyman MB, Mahadevan U. Transitioning the adolescent inflammatory bowel disease patient: Guidelines for the adult and pediatric gastroenterologist. Inflamm Bowel Dis. 2011;17(10):2169–73.
23. Escher JC. Transition from pediatric to adult health care in inflammatory bowel disease. Dig Dis. 2009;27(3):382–6.
24. Sawyer SM, Blair S, Bowes G. Chronic illness in adolescents—transfer of transition to adult services? J Paediatr Child Health. 1997;33:88–90.
25. Suris J. Chronic illness and emotional distress in adolescence. Pediatr Clin North Am. 1996;19:153–6.
26. LeBlanc L, Goldsmith T, Patel D. Behavioural aspects of chronic illness in children and adolescents. Pediatr Clin North Am. 2003;50:859–78.
27. Charlton A, Lacombe I, Meller SA. Absence from school related to cancer and other chronic conditions. Arch Dis Child. 1991;66:1217–22.
28. West C, Brodie L, Dicker J, et al. Development of health support services for adults with spina bifida. Disabil Rehabil. 2011;33(23–23):2381–8.
29. Liao L, Tacconelli E, Wood D, et al. Adolescent girls with disorders of sexual development: a needs analysis of transitional care. J Pediatr Urol. 2010;6:609–13.

The Psychological Impact of Lower Urinary Dysfunction

22

Jackie Gordon and Marcus J. Drake

Body image can be defined as 'what we think and feel about our body' [1]. Unsurprisingly, the Royal College of Obstetricians (2006) states 'Incontinence may seriously influence … the psychological and social well-being of affected individuals' and have a profound impact on families and carers [2]. It is common to hear patients report reduction of previously pleasurable activities, such as exercise [3]. Issues around body image are likely to occur with urinary incontinence or nocturnal enuresis, self-catheterisation, undergoing surgery and particularly having a stoma. At several stages, the impact of these processes need to be handled sympathetically and dealt with frankly and openly. For a patient initially presenting with incontinence or nocturnal enuresis, they have often lived with these problems for some time. Commonly they will have tried to keep the symptoms secret and will not have been able to confide to relatives or friends, therefore lacking the benefit of support which is valued by patients in other health contexts. They may also be suffering anxiety at times of hospital contact, since this will be potentially a time that

relatives could 'discover' the patient has a problem they are trying to keep secret. The patient may also have a sense of shame, since attaining continence is a life event in childhood associated with a sense of achievement and pride; loss of continence can thus have a substantial impact. People may have a feeling of incontinence as 'bad' behaviour from childhood, something to feel shame about.

The shame and embarrassment in the context of incontinence and urinary dysfunction is compounded where the symptoms are evident in sexual activity. Urinary incontinence may also affect sexual functioning. One study reported that 43 % of study participants with urinary incontinence felt that their urinary disorder had adversely affected sexual relations [4]. Incontinence during sexual intercourse may be the event that triggers medical consultation, since it is impossible for the patient to keep secret, and may threaten maintenance of relationship with the partner. The necessity to discuss sexuality alongside issues of incontinence magnifies the embarrassment and sense of shame, such that the anticipation of consultations is very stressful for patients. Dealing with these issues is an essential element of establishing an environment that will enable the clinician to ascertain the full scope of the symptoms and their impact and is effectively the initial step in therapy.

Treatment of lower urinary tract dysfunction can have additional psychological implications. Undergoing surgery is a major event for patients in its own right, and the potential for suboptimal

J. Gordon, M.A., M.B., B.Chir., M.R.C.Psych.
Mental Health Liaison Service, Worthing Hospital, West Sussex, UK

M.J. Drake, M.A. (Cantab), D.M. (Oxon.), F.R.C.S. (Urol.) (✉)
University of Bristol and Bristol Urological Institute, Bristol, UK
e-mail: marcus.drake@bui.ac.uk

outcomes or adverse events compels a fully informed patient to make a value judgement on the appropriateness of proceeding in a context of a health issue that is not life-threatening. Long-term outcomes may require considerable changes to which the patient has to adjust, for example, the need for intermittent self-catheterisation or adjust to the presence of surgical scars, even a stoma. When the patient is first informed about such possibilities, they will typically not have anticipated ongoing lifelong adjustment to be necessary; in most cases, patients will envisage solutions that 'cure' the problem so they can put the issues behind them once and for all. Self-catheterisation unavoidably constitutes a regular reminder of urinary dysfunction and an intrusive, often unpleasant process which can come to be regarded as being as bad as the original presenting symptoms—replacing one problem with another. If efficacy of treatment is suboptimal, such that incontinence only partly improves (or later returns, as in botulinum treatment of detrusor overactivity), the situation is particularly difficult. The patient may then come to regard the treatment as having introduced an additional problem.

Research has also looked at the possible link between depression and urinary incontinence [5–8]. Urinary incontinence and major depression disproportionately affect women and both are associated with significant social stigma. Comorbid depression may compound a woman's sense of embarrassment from incontinence and lead to increased shame and isolation [9].

Contributions of Healthcare Professionals

Primary care physicians may have only limited training in lower urinary tract symptoms and their treatment. Accordingly, the secondary care referral may represent the first occasion on which the symptoms are talked through openly and in detail by the patient. The specialist needs to ensure a sympathetic and attentive consultation, gently raising issues the patient may not volunteer

spontaneously, such as effect of symptoms on sexual function. Likewise, implications of treatment, such as partial response, adverse consequences and influences on body image, must be dealt with appropriately. Since medical consultations are typically of limited duration and patients need time to consider and adjust to what they have been told before they can think of the questions they need answered, follow-up discussion is often needed before committing to irrevocable treatment. Probably most important are the urology specialist nurses who work closely with this patient group and who not only understand the nature of the conditions and their treatments but also more likely to know, empathise and be trusted by their patients. It is the nurse specialist to whom the patient is most likely to express fears and concerns about their condition and who therefore is in the best position to identify psychological issues. He or she may feel able to support and manage the patient through what is likely to be a period of adjustment. An important part of the nurse specialist role is around careful nursing to help re-establish the patient's body image. He or she (used to seeing the psychological 'norm') is also likely to identify where their psychological skill and competence ends and when they will need other psychological or psychiatric specialist input.

Health psychologists are potentially important professionals in this area—though they are a scarce resource and may be difficult to access. 'Liaison' psychiatrists are general hospital based, working at the interface between physical and mental health, and are more likely to be called upon for advice. Referrals from urology to liaison psychiatry are unusual, but this may reflect a failure on the part of the urological and gynaecological professions to recognise the need to involve specific assistance, rather than lack of impact of the condition and/or treatment on individual patients. 'General' psychiatrists are less likely to be involved with this patient group as they work with what is termed 'severe and enduring mental illness' (e.g. schizophrenia and bipolar affective disorder).

Specific Situations

Clean intermittent self-catheterisation (ISC) may be associated with patients feeling grief and a sense of loss, stigmatised and embarrassed, and the loss of normal bladder function is seen as a 'devastating event'. Specialist nurses and doctors should be aware of the range of these difficult emotional responses and help patients to assimilate ISC into their lifestyle for long-term psychological well-being [10]. Teaching ISC has to go beyond mere instruction in the physical process; healthcare professionals responsible for training a patient in ISC have to tackle the psychological issues of anxiety, embarrassment, uncertainty, ambivalence and fear of discomfort in full to achieve successful introduction of the technique. ISC should be discussed in light of opening out possibility of treatment which would otherwise potentially not be possible and beneficial compared with alternatives such as indwelling catheterisation. Training can successfully be achieved with prior provision of written information followed by unhurried face-to-face discussion with a suitably trained nurse. These need to precede the process of physical demonstration, and the patient then needs to attempt the technique under supervision. A follow-up phone call to go over issues once the patient has attempted ISC unsupervised at home helps reinforce best practice and compliance and reassures the patient to their psychological benefit. Taking this approach can achieve successful training in ISC in 84 % of patients regardless of age [11].

Ileal conduit urinary diversion places a stoma which is permanently visible and consequently impacts on sense of privacy. The healthcare professional needs to assist with practical measures to disguise the presence of the stoma. This requires planning preoperatively to help with stoma placement in a location suitable for the patient's typical clothing and day-to-day context (such as physical position for wheelchair users).

Additional post-operative support is needed, since the final location and structure of the stoma may not have achieved what was intended due to surgical issues. Leaking bags and containment issues are a major concern, and fear of minor leaks or soaking from bag disconnection is a considerable psychological issue. Finally, self-image and sexual attraction anxiety [12] are profound, requiring considerable need for emotional adjustment.

References

1. Price B. A model for body-image care. J Adv Nurs. 1990;15:585–93.
2. National Collaborating Centre for Women's and Children's Health (UK). Urinary incontinence: the management of urinary incontinence in women. London: RCOG Press; 2006.
3. Nygaard I, DeLancey JO, Arnsdorf L, Murphy E. Exercise and incontinence. Obstet Gynecol. 1990; 75:848–51.
4. Sutherst J, Brown M. Sexual dysfunction associated with urinary incontinence. Urol Int. 1980;35:414–6.
5. Zorn BH, Montgomery H, Pieper K, Gray M, Steers WD. Urinary incontinence and depression. J Urol. 1999;162:82–4.
6. Wyman JF, Harkins SW, Choi SC, Taylor JR, Fantl JA. Psychosocial impact of urinary incontinence in women. Obstet Gynecol. 1987;70:378–81.
7. Dugan E, Cohen SJ, Robinson D, et al. The quality of life of older adults with urinary incontinence: determining generic and condition-specific predictors. Qual Life Res. 1998;7:337–44.
8. Robinson D, Pearce KF, Preisser JS, Dugan E, Suggs PK, Cohen SJ. Relationship between patient reports of urinary incontinence symptoms and quality of life measures. Obstet Gynecol. 1998;91:224–8.
9. Melville JL, Walker E, Katon W, Lentz G, Miller J, Fenner D. Prevalence of comorbid psychiatric illness and its impact on symptom perception, quality of life, and functional status in women with urinary incontinence. Am J Obstet Gynecol. 2002;187:80–7.
10. Ramm D, Kane R. A qualitative study exploring the emotional responses of female patients learning to perform clean intermittent self-catheterisation. J Clin Nurs. 2011;20:3152–62.
11. Parsons BA, Narshi A, Drake MJ. Success rates for learning intermittent self-catheterisation according to age and gender. Int Urol Nephrol. 2012;44:1127–31.
12. MacArthur A. Sexuality and the stoma: helping patients to cope. Nurs Times. 1996;92:34–5.

Index

A
Abnormal adult bladder function
  emptying/voiding, 21, 22
  functional categorization, therapy, 23, 24
  lower urinary tract, 22
Acute urinary retention (AUR)
  bladder and symptom relief, 113
  lower tract symptoms, 163–164
  medical therapy, 238
  pain relief, 53
  women, 51
Adolescence
  females, 285
  and urology (*see* Adolescent urology)
Adolescent urology
  chronic illness, 283
  social relationships, 283
  and transitional care (*see* Transitional care)
  urethral reconstruction, 284
α-Adrenoceptors (ARs)
  bladder afferent activity, 9
  detrusor muscle, 9
  rat urinary bladder, 10
  sympathetic noradrenergic control, 40
β-Adrenoceptors (ARs)
  β_3-ARs, 10
  bladder relaxation, 11
  human detrusor, 10
  mRNA, 11
Ambulatory urodynamics, 92
Anatomic outlet obstruction
  BOO (*see* Bladder outlet obstruction (BOO))
  DUA, 37
  muscle hypertrophy, 39
  neurones, 39
  outlet obstruction, 38
  urethral stricture and contracture, 42–45
  voiding symptoms, 38
ANS. *See* Autonomic nervous system (ANS)
Antepartum PFMT, 106, 107
Antidepressants, 136–137
Antimuscarinic (anticholinergic) drugs
  α_1-AR antagonists, 144–146
  β_3-AR antagonists, 146
  and 5α-reductase inhibitors, 147
  bladder urothelial cells, 123

  clinical use, 125–127
  intravesical application, drugs, 147
  muscarinic receptor, 122, 123
  treatment, OABs/DO, 122, 124
  trospium, 184–186
Anxiety
  hospital contact, 289
  self-image and sexual attraction, 291
  and sleep disorders, 154
β-AR agonists
  β_3-AR, 131, 133, 146
  membrane channels, 130–133
  stress incontinence, women, 157–158
α-AR antagonists
  antimuscarinics, 144–146
  5a-reductase inhibitors, 147–148
  membrane channels, 129–130
  stress incontinence, women, 156–157
Atropine, 122, 125, 171
Augmentation cystoplasty, 251–252, 265
AUR. *See* Acute urinary retention (AUR)
Autonomic innervation
  nervous system, 7
  and somatic efferents, 11
Autonomic nervous system (ANS), 28

B
Baclofen, 143–144
BCR. *See* Bulbocavernosus reflex (BCR)
BDNF. *See* Brain-derived neurotrophic
    factor (BDNF)
Behavioral modification, 103, 104, 173
Behavioral therapy
  bowel function, 105
  BT, 103
  dietary bladder irritants, 105
  fluid intake and urine volume, 105
  lifestyle modifications, 104
  modification, 103, 104
  obesity and weight loss, 106–112
  PEM, 103
  PFMT, 104
  scheduled voiding, 103
  smoking, 106
  TV, 103

CPSIA information can be obtained at www.ICGtesting.com
Printed in the USA
LVOW02*1450290714

396575LV00003B/7/P

9 781493 908523